Aging,
Society, and The
Life Course, 3rd
Edition

Leslie A. Morgan, PhD, is Associate Dean at the Erickson School of Aging Studies, Codirector of the Gerontology Doctoral Program, and Professor in the Department of Sociology and Anthropology at the University of Maryland, Baltimore County. Dr. Morgan has 27 years of experience in teaching and research in aging and has published on a variety of topics from economic well-being and family relationships to assisted living. She has authored or coauthored three books and numerous articles. Dr. Morgan has been principal or coprincipal investigator on several NIH-funded studies of life in assisted living, examining the quality of resident experience, and transitions among residents.

Suzanne R. Kunkel, PhD, is the Director of Scripps Gerontology Center and Professor in the Department of Sociology and Gerontology at Miami University. Dr. Kunkel has 20 years of experience in research and teaching in gerontology. She is the recipient of the 2006 Outstanding Gerontology Educator Award from the Ohio Association of Gerontology in Higher Education. She has authored or coauthored more than 35 articles, book chapters, and research monographs, and has recently coedited with Valerie Wellin, *Consumer Voice and Choice in Long-Term Care* (Springer Publishing Company, 2006). Her research focuses primarily on demography of aging, health and disability, and innovations and quality in long-term care systems.

Aging,
Society, and The
Life Course

3rd
Edition

Leslie A. Morgan, PhD
Suzanne R. Kunkel, PhD

SPRINGER PUBLISHING COMPANY

New York

Springer Publishing Company, LLC.
11 West 42nd Street
New York, NY 10036

Acquisitions Editor: Sheri W. Sussman
Managing Editor: Mary Ann McLaughlin
Project Manager: Carol Cain
*Cover design b*y Joanne E. Honigman
*Typeset b*y Apex Publishing, LLC

08   09   10/   5   4   3   2

Library of Congress Cataloging-in-Publication Data

Morgan, Leslie A.
Aging, society, and the life course / Leslie A. Morgan, Suzanne R. Kunkel. — 3rd ed.
   p. cm.
   Includes index.
   ISBN 0-8261-0212-3
1. Older people--United States.   2. Aging--United States.   3. Gerontology--United States.
I. Kunkel, Suzanne.   II. Title.
   HQ1064.U5M6818 2006
   305.26--dc22

Printed in the United States of America by Bang Printing

Contents

Acknowledgments

With any project of this scope, there are many people who make important contributions to its completion. We would like to acknowledge the technical support provided by the staff at Springer Publishing Company, LLC. We also need to thank our support systems on our campuses. For Leslie Morgan this includes the Department of Sociology and the Erickson School at the University of Maryland, Baltimore County, most especially the support of David Hamilton, graduate research assistant. For Suzanne Kunkel appreciation is extended to a long list of colleagues, graduate assistants, and undergraduate student assistants at Miami University's Scripps Gerontology Center. Special thanks to Arlene Nichol for overseeing the production of the manuscript. E. J. Hanna and Mike Payne contributed all of the photos in the book; an added thanks to Mike Payne for preparing photo captions.

We would also like to acknowledge our mentors and colleagues (both proximate and remote) who have shaped our professional lives and perspectives. These include Robert Atchley, Vern Bengtson, Kevin Eckert, William Feinberg, Joe Hendricks, Norris Johnson, Matilda White Riley, Neal Ritchey, Mildred Seltzer, and Judith Treas, among others. Finally we would like to acknowledge our families and closest friends; these are the people who give us our roots and our wings, help us keep perspective, and remind us of the importance of balance in our lives.

Each new edition of a textbook provides authors new opportunities to sharpen, update, and extend the material and to include emergent issues that have come to the forefront in recent years. This edition reflects a major reorganization of material, focusing more on the social and sociological aspects of aging. We have moved away from our earlier approach of including separate chapters on the biology and psychology of aging, instead examining these issues as they integrate with the social aspects of the life course and human aging within a social context. In rethinking our organization of content, we recast some larger chapters into two (separating material on working from that on retirement, for example), which give somewhat shorter, more focused chapters. The resulting 13-chapter book is also better attuned to most academic schedules for a "one chapter a week" reading assignment.

Continuing Themes

In presenting knowledge about aging in social context, we continue to focus on four major themes. The first theme is emphasizing the diversity of the older population; this "stereotype-busting" focus carries throughout all of the chapters, emphasizing how notably diverse the older population has become. Material highlights diversity by gender, social class, race/ethnicity, and even age differences among older adults. A second major theme is the micro/macro distinction in understanding aging as a social phenomenon. Human aging occurs within layers of social context from the family to the political and economic systems. Understanding the complex dynamics among these multiple levels is a key to a deep understanding of aging processes and outcomes. The third key theme is social construction. Through this approach, which is described further in chapter 1, we hope to highlight how aging is much more than an individual journey through time; aging is a complex social process that influences each of us on the journey and is, in turn, influenced by those making the journey.

The final key theme of our approach is integrating the learning of theory with content about aging. Reading theories without much substance attached is challenging for many students. Instead, scattered throughout our chapters are "Applying Theory" segments that describe a particular theory as it relates to content such as health care, family caregiving, or retirement. In this way the theory is grounded with some application that makes it more relevant and memorable.

Pedagogical Features

We have continued three features from earlier editions. First, we have updated our "Web Wise" listings at the end of each chapter. These reflect selected Web sites that students may find useful in connection with the material presented in the chapter. A second feature that is helpful to learning and retention is highlighting key terms used at the end of each chapter. The terms are presented in bold type, with a definition, within the body of the book and are among the essential elements of understanding the content presented. They are useful for review and discussion.

In our teaching experience, most students relate easily to aging through their personal or family experiences. Seldom do they come to a course understanding the implications of an aging society for major social institutions. Based in the fundamental expansion of the "sociological imagination" into the "gerontological imagination," we hope to expand students' perspectives to a bigger picture of aging as a social phenomenon that will reshape their lives well before they themselves are older adults. One way that we expand one's view of aging is through our third continued feature, a series of Topical Essays, which are scattered between chapters throughout the book. Our intention with these essays is to take the lens of aging and look at an array of contemporary issues, reflecting a more engaging way to "think outside the box" regarding the implications of aging for persons and the larger society. Interesting ideas, such as the role of music in the life course and anti-aging medicine, are employed to provide opportunities for discussion, take a further step with knowledge gained in the prior chapters, and connect concepts to real-world experiences we share.

Our original and continued purpose in writing this book has been to provide a new type of textbook on the social aspects of human aging—one that is neither encyclopedic in its coverage of research findings nor overly weighted down with jargon. We hope that we have more closely approached these goals in this third edition.

Aging,
Society, and The
Life Course, 3rd
Edition

Aging and Society

The individual does not act alone, although conscious beings will do and act as if they had control over their lives and could do what best pleased them.... No person really acts independent of the influences of our fellow human beings. Everywhere there is a social life setting limitations and influencing individual action. People cooperate, compete, combine, and organize for specific purposes, so that no one lives to him/herself. (Blackmar, 1908, pp. 3–4)

ging is something that happens to all of us. It is a natural and virtually inevitable process. Yet older people are often the subject of bad jokes and negative stereotypes, and many people in our society dread growing old. A quick visit to the birthday card section of your local card shop will confirm our preoccupation with negative views of, and jokes about, aging. Despite this preoccupation, our ideas about what aging really means and why it matters are notably diverse. Consider:

- At age 40, people in the labor force are legally defined as "older workers" by the Age Discrimination in Employment Act.
- Most of us know, or know about, people who became grandparents in their 40s; we also know people who became parents in their 40s.
- In January of 2005, Adriana Iliescu of Romania became the world's oldest recorded mother; she was 66 when she gave birth to a baby girl.
- In 1989, United Airlines Captain Al Haynes was credited with saving the lives of over a hundred people in a plane crash in Iowa. His years of experience were

The authors would like to acknowledge Robert C. Atchley for the contributions he made to the earliest version of this chapter.

cited as the major factor in his ability to respond so effectively to the emergency. A few months after this dramatic event, Captain Haynes turned 60 and was forced to retire.

■ "Until the mid-sixteenth century … few people knew exactly how old they were" (Cole, 1992, p. 5).

■ Most people who are age 75 do not think they belong in the "old" age category.

■ At age 16, people are "old enough" to be licensed drivers, at age 18 they are "old enough" to vote, and at age 21 they are "old enough" to drink alcohol. Why do we say "old enough"? Can you think of examples when we say someone is "too old" to do something?

■ Men can join the senior professional golf tour at age 50. The senior tour in men's tennis is for those age 35 and older.

■ Members of the armed forces can retire as early as age 37.

■ At age 90, Ludwig Magener won the national swimming championship in six masters' swimming events.

■ The human genome project could potentially extend life expectancy significantly. What will it mean to be 75 if life expectancy is 200? What will happen to our ideas about education, careers, and grandparenthood?

These examples illustrate two very important points. First, our society has many different formal and informal social definitions of age and aging. Second, the meanings, definitions, and experiences of aging vary across situations, cultures, and time. So, questions about when aging begins, what it is, and why it matters can only be answered by paying attention to the social contexts in which aging takes place.

Dimensions of Aging

If you ask anyone to define "aging," she might reasonably respond that it means growing older. But what does growing older mean? Is it simply the passage of time, having another birthday? Increasingly, scholars argue that chronological age is a relatively meaningless variable (see Ferraro, 1997; Maddox & Lawton, 1988). Age is only a way of marking human events and experiences; these events and experiences are what matters, not time itself (Botwinick, 1978). Time's passing is of concern only because it is connected, however loosely, with other changes: physical, psychological, and social.

Physical Aging

The passage of time for humans is related to a large number of specific physical changes such as gray hair; wrinkling of skin; and changes in reproductive capacity, immune system response, and cardiovascular functioning. An interesting question about these physical changes is whether they are inevitable, natural consequences of growing older. In fact, research shows that some of the changes we think of as normal are modifiable, preventable, and related to socially influenced life-style choices and cultural practices. For example, while some wrinkling of the skin and some loss of arterial elasticity appear to be related to physical aging processes, the magnitude of change and speed of deterioration are affected by life-style choices and culture. We know that wrinkling of the skin is acceler-ated and accentuated by sun exposure and by smoking, and some of the changes over time in cardiovascular functioning are related to diet, exercise, and smoking. Similarly, most of us know 70-year-olds who are as active, healthy, and vigorous as an average 40-year-old. Increasing evidence shows enormous variability in physical aging among individuals; this growing evidence of variability has resulted in new ways of thinking about aging.

In the past, researchers searched for the "normal" changes that accompanied aging; an important part of this search was to distinguish normal age changes from pathological or disease processes that became more prevalent with age but were not caused by aging. Knowledge about the modifiability and variability of physical aging processes resulted in a new way of thinking about aging. Rowe and Kahn (1998) offered the concept of successful aging, drawing distinctions among "usual," "optimal," and "pathological" aging. Optimal aging is characterized by minimal loss of physical function and a healthy, vigorous body; pathological aging is aging accompanied by multiple chronic diseases and negative environmental influences. Usual aging refers to the typical or average experience—somewhere between pathological and optimal. Exhibit 1.1 illustrates this view of the variability of physical aging (Machemer, 1992). The concept of successful aging is undergoing continual refinement (see Rowe & Kahn, 1997), and research about successful aging—how it is defined and measured, who achieves it, how it is attained—is still in its early years (Blazer, 2006). Even with continuing debate and the need for fur-ther research, the distinctions among usual, optimal, and pathological aging reflect new ways of thinking about physical aging as a variable and sometimes modifiable set of processes that often have important social components.

As we continue to find that the changes we call physical aging are merely age-*linked* and not age-*caused* and that many are, in fact, modifiable, we are forced to reconsider the question of what aging means as a physical process. The ever-increasing evidence that individuals vary greatly in their experience of physical aging suggests that few, if any, of

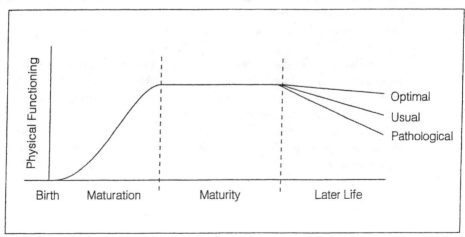

Variability of Physical Aging
Adapted from Machemer, 1992.

the significant aspects of aging are purely or even primarily physical. These issues are discussed further in chapter 10.

Psychological Aging

Psychological aging processes include changes in personality, mental functioning, and sense of self during the adult years. Some changes are considered a normal part of adult development, some are the result of physiological changes in the way the brain functions, and some psychological dimensions show little change at all in later years. As in the case of physical aging, a wealth of research has explored the complexities of these processes and ways to distinguish disease processes such as Alzheimer's disease from normal aging changes.

For our purposes, several generalizations are important. First, humans do continue to develop and grow throughout their lives. Some researchers in gerontology are interested in the unique nature of human development in the later years—the tasks, growth, and adaptations that take place. Much of this work focuses on opportunities for personal development and contributions to the world around us that can emerge in later life. Concepts such as "gerotranscendence" (Tornstam, 1997, 2005), serving from spirit (Atchley, 2004), "sageing" (Schacter-Shalomi & Miller, 1995), and "elderhood" (Thomas, 2004) offer a glimpse into the developmental stage that may characterize late life. We will explore these ideas further in chapter 4. For now it is sufficient to recognize that human development occurs throughout our entire lives; it does not end with adolescence or early adulthood.

A second broad statement related to psychological aspects of aging is that personality does not undergo profound changes in later life; most personality traits, self-concept, and self-esteem remain fairly stable from mid-life onward. For example, people do not become wise, grumpy, or rigid in their thinking as a result of growing older; the grumpy old man was very likely a grumpy young man. Although the developmental challenges and opportunities we encounter do vary through our lives, the strategies we use to adapt to change, to refine and reinforce our sense of self, to work toward realizing our full human potential are practiced throughout our adult lives. The simple passage of time seldom requires or causes fundamental changes to these basic personality structures and strategies.

Similarly, loss of cognitive functioning is not an inevitable result of aging. Just as significant loss of physical function is not inevitable or universal, so too memory and other cognitive skills may remain stable or even improve with age. However, it is important to be accurate here. Research on the physiology and psychology of aging shows that, in the absence of disabling disease, aging causes only minimal declines in functioning until around age 85, at which point about 25% of elders begin to show frailty even in the absence of disease.

Social Aging

If aging brings only relatively small universal and inevitable changes in physical or cognitive functioning, in the basic structure of personality, and in the trajectory of adult development, why does it matter in people's lives? In this book, we argue that, at least before age 85, age is significant primarily because of the social meanings, structures, and processes attached to it. Gray hair, wrinkles, longer reaction time, and even some short-term memory loss matter only because the social world in which we live has defined those characteristics as meaningful. Much of the social meaning of aging is tied to erroneous beliefs about the effects of aging on physical and mental capabilities. Aging does not inevitability cause us to become rigid in our thinking, forgetful, or unable to carry out our favorite physical or intellectual activities. For most people, aging is a process of change that is so gradual that we compensate for most of it so that it has little impact on our everyday lives.

However, society uses age to assign people to roles, to channel people into and out of positions within the social structure, as a basis for allocation of resources, and as a way to categorize individuals. In its most benevolent form, using age to allocate opportunities is a reasonable mechanism. For example, our society has rules about minimum ages for employment; these laws were designed to protect young people from being exploited, and, according to some, they are good for the labor force because they control the flow of new workers into the labor market. In a more constraining way, however, age artificially and unevenly limits the opportunities of people. Gray hair and wrinkles, perhaps the most visible signs of aging, and the chronological age of 65—the most often-used criterion of old age—have no effect on physical functioning or cognitive capability. They do, however, have profound effects on social interactions and opportunities for individuals in the social world. Whether we would seriously consider someone as a possible candidate for a job or as an interesting partner in social interaction is, in fact, influenced by our assessment of the age of that person and what that person's age symbolizes to us. Again, it is not because age 65 or gray hair are symptomatic of competence or incompetence or of a boring or dazzling personality, or even that visible signs of aging are inherently unattractive or attractive. We make these assessments because we live in a society that has constructed the meaning of aging in particular (primarily negative) ways.

It is important to think about the extent to which the very same processes work at other ages and stages of life. In our culture, it is possible to be "too young" just as it is possible to be "too old" for certain roles and opportunities. We have very clear social prescriptions, often in the form of federal and state laws, about when a person is old enough to drive a car, get married, and be president of the United States. In these examples, "old enough" seems to imply the window of opportunity between legally too young and socially too old.

X **Social aging**, then, refers to the ways in which society helps to shape the meanings and experiences of aging. Social aging includes the <u>expectations</u> and <u>assumptions</u> of those <u>around us about how we should behave,</u> what we are like, <u>what we can do</u>, and <u>what we should be doing at different ages</u>. The concept of social aging also refers to the ways in which those expectations influence what opportunities are open to us as we grow older. Chapter 4 explores these issues in detail, and later chapters in the book apply the concepts of social aging to the major dimensions of our social lives.

Social Construction of Aging

The preceding discussion about how the experiences of aging are largely constructed by society is an example of an important sociological idea: the so-called **social construction of reality**. This concept suggests that reality does not exist "out there," waiting to be measured and understood by us. Rather, reality is created out of interactions among humans and by the social institutions in which people live their lives. For an illustration of the gap between physical reality and people's lived experience of aging, think about witnesses to an unusual event, such as an auto accident. While we know that there are "facts" in such a situation—for example, the color of the cars, the direction and speed they were traveling—eyewitness accounts often vary greatly on even these details. Humans pay attention to different things, remember different things, and report different things. If one of the people in the accident is an older person, the witness might be motivated (consciously or unconsciously) to notice and report details based on their assumptions about that driver's capabilities. You can probably think of many examples from your everyday life in which a conversation, phrase, or gesture has been interpreted very differently, depending on the perspectives of the people involved.

Societal Aging

Beyond the social construction of aging, social forces influence the experience of aging in another important way. Societies themselves age. As the proportion of a population in the "older" age categories increases, profound changes in the social structure take place. Societal aging—these demographic, structural, and cultural transformations—affects every aspect of social life, from social institutions to the experiences of aging individuals. We can define societal aging as the demographic, structural, and cultural transformations a society undergoes as the proportion of its population that is aging increases. Education and the economy are good examples of social organizations and institutions that are affected greatly by the growth of the older population. The impact of population changes on the educational system in the United States can be seen in the growing number of attempts to address the needs of mature learners and in the growing number of college and university programs targeting the older population. Some institutions host summer Elderhostel programs or offer free tuition for students over age 65. The University of Massachusetts at Boston has a certificate program in gerontology; over half of the hundreds of people who have earned that certificate are over the age of 60. The impact of population aging on our society is discussed in greater detail in the later chapters of this book.

Another impact of the growth of the older population is the increased visibility of aging and increased exposure of the general population to the diversity and uniqueness among older individuals. As older people become more numerous and visible, stereotypical attitudes and discriminatory practices that disadvantage older people are more likely to be challenged. For example, in comparing magazine advertisements in the year 2005 to those from 1980, there is a definite increase in both the number of ads that feature older people and in the average age of many models (other than the supermodels, who still are very young). While most people in ads are young, the increased visibility of older people begins to change our images of aging and general awareness of the aging of society.

The aging of a population influences how aging itself is socially constructed. As **cohorts** of different size and with unique characteristics move through the age structure, they are affected by, but also have an impact on, the experience of being older. The baby boomers will experience aging in a very different way than the current generation of older people. Negative stereotypes are being challenged, age discrimination is illegal, and a growing diversity among older people and recognition of the expanding mature market for goods and services are part of this change. When these social changes combine with the political activism that has historically characterized the baby boomers, and with their potential power in the marketplace and in the polling booths, their experiences and definitions of aging are being altered.

The movement of cohorts born at different time periods into later life also has an impact on social institutions such as the economy and health care. For example, the current generation of older people grew up during the Great Depression. Their investment, purchasing, and savings habits have been shaped by that experience; they tend to save at higher rates than other groups of adults, especially the baby boomers, and they are less likely to make risky investments or purchases. The baby boomers grew up during relatively comfortable economic times, are not good savers, and are more likely to make nonessential purchases. The past decade has seen tremendous growth in the "games for adults" industry; toy stores now carry a large number of board games designed for adults, far beyond the number available just 10 years ago. This trend is related to the purchasing power, leisure preferences, and buying habits of baby boomers. You can use your imagination to think about new leisure, health care, and convenience products for aging baby boomers. Thus the aging of cohorts (groups of people born at the same time) as a dimension of population aging has an impact on the economy—on product and service development, on savings, and on consumer demand patterns.

These examples are not meant to oversimplify societal aging or social change in institutions such as the economy. Rather, these examples are intended to illustrate how the experiences of aging, and the social contexts in which they take place, change over time as a result of the aging of unique cohorts. As new groups of people go through stages of growing older, they bring with them a unique historical profile, and they alter the meanings and values associated with growing older. The movement of new groups into old age also places new demands on the social system. Changes to the social structure emerge in response to the size, characteristics, and demands of each new group of older people. The intricacies of this dynamic between cohorts and social change are discussed in further detail in later chapters. For our purposes at this point, it is important to acknowledge that societal aging is a significant dimension of the social processes of aging.

Ways of Categorizing People by Age

As we consider the many dimensions of social aging, we need a way to mark or measure the age of individuals. Most often people are categorized in one of three ways: chronological age, functional status, or life stage. Each way of expressing age has advantages and disadvantages, and the decision to use any one of them should be based on the goals of examining age. Keep in mind that whether we use chronological age, functional status, or life stages, we are applying socially constructed labels and definitions that allow us to treat people as members of meaningful social categories. We use these definitions in many ways. We sometimes make implicit judgments about whether we are likely to have anything in common with someone based on the age group they appear to belong to, and we explicitly use age to select a specific target for social action or policy or to define a subject of study. Remember, all these definitions, including chronological

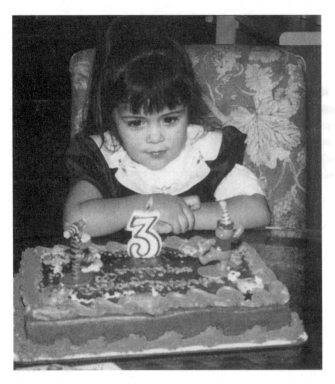

Like most cultures, ours places a big emphasis on chronological age—for both young and old alike. (Credit: M. Payne)

age, are human creations. In selecting definitions of aging or age categories, we need to be conscious of our underlying purpose and select our definitions accordingly.

Chronological Age

This is one of the simplest assessments of age and thus it reduces administrative complexity. Chronological age is used in our society as the basis for determining many social roles (voting, driving, marrying, holding public office), for eligibility in social programs (such as Social Security, AARP membership, or Older Americans Act services), and inclusion in research projects.

The use of chronological age to mark major life transitions is taken for granted in modern urban societies. However, it is a relatively recent development coinciding with the rise of large-scale industrialism in the early twentieth century (Moody, 1993). The industrial economy required that human lives be ordered efficiently so that work years coincided with the years assumed to be associated with peak productivity. Chronological age was adopted as a simple way to define a worker's life stage.

The meaningfulness of chronological age is questioned in many ways today, however. The number of birthdays an individual has had tells us little in and of itself. The fluidity and multiplicity of today's life-styles defy the use of boundaries as rigid as numerical age (Moody, 1993). When it is possible to have two career peaks—one at age 40 in a first career and a second at age 60 in a second career—when it is increasingly common to find people having children when they are 40—about the age at which others are becoming grandparents—the usefulness of chronological age as a life stage marker is indeed questionable.

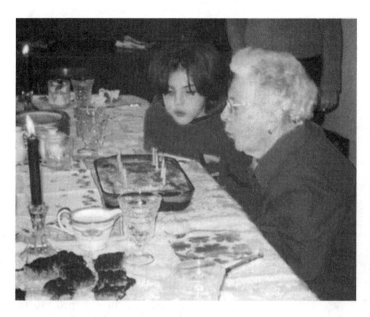

For many, each birthday is a blessing, bringing more to celebrate with each passing year. (Credit: Courtesy of Julia Wing)

In the world of social policy and programs, the validity of chronological age is being questioned at another level (Torres-Gil, 1992). Even though "age has long stood as a formidable proxy for demonstrable need and, in turn, the receipt of support from the larger society" (Hudson, 2005, p. 1), there are political and ideological debates about the usefulness of age-based policies. The age for eligibility for full benefits under Social Security is gradually being raised, so that by the year 2027 workers will need to be 67 to retire with full benefits. Older Americans Act services, for which people become eligible at age 60, are increasingly being targeted to groups within the older population with the greatest need—frail, low-income, and minority groups. In general, policies seem to be moving away from such a central focus on chronological age. These policy issues are discussed in greater detail in chapter 12, but the policy shifts are further examples of the challenges to the meaningfulness of chronological age.

Functional Age

What marker of age will we use if chronological age continues to lose its significance and usefulness? There is considerable difference between 65-year-olds and 95-year-olds, yet all are considered to be older adults. In the case of policies and programs, targeting services to specific subgroups is increasingly common, not simply on the basis of age but on the basis of need. For example, to identify people who have physical limitations that require regular assistance, we can use measures of functional status such as Activities of Daily Living, a generic term for several scales that measure an individual's ability to accomplish, without assistance, routine personal care activities such as bathing, eating, dressing, and getting in and out of bed. Such measures are useful for targeting home care programs to those who need them because of physical frailty.

When we use chronological age as a convenient way to determine eligibility for benefits such as Medicare, we are assuming that age is a proxy for the need for those services. Functional status is a way to move beyond that generalized assumption about age,

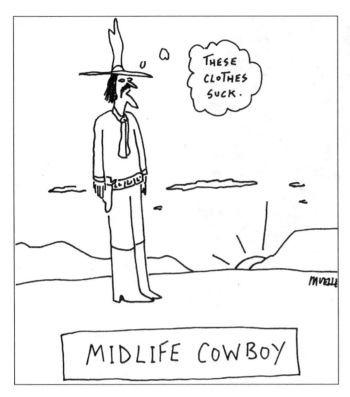

but it is obviously a much more complicated way to grant access to programs and services.

Life Stage

As lives progress, people tend to reach certain plateaus of stability (life stages) punctuated by periods of change or transition. Thus, people can be categorized as being in roughly comparable circumstances, such as adolescence, young adulthood, middle age, and later maturity. We can assume that people going through the "empty nest" transition have adult children and are in the process of launching them into lives as independent adults. We can assume that people in very old age (sometimes call "old-old" age, referring to people 85 and above) are probably physically frail and live simple lives. **Life stages** are thus broad social categories that describe particular times of life involving new social roles (such as grandparenthood), physical changes (such as physical frailty), or transitions (such as leaving one's job to retire).

Life stages roughly correspond to chronological age ranges but are much more socially constructed and culturally based than chronological age. For example, when is someone an adult? When they move out of their parents' home, reach age 18 or age 21, have a child, have a full-time job, or act mature? Life stages rely on some information about physical changes but are much more attentive to other traits such as the roles (e.g., parent, employee) that people play. For example, the "empty nest" described above implies something about chronological age but derives its meaning from the new family roles and relationships emerging during that stage. The concept of life stage is discussed further in chapter 4, when we explore the sequences of roles people move into and out of during their lives. We will specifically discuss life stages within the family and within the economy, emphasizing the shared expectations about what roles people should be playing at what ages.

Ageism

With all of the possible ways to assess and define age, and the limitations of any single approach, it is fair to ask why we continue to use age in so many aspects of social life. In part, we use social categories to help organize our world so that every situation is not completely new and confusing. Unfortunately, our use of social characteristics such as age, gender, and race to categorize people often leads to stereotypes, prejudice, and discrimination. **Ageism** is "a systematic stereotyping of and discrimination against people because they are old, just as racism and sexism accomplish this with skin color and gender" (Butler, 1989, p. 243). At the heart of any kind of "ism" (ageism, racism, sexism, classism) is the creation of an "other"(grouping together people identified as different because of some characteristic they do or do not possess (e.g., gender, race, class, or age). Ageism and other "isms" can lead to the use of sweeping generalizations about members of that "other" category, stereotyping them (often incorrectly) as sharing common traits or attitudes. These stereotypes often extend to excluding the "others" from aspects of participation in social life or limiting their opportunities. We are all familiar with the views of older people as lonely, frail, poor, and deserving of help. This "compassionate ageism" (Binstock, 1991a) exists side by side with other stereotypical views: older people are cute and interesting; older people are wise and funny; older people are greedy and selfish and economically advantaged. While the content of these ageist views varies considerably, the impact is the same. Older people are seen as "other"—in either positive or negative light—different from us, but all like each other.

We often use visual, informal assessments to decide whether a person is "old." However, such categorizations limit the opportunities available, both for formal social participation and for informal interaction, to the person assigned to the "older" category. For example, think about your reactions to someone who seems "old" and strikes up a conversation with you as you wait to cross the street. If you have any kind of automatic negative reaction to that person, you may unconsciously limit the possibilities for interaction. As further illustration of the power of these visual assessments, think about why it is considered such a compliment to say to someone, "You don't look 50 (or 30 or 80)." Why is it so desirable to look younger than your age? And what "should" 50 look like?

The Rise of Old Age as a Social Category

We tend to take for granted the idea of categorizing people by age. We sometimes are not conscious of the many ways in which this categorization takes place, or of its impacts. It is often difficult to take a step back from our everyday lives in order to reflect on why we organize our social lives the way we do. Social science, especially sociology, helps us to gain a more reflective attitude. The notion of systematically studying society and its dynamics developed at the time of the industrialization of Western Europe in the mid- to late nineteenth century. The era's grand masters of social theory—Comte, Spencer, Durkheim, Weber, and Marx—focused on the ideological and cultural shift that transformed Europe from agricultural, small-scale societies to urban mass societies. They also observed the shift from the family as the basic economic unit to individual achievement and performance in a complex division of the labor market. They either said nothing at all about age, aging, or generations or referred to these topics only in passing, perhaps because they were more interested in society as a whole than in the details of individual life structure. Populations in these societies were much younger then, before the significant changes discussed in chapter 3 that brought about societal aging.

Generational Consciousness

By the 1950s, social theorists began thinking and writing about age, aging, generations, and the life course. Their work remains relevant today. The first serious attempt to look at the social importance of age groups was made by the German sociologist Karl Mannheim in an essay titled "The Problem of Generations," which was first published in 1927. Mannheim defined **generation** as a category of people born within a specific historical era or time period. For Mannheim, a generation was also characterized by common world views that distinguished it from other generations. Mannheim was keenly aware that accident of birth timing did not automatically create these common understandings and worldviews; he observed that social and social psychological processes led some members of a generation to develop an identity and consciousness with their age peers. Mannheim suggested that generational consciousness arose not from merely being born at the same time but from being exposed to the same kinds of experiences and historical events in a common social and political environment. According to Mannheim, belonging to a generation is a combination of a *state of mind* and an age grouping.

Each generation reacts to its social and historical time. Today's teenagers, called the "multitasking generation" or "Generation Tech," are categorized as technologically savvy, cynical about the materialistic values of preceding generations, and jaded by growing up in a world of violence, but there are certainly different subgroups within "Gen Tech." The idea that each generation has its own identify is intuitively appealing, but it is easy (and dangerous) to overgeneralize. Mannheim suggested that each generation may comprise a number of specific units, each with a unique consciousness. For example, the 1980s saw the young adult cohort split between the *yuppies* (young, upwardly mobile professionals) with a self-centered life philosophy that influenced social change in the economy particularly, and the *environmentalists*, with their concerns about creating an economically and physically sustainable future for life on earth. These generational units, although of the same age, were quite distinct.

Mannheim proposed that much of the potential for conflict between generations stemmed from the tendency of older generations to hold on too long to their generational philosophy.

> Any two generations following one another always fight different opponents.... While the older people may be still combating something in themselves or in the external world in such a fashion that all their feelings and efforts and even their concepts and categories of thought are determined by that adversary, for the younger people this adversary may simply be nonexistent. (Mannheim, 1952b, pp. 298–299)

For example, the defining theme of needing to be free from want that drove the Great Depression generation was not the defining theme of the generations that followed, such as the World War II generation or the 1960s generation.

Generational tensions are not inevitable. Mannheim suggested that intergenerational conflict is minimized by the fact that each generation spends much of its time interacting with the generations just before or after it and little time interacting with distant generations. The adjacent generations serve as mediators and interpreters of the much older or much younger generations. Much of Mannheim's commentary about

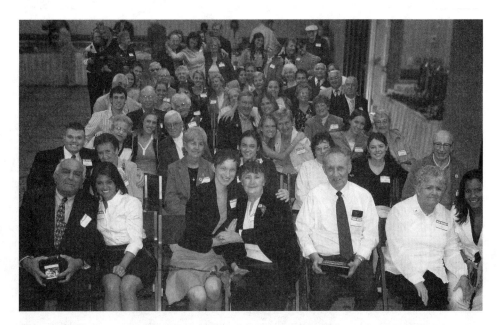

There is often a very special, loving bond between grandparents and their grandchildren that immensely enriches both generations. (Credit: E. J. Hanna)

intergenerational dynamics is relevant to today's debates about generational equity and intergenerational conflict, which are discussed in chapter 12.s

Mannheim's ideas about generations, generational consciousness, and the succession of generations remain useful and have served as major building blocks for sociological theories of aging. However, Mannheim sidestepped the central question of aging. He acknowledged that aging is part of the dynamics of generations, but he does not explicitly consider what that part might be.

The Aging Population as a Social Force

Warren Thompson and P. K. Whelpton, like Mannheim, drew attention to issues related to aging in the late 1920s and early 1930s. However, Thompson and Whelpton used a demographic perspective to ponder the effects of population aging on society. As a student, Thompson had become interested in the interplay between population and social structure. In 1930, the President's Research Committee on Social Trends gave Thompson and Whelpton the assignment of projecting the population of the United States from 1930 to 1980 and identifying significant population trends that should be taken into account in national planning.

The rapid growth of the older population and societal aging (discussed further in chapter 3) were identified by Thompson and Whelpton (1933) as perhaps the most fundamental expected change in the population of the United States. Exhibit 1.2 shows how dramatically Thompson and Whelpton expected the population age structure to change in what, for a large population, was a very short period of time. Even though Thompson and Whelpton had no way to anticipate the post–World War II baby boom, their projections concerning growth in the older population were very much on target.

The actual proportion of people age 65 and over in the United States in 1980 was 11.9% compared to their projection of 12.1%.

Thompson and Whelpton assumed that retirement would continue to occur at age 65 and speculated that funding retirement pensions would be a major social challenge for the future.

> [T]he problem of old-age pensions is one thing in 1930 with 5.4 percent of the population over 65 years of age but will be a different thing in 1980 when the proportion over 65 years of age will probably be more than twice this large (over 12 percent). (Thompson & Whelpton, 1933, p. 165)

Writing before Social Security was enacted, they were understandably concerned about the potential social disruption that might come when a large proportion of the population would be retired but with no broad-based programs in place to provide continued retirement income. They were also concerned that poverty at older ages could be even greater than they anticipated "if, as is quite commonly believed, industry and commerce are scrapping men at earlier ages than formerly and if they hire older men only at very low wages" (Thompson & Whelpton, 1933, p. 170). (The use of "men" in this quote reflects a very different era; in the 1930s, the vast majority of middle-class workers were, indeed, men.)

Making an assumption that elders are more politically and socially conservative than the average American, Thompson and Whelpton suggested that an increase in the proportion of older adults in the population might lead to stronger defense of the status

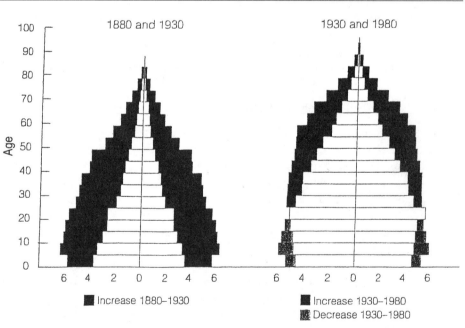

Distribution of the Population by Five-Year Age Periods: 1880–1930 and 1930–1980
Source: Thompson and Whelpton, 1933.

quo in politics and less innovation and risk-taking in business. Older people would, they argued, be less ready to abandon outdated social policies and business practices. To their credit, however, Thompson and Whelpton pointed out that social innovation could still be fostered through intentional planned effort by middle-aged and older members of society to search for creative and more efficient business methods.

In their discussions of employment and income problems for an aging population, Thompson and Whelpton tended to portray the growing population of older Americans as an imminent social problem. However, social problems refer to difficulties that categories of people encounter not because of their own qualities but because of the way they fare in the operation of the social system. C. Wright Mills (1959) spoke of the distinction between private troubles that arise from accidents of personal history and social problems that arise from inequities built into the concepts, laws, rules, and procedures we live by. Thompson and Whelpton were writing specifically about the social problem of poverty arising from the practice at that time of compulsory retirement at age 65 in the absence of retirement pensions. But in an entirely different vein, they noted that the processes of adult development could have a beneficial influence on social cultural trends. They wrote:

> Youth is more concerned with doing things, forging ahead, and making a place in the world. Age is apt to be more reflective, perhaps because the spur of poverty is less sharp, the inner drive is weaker, or time and thought have brought about a change of ideas as to the goal of life. The mere shift in age distribution, therefore, may lead to more interest in cultural activities and increased support for the arts. Such developments in turn will influence the outlook and taste of the whole population. (Thompson & Whelpton 1933, p. 168)

Here they acknowledged that elders were not simply a social problem or a category toward which policy might be directed, but also people who were continuously evolving and could become social resources and agents for change. This potential role for the older population sounds very similar to an idea that is currently receiving a great deal of attention. **Civic engagement** refers to the involvement by people of all ages in actions and efforts designed to make a difference in communities; it is both an activity and a value. As a social value, civic engagement implies a commitment to solving problems and making a difference (Ehrlich, 2000). Recognizing and encouraging the many ways that older people can contribute skills, knowledge, and energy to the common good is a growing topic of research, advocacy, and public policy in gerontology. Thompson and Whelpton foreshadowed this movement with their observation that aging populations might benefit from the unique contributions that older people can make to civic life.

The Life Course and Old Age

A further key step in the development of old age as a social category came with the comparative, cross-cultural work of an anthropologist Ralph Linton (1942). Social anthropology is concerned with identifying cultural universals, patterns that appear in all human cultures, as well as links between culture and personality. Linton advanced the thesis that all known societies have been stratified by at least two human characteristics, age and sex. The definitions of age and age categories, the number of age categories, and the rules governing transitions from one age to another have varied considerably across societies, but in all societies old men and old women have been differentiated from one another and from adult men, adult women, boys, girls, and infants. Linton's simple and basic statement of fact is still true over 60 years later.

Linton suggested that the modernization of society has affected the status of the old by transforming age from a key status location in the social structure to just one of many individual attributes. Thus, *old* shifted from a meaningful adult category with rights and duties to simply a qualifying adjective used to make other role expectations more precise—for example, older worker.

Another important concept that permeated Linton's work was the idea of a **life course,** formed by a succession of age-sex categories. In all societies, males who survived infancy would go on to experience boyhood, ascend to adult manhood, and then become either elevated to or relegated to the position of old man, depending on whether the society was accepting or rejecting in its treatment of old men. A parallel sequence existed for females.

Linton believed that these life course age-sex categories are arranged in a hierarchy of social influence. In most societies, the adult males have been the most influential, although occasionally Linton discovered cases where elder men have had the most influence. He found another kind of variability. In many cases, elder women experienced increased freedom and status when they went through the transition from adult to older woman.

> Even in societies which are strongly patriarchal in theory it will be found that a surprisingly large number of families are ruled by strong willed mothers and grandmothers.... [Among the Comanche,] old women ... could acquire and use "power" on exactly the same terms as men and were treated as equals by male "power" holders. (Linton, 1942, p. 594)

In addition to looking at life stages and age-sex categories, Linton discussed transitions from one age-sex category to the next. He was impressed with the capacity of humans to make sometimes quite abrupt and substantial changes without showing signs of mental distress. Linton suggested that the transition from adulthood to old age was a particularly difficult one, because the loss of power is not satisfactorily offset by a decline in obligations and because formal values about respect and authority granted to older people may not be carried out in actual practice.

Linton's work has been an extremely important resource for the social perspective on aging. He drew attention to the process that connects age to social position and influence and used the sociological concepts of status and role to explicate a complex social structure made up of interconnected role obligations and opportunities. Linton's work presented the life course as a progression of age grades, thus linking the issue of aging with life stages. The life course perspective is, in fact, one of the most important frameworks in social gerontology today. Finally, Linton drew attention to the importance of life course transitions and hinted at a human adaptive capacity to deal with life changes.

Social Perspectives on Aging

The social scientists described above provide excellent illustrations of understanding age as a social category. Throughout our discussion of old age and aging, we have referred to the way society creates and perpetuates ideas about who is old, how they should act, and how we treat them. We will continually return to the ideas of social construction as we discuss the many aspects of aging. While many fields of study discuss society, social changes, and peoples' lives, two perspectives in particular are helpful frameworks for understanding the social context of aging: *social gerontology* and the *sociology of aging*.

Social Gerontology

Many social gerontology courses are taught in departments of sociology by sociologists, and much of the material included in social gerontology courses consists of research on aging by sociologists. However, social gerontology has a broader range of interests than the sociology of aging. **Social gerontology** is a multidisciplinary field that includes research, policy, and practice information from all of the social sciences and the humanities (see Exhibit 1.3). A specific example describes its scope.

More and more families are facing the challenge of deciding about long-term care arrangements for relatives or friends who need increasing amounts of help throughout each day. Decision-making about long-term care is a topic that has implications for individuals, families, health care systems, and public policy. How, when, by whom, and with what outcome are different questions related to the long-term care decision; each of these topics can be approached from many different angles, with many different disciplinary perspectives. Psychologists might be interested in the communication and cognitive processes that are involved in negotiations and decisions of this type. Sociologists could

Exhibit
1.3

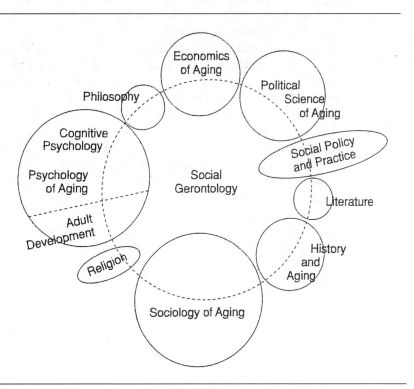

In Social Gerontology, the Sociology of Aging Is But One of Many Disciplines.

consider the hierarchy or differences in power that might come into play as family members, the older person, and professionals negotiate the decision. Professionals from the world of long-term care practice might be interested in ways to more effectively describe options to families; they might also be concerned about making sure that the older person whose life is being discussed has a say in the planning and decisions. Researchers interested in public policy might focus on how the timing of long-term care decisions might be affected by the service options available and an effect on costs to the long-term care system. Social gerontologists would draw on all of these perspectives to fully understand the processes and outcomes of decisions about long-term care.

Both social gerontology and the sociology of aging share an interest in sociological work applied to aging. The **sociology of aging** is concerned with understanding aging from sociological perspectives and applying that understanding to sociology in general. Social gerontology is concerned with understanding aging from a variety of perspectives and integrating information from various social science and humanities disciplines to achieve an understanding of aging in general, and to apply that understanding to resolving problems and creating policy. Increasingly, social gerontologists are seeking to more fully benefit from the multiple disciplinary perspectives that can be brought to bear on any topic related to age, aging, and the life course by moving to an **interdisciplinary** approach. While social gerontology is, by definition, multidisciplinary (drawing on multiple perspectives), interdisciplinary research would involve more than working together with respect for, and being somewhat conversant in, other disciplines. Interdisciplinary research would mean active collaboration and new ways of formulating the questions we are asking, and new methods for exploring those questions. The study of the genetic, behavioral, social, and cultural factors that contribute to longevity could be an example of interdisciplinary research. Does this mean that every member of the research team must be trained in all of these specialties, or does it mean that the team works together with new methods and techniques? This question does not have a clear answer yet. In the meantime, social gerontology is continuing to develop as a truly productive multidisciplinary field.

Although the sociology of aging and other disciplinary perspectives can be differentiated from social gerontology, in the actual study of aging the boundaries among them are often blurry. Often studies focus on a topic that falls both within the domain of social gerontology and within the traditional domain of sociology and economics or psychology. However, as a field, sociology has not been particularly interested in the sociology of aging. Until recently, aging has generally been seen as a fringe topic rather than a serious area of scholarship dealing with one of the most important social trends societies will confront over the next 50 years. By contrast, the field of aging (gerontology) has been very interested in the sociology of aging. Some of the unique contributions of sociology are presented here.

The Sociological Imagination

The promise of the sociological perspective has nowhere been more powerfully and eloquently expressed than in C. Wright Mills's classic presentation of the sociological imagination. He suggested that the promise, and the responsibility, of sociology lies in giving individuals the tools to make the distinction between, and see the connections between, concerns we face in our own lives and problems that are rooted in society. Mills (1959) advises,

> Know that many personal troubles cannot be solved merely as troubles, but must be understood in terms of public issues—and in terms of the problems of history. Know that the human meaning of public issues must be revealed by relating them to personal troubles—and to the problems of the individual. (p. 226)

We can make this distinction if we have a social context and a sense of history from which to understand personal experiences. The ability to shift perspectives, to analyze an experience or an issue from many levels of analysis, and to see the intersection of these many levels of mutual influence, is the fruit of the sociological imagination. If you develop a new understanding of your attitudes about older people because of what you learn about how societies construct meanings of age, you will have experienced the sociological imagination. If you understand how an older individual's situation of economic disadvantage is a product of social forces rather than simply personal choice or chance, you are applying the sociological imagination.

"No social study that does not come back to the problems of biography, of history, and of their intersections within a society has completed its intellectual journey" (Mills, 1959, p. 5). Mills suggests that there are three basic questions we must continually ask in exercising the sociological imagination. First, what is the structure of this particular society as a whole? How does it differ from other varieties of social order? Second, where does this society stand in human history? What are the essential features of this period? Third, what "varieties" of people prevail in this society and in this period? How are these types "selected and formed, liberated and repressed, made sensitive and blunted?" (p. 7).

Note particularly Mills's third question, which suggests that social order and historical period select in favor of certain kinds of people. This is a profoundly different view of human nature than most of us are familiar with. Yet, armed with this understanding, we can go on to understand how, "by the fact of our living, we contribute, however minutely, to the shaping of our society and to the course of its history, even as we are made by society and its historical push" (Mills, 1959, p. 4). Also, defining an issue as "public" creates new ways to seek answers beyond adopting an "every person for him- or herself" approach. Age-based policies developed as a consequence of seeing aging as a public issue. Social Security developed as a consequence of the Great Depression, when poverty became seen as a public matter, not an individual problem.

Micro and Macro Perspectives

Mills' discussion of history, society, and biography draws attention to the intersection of individual life experience and broad social forces, and in doing so points to the micro-to-macro range of perspectives on any topic. A **micro perspective** focuses on the individual level, while a **macro perspective** focuses more broadly on society. Behaviors, attitudes, and feelings are shaped partly by personalities and partly by one's social situation. There is an interplay between individual responses to social influences (**micro concerns**) and the social structures—organizations and institutions—that create the conditions requiring a response from individuals (**macro concerns**). The camera lens is in many ways an apt metaphor. A standard lens depicts a modest visual field and a modest amount of close-up detail. The wide-angle lens captures a much wider visual field, but the images of specific objects within the field contain less detail than images produced by the standard lens. A telephoto lens can focus on distant objects in greater detail, but the width of the visual field is very narrow. Three photographs of the same general visual field taken with different lenses will not capture everything that the human eye is capable of seeing. Which photograph is the most useful depends on the purpose to which the photograph is to be put. Similarly, different questions about the social context, meanings, and experiences of aging require different perspectives along the micro–macro continuum.

Several major streams of research are concerned with understanding micro–level issues such as the adaptation of individuals to the changes that accompany aging. This work considers the individual's adjustment to changes in his or her social situation, such as retirement. A more macro perspective seeks to understand, explain, and predict the social construction of those conditions to which the individual must respond: what is the status attached to being retired, what provisions does society make to support economic and other needs of retirees, and what are corporate rules regarding eligibility to retire? Other questions look at larger macro–level questions without considering the individual (micro level). How does retirement affect companies? How is retirement related to over-all societal patterns of employment and unemployment? How does retirement reflect and affect the overall economy of a society?

This micro–macro distinction is one of the energizing tensions in the study of aging; each perspective enriches the other and can push the other to greater clarity and applicability. There are many ways of classifying and organizing our experiences of the social world. The micro–macro distinction is one important way of categorizing ideas and information, directing us to different, but equally important, questions about aging in the social world.

Patterning of Experience: Diversity and Heterogeneity

Looking more deeply and critically at the ways in which society influences the meanings and experiences of aging, some sociologists have focused on how, why, and to what extent the experiences of aging are different for different groups of people—looking for a **patterning of experience**. For example, poverty is substantially more prevalent among Black women who live alone than among any other group of older people. Why does this pattern exist? What social forces have produced this structured disadvantage for older Black women?

Many scholars have warned against using averages to describe the older population, because there is more variation among older people than among younger people on some variables. This heterogeneity is very often acknowledged but not thoroughly examined. Arguing for the need to analyze patterns of difference, Dannefer (1988) suggested that research should begin to look for the extent, nature, and patterns of heterogeneity on a wide range of variables. Is the older population as heterogeneous on life satisfaction as they are on income? Are the political attitudes of older people as varied as health status in later life? Does the amount of heterogeneity on health status change as people grow older? What is the pattern of that change? Does heterogeneity increase, decrease, or fluctuate over time? Finding out more about how much heterogeneity exists among the older population, on which variables, and in what pattern is an important first step in understanding the different experiences people have as they age.

But we need to go even further to really understand the many different realities of aging. Dannefer (1988) suggests that the next step is to analyze the sources of heterogeneity. How is heterogeneity produced, and what should be done about it? Calasanti (1996b) further refines this position by distinguishing between heterogeneity as variation among individuals and diversity. Heterogeneity—the extent to which older individuals are different from each other—as discussed in the preceding paragraph might also be called individuality. **Diversity** refers to patterns of difference among *groups of people* in different social locations. The most common indicators of these social locations are gender, race, ethnicity, and social class. Scholarship on diversity searches for the nature, extent, and causes of differences among groups of older people. It acknowledges that the realities of aging are not the same across all groups. Throughout this text we present information and ideas about the diverse experiences of aging, focusing on race, ethnicity, gender, and social class. Race and ethnicity are extremely complex, personal, and significant identities. In the most recent U.S. census (2000), six race categories were listed and people could check more than one. In addition, there were questions about Latino or Hispanic identity. Hispanic/Latino respondents can be of any race, so many combinations of race and ethnicity are possible. The complexities and importance of race and ethnicity are far-reaching. For the purposes of this book, we focus on two major categories of race, and Hispanic or Latino for ethnicity. We use Black and White for much of the race data and Hispanic/non-Hispanic in the discussion of ethnicity.

Studying diversity can take one of two directions. We can compare groups to try to understand their different experiences of aging. A fair amount of research takes this approach, and some of it is referred to in later chapters. This is a useful but limited approach. The disadvantage of the "comparison" model for studying diversity is that there is always a reference group to whom everyone else is compared. For example, we can say that women have higher rates of diabetes than men, or that older Black women have the highest rates of poverty among adults. While this information is instructive, the implicit use of a dominant group as a point of comparison reinforces the reference group's experience as "normal" and minimizes the different social reality inhabited by the "other" groups (Calasanti, 1996b). Most typically the comparison group is White males, even though women outnumber men at later ages because of the differential in life expectancy by sex.

The limits of the comparison approach are well illustrated by the fact that such analyses often categorize people as White/non-White or male/not male. This approach assumes that the complexities of life in a particular social category (Black, female, working class) are somehow captured by not being a member of the reference group. But it is clear that being female is not the same as not being male (Kunkel & Atchley, 1996).

By focusing on groups of people in particular social locations, we can better understand the different worlds of aging. We would ask different questions that delve more deeply into the lives of the members of the group we are interested in. Instead of comparing men's and women's rates of diabetes, we might ask how the rates of diabetes vary among women, by social class and race; or we might attempt to specify exactly how social forces affect the lives of members of a particular group. Listening to the "voices" of specific groups better illuminates their situation than focusing on how they are different from the dominant group. The questions asked, the concerns attended to, and the items included on a survey will be more insightful if we begin with a conviction that reality is different for groups in different social positions. For example, Gibson (1996) writes about the retirement experience of older Blacks. She introduces the "unretired-retired" status to describe individuals who are 55 or older and not working, but who do not consider themselves retired. This status is most common among poor Blacks. They do not meet traditional criteria for retirement and therefore are not included in studies of retirement. This example clearly illustrates how using the experiences and meanings that are relevant for one dominant group completely undermines the ability to understand the experiences of other groups.

As social research on diversity in aging matures, more attention is given to diversity as an approach to reality rather than a kind of comparative content. Calasanti (1996b) argues for an acknowledgment of the constructed and contextual nature of social reality in all theorizing and research. "Being inclusive requires acknowledging the unique configuration of a group within the matrix of power relations, being sensitive to the importance of these cross-cutting relations, and not making undue generalizations" (p. 15).

SUMMARY

Aging is a broad and diverse field of study. In recent decades, as the population has aged, aging has steadily become an important topic addressed by many disciplines and perspectives. It is an exciting time to be using sociology and social gerontology to study age, aging, and the life course. Enormous social changes are underway—changes that both affect older people and are affected by the aging of society. Public policy, families, health care, education, and the economy are all changing as society ages.

The very large baby boom generation is on its way to joining the ranks of the older population; the oldest baby boomers turned 60 in January 2006. The sheer size of this group, and its unique generational experience, will doubtless change the meanings and experiences of aging for those to follow. Two recent publications suggest the transformations that are underway. *Reinventing Aging* (Center for Health Communication, Harvard School of Public Health, 2004) describes the opportunities for, and promise of, the baby boom generation to continue to be involved in society well into old age. *Reimagining America* (AARP, 2005a) summarizes the challenges that the United States faces as baby boomers enter old age and offers suggestions for innovative solutions to those challenges.

Our goal in this book is to illustrate the kinds of work leading us to a new understanding of the social context and social constructions of aging. An understanding of how social theorists and researchers think about, analyze, critique, and investigate questions related to aging is our major focus. In the process we will note areas that have not received adequate attention and offer some suggestions about why some questions and issues have remained unasked and unexamined. This latter course requires some speculation, but we decided it would be more challenging and interesting and might inspire some readers to fill in the gaps in our understanding of aging.

In the chapters that follow, we delve more deeply into the social aspects of aging at both the micro and macro levels, focusing on the changing face of later life within the dynamic context of the social world. Since aging is reshaping the future for us all, we expect you will find compelling issues for yourself, your family, and for the larger society.

WEB WISE

At the end of each chapter we present a number of Web sites that may be relevant to further investigation of select topics presented in that chapter. Some are oriented toward research, while others focus on policy or practice. For each site we provide the address and a brief description of what is included or tips on links you may wish to pursue. To get you started, we have included a "how to" Web site that describes how to access, use, and cite information from the Internet. Another included site contains a directory to many other useful Web sites on topics for which we did not list a particular site.

Columbia University Press

The Columbia Guide to Online Style
http://www.columbia.edu/cu/cup/cgos/idx_basic.html

This site outlines both the MLA (humanities) and APA and CBE (scientific) methods for citing online references within text and for correct bibliographies at the end of papers. Provides formats for materials cited from nontraditional sources, such as online materials.

Sites To Help Locate Other Sites on Aging

AOA Internet and E-mail Resources on Aging: An Online Directory
http://www.aoa.dhhs.gov/aoa/pages/jpostlst.html

Joyce Post, a librarian at the Philadelphia Geriatric Center, has compiled and categorized electronic resources related to aging. This site, maintained in cooperation with the Administration on Aging, includes over two thousand sites and listservs related to aging and can be searched to find more specific information. We suggest going to "General Resources" or checking items marked as "Best Bets."

AARP Policy & Research Page
http://www.aarp.org/research

This page provides a guide to a wide array of information collected by AARP on topics ranging from individual health, mobility, and housing to public policy and law. It includes links to pages where more detailed headings connect to resources of interest. AARP opinion pieces and research reports on many topics can be accessed.

KEY TERMS

ageism	life course	patterning of experience
civic engagement	life stage	social aging
cohort	macro perspective	social construction
diversity	macro concern	social gerontology
generation	micro perspective	societal aging
interdisciplinary	micro concern	sociology of aging

QUESTIONS FOR THOUGHT AND DISCUSSION

1. Browse through a birthday card selection, taking note of cards that are designed for different ages. What is your reaction? How are the messages of the cards different, based on the age group for whom they are intended? What makes a birthday card funny?

2. John Glenn recently completed his much publicized return to space. His age (he was in his 70s) was a major topic of conversation. Why is the American public so amazed, and possibly wary, of a 75-year-old astronaut?

3. Respond to the statement that "You are only as old as you feel." Do you agree or disagree? What are some of the things that influence how old we feel?

4. What are some of the causes, consequences, and solutions to ageism?

Studying Aging

[N]ever begin a sentence with "The elderly are ..." or "The elderly do ..." No matter what you are discussing, some are, and some are not; some do, and some do not. The most important characteristic of the aged is their diversity. The average can be very deceptive, because it ignores the tremendous dispersion around it. Beware of the mean. (Quinn, 1987, p. 64)

Despite the perennial desire to understand how and why people age in a physical sense, the study of the social aspects of **aging** is a relatively recent phenomenon; the vast bulk of research has been done in the past 40 years. The research techniques that were initially applied to the study of aging in a social context were borrowed from the disciplinary research traditions of sociology, economics, history, and other fields and then applied to the study of processes and products of aging in social life. The traditions and assumptions of these transplanted analytical frames of reference have shaped both the types of questions that are asked and the manner in which we seek answers to them. More recently, however, the study of aging has matured and developed its own unique approaches to answering the key questions. These new approaches were necessary because of the kinds of questions that research on aging seeks to answer and because of the interdisciplinary nature of the field. The innovative methodological frames of reference, the unique questions and challenges of gerontological research, are the subject of this chapter.

Mainstream social science research has dealt with "age" for years as a variable in research, often as an important background variable along with race, ethnicity, social class, and gender. The study of aging, however, redirects our attention to age as the central variable of interest, with the correlates and consequences of aging the focus of attention. The earliest research on social aspects of aging focused on the aged as a group, considering their circumstances (such as poverty and ill health) as social problems and examining ways to intervene on both the individual and societal levels. More recently, however, the focus has shifted from studying "the aged" as a population category to studying *aging* as a social process (Campbell & O'Rand, 1985). This shift has prompted a move away from research methods that focused on analysis of a static group (those over 65 or some other arbitrary age) to studies of dynamic processes in society as groups of individuals move through life's various stages to later life. The addition of this dynamic view and application of the life course perspective have raised a whole range of new questions and prompted the development of new methodological approaches to answer them. So, although the roots of research in aging reach into the most enduring traditions of several social science disciplines, researchers are constantly struggling to find new and better ways to examine the dynamics of aging in an ever-changing society.

Why Do We Conduct Research?

There are a number of important reasons to conduct research on our social world. The most central motive is a deep curiosity. Most of us are curious about how our world works. Social research helps us to understand how the various facets of our social world interact to shape the lives of individuals, groups, and major social institutions such as the economy, contributing to the stream of social change that we all encounter during our lives (Schutt, 2004). Thus, the first impulse of research is to generate accurate knowledge about the social world in which we live.

The interest in research goes deeper than this curiosity and desire for knowledge. Social scientists, like all scientists, are committed to a fuller understanding of how and why things (in our case, the social world) work the way they do. This understanding requires building theories that both explain and predict social behavior on the micro level of the individual, on the macro level of the social institution or society, or on any intermediate level between these two extremes. The second major purpose of doing research, then, is to generate, test, and refine theories. Ironically, the purpose of any specific piece of research is not to validate a theory, but to refute it. Because most theories are created and promoted because they seem logical and plausible, it can be easy to accept their propositions as intuitively appealing. As with many other scientific fields, the study of aging has had theories that seemed intuitively appealing when first proposed but that were subsequently proved to be inadequate or false. Some examples of both successful and unsuccessful theories are described in subsequent chapters. Scientific method requires that we do as much as we can to test a theory by trying to prove it to be wrong, thereby invalidating it and prompting us to develop new or alternative theories to explain what we see. In this way, progress is made toward understanding social phenomena, including the processes of aging.

A third and increasingly compelling reason for conducting research on aging is to provide input for public policy and intervention. This type of study, referred to as applied research or evaluation research, uses scientific methods to provide answers to important questions of policy and practice (McAuley, 1987; Schutt, 2004). Studying a particular service-delivery technique to support family caregivers of older adults with physical or cognitive health problems, for example, would be an applied evaluation study with direct implications for policies and programs. Such research typically looks at the effects of programs, services, and policies on those they are intended to serve. Studies with this purpose, known as evaluation research, have long been commonplace in the fields of education and public health (Rossi, Lipsey, & Freeman, 2004). In these areas of policy and practice, the demonstrated effectiveness of an intervention (such as a special program for educationally at-risk students or a falls-prevention program for older adults) helps to decide its fate—whether it should be refined, funded, and continued. Similar research—about whether programs and services for older people are working in the way and to the extent expected—is becoming increasingly visible in the field of gerontology, as is a commitment to translating research findings into practice.

In an aging society and an aging world, the fate of individuals and groups as they grow older becomes inextricably linked to the well-being of the overall society. For example, older women are much more likely to be poor in later life, with many of them relying on modest Social Security survivor benefits as their sole source of income (Beedon & Wu, 2005). As society changes and more women are employed throughout adulthood, however, the plight of this group may improve as more aging women have their own pensions, savings, and Social Security benefits (Morgan, 1991). Making plans and policies based on current situations, without research insights on elders of the future, might lead to serious mistakes. More and more aging research is applied in the sense that its findings are directly translatable to strategies for intervention in the lives of older persons or policy recommendations on the local, state, or federal level.

Each of these goals—generating knowledge, refining and testing theory, and shaping policy—requires research that is systematic and rigorous. Social research represents a significant improvement over everyday observations that can be affected by errors such as selective perception (only seeing part of the picture), or overgeneralization (assuming that what we are observing is true for all people or in all similar situations) (Schutt, 2004). Research that is carefully designed and rigorously executed will provide knowledge that is more valid and understanding that is richer and more trustworthy than casual observation. Social science research design involves many complex decisions that are beyond the scope of this chapter. Designing good research about aging involves some unique challenges that we explore in this chapter. As a starting point, let us consider the link between theory and research. This link is important for all research.

The Role of Theory

Theories are often described as the driving force behind research, dictating both the specific questions that need to be asked and the choice of the most appropriate analytical techniques to answer them. For example, during the 1960s and 1970s, the theoretical contention between disengagement and activity theories led to considerable research on the concept of life satisfaction among the elderly. Today, these theories are seldom discussed, and contemporary research gives only minimal attention to life satisfaction (Markides, Liang, & Jackson, 1990).

Research methods are sometimes viewed simply as tools to enable the testing of theoretical propositions, allowing them to be supported or refuted. But the relationship between theory and methods is more complex than that. Both theory and methods are shaped by dominant ideas about what kinds of questions are interesting and appropriate and what tools are appropriate to answer them (Biggs, Lowenstein, & Hendricks, 2003). This argument is compellingly presented by Thomas Kuhn, who describes the ways in which our views of the world are necessarily limited. We cannot consider, see, or explore every possible aspect of reality. The work of other researchers and scholars provides a map of our destination and possible paths; that is, a model of the questions we are trying to answer and the methods we use to explore them. Kuhn called these maps "paradigms." Paradigms are conceptual lenses or models that influence what we define as a problem and what we can consider as solutions. "In learning a paradigm, the scientist acquires theory … and methods together, usually in an inextricable mixture" (Kuhn, 1996, p. 109). To illustrate, we can return to the tension between disengagement and activities theories mentioned above. These theories propose different explanations for aging; disengagement theory suggests that aging individuals and society mutually withdraw, while activity theory proposes that maintaining activity levels and involvement in social roles explain high life satisfaction in later year. Even though these theories propose different solutions to the "problem" of aging, they both focus on how individuals should and do adapt. The methods used to examine these competing theories involve the measurement of individual circumstances, attitudes, and adaptation. A different paradigm might shift our focus to very different questions: Why does aging require adaptation? What is the source of the problems that people must adapt to as they age? This paradigm would lead to theories and methods that consider the ways in which societies and social institutions cause the problems of aging, rather than the ways in which individuals might cope.

Given their common roots in dominant paradigms, the relationship between theory and methods is very dynamic. By constraining what the researcher is able to do, the methods available often stimulate the development of theory in certain areas while blocking it in others. A theory that cannot be tested through research, although it may be intriguing, is not scientifically viable (Achenbaum & Bengtson, 1994). Again, a good example is disengagement theory (discussed in detail in chapter 7). The theory was compelling, but it could not be tested effectively in research. For this and other reasons, interest in the theory soon waned, and researchers looked to other theories that provided more productive avenues for advancing knowledge. Although theory shapes methodology, the relationship is actually a reciprocal one, with feedback from methodology to theory development, as shown in Exhibit 2.1. Theory can be research-driven (Campbell & O'Rand, 1985), just as research is often theory-driven. Theory can even arise from research, as in the case of grounded theory (Glaser & Strauss, 1967). The link between research and theory is further discussed later in this chapter when we present qualitative and quantitative approaches to understanding our social world.

How Do We Conduct Research on Aging?

Research on aging can be driven by theories, curiosity about the surrounding world, or other research. One of the interesting and challenging features in aging research is that it seeks to answer a dazzling array of questions, covering topics related to the aging of cells to the aging of societies. What is it like to be old? What does aging "do" to us physically, emotionally, or socially? How do different cultures or societies treat people differently on the basis of their age? How, why, and in what ways does age make a difference in our lives? What are the costs and impacts of programs and policies serving older people? How do families adjust to the changes throughout the life course, including the onset

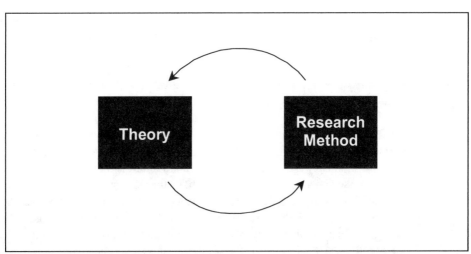

Synergy Between Theory and Research Methods

of disability and need for help from other family members? Each of these broad areas of curiosity could lead to a seemingly endless list of possible research questions.

The range of questions we might explore in research on aging relates to the micro–macro continuum discussed in chapter 1. To some extent, the kind of question a researcher might investigate will be influenced by her or his academic tradition. For example, biologists may examine aging in units as small as chemical compounds and components of the cell, whereas the macro level for a biologist may include entire complex organisms, such as mice or humans. Within the social sciences, the continuum also differs by discipline. Psychologists move from within-individual phenomena such as changes in cognitive or sensory functioning (micro) to the complex behavior of the person in social interaction (macro); sociologists take the individual as the micro end of their disciplinary continuum and entire societies as the macro end.

Often the same topic can be addressed using many different units of analysis to examine different aspects. For example, the social phenomenon of early retirement can be examined with the individual as the unit of analysis (addressing questions such as the effects of early retirement on economic well-being, friendship patterns, or marital satisfaction), on the company level (how does early retirement affect the quality of the pool of workers?), or on the societal level (how do the economies of Western societies fare when there is large-scale early retirement?).

The first step in any research process is to think through exactly what we want to explore. Before researchers can work through the details of how to design and conduct a study, they must be very clear about the scope, level, and unit of analysis implied in their question. One of the unique challenges in aging research is specifying exactly why and how age is included in a study.

Age as a Variable

As discussed in chapter 1, age can have many different meanings. Similarly, when we say that we want to study aging, we can be referring to very different kinds of questions related to age, aging, or the life course. Consider these three related examples: (1) a study of the impact of aging on physical health; (2) a study of older people who are participating in an exercise program; and (3) a project designed to find out whether an exercise program has the same effects for older people as for younger people. Although all of these topics are similar, the role that age would play in the research would be very different. In the first study, where the aim is to find out how age affects health, age is treated as an independent variable. An **independent variable** is assumed to cause, or have an impact on, another variable (the dependent variable). In the second study, to see if participating in an exercise program has a positive effect on the health of older people, age is simply a selection variable. We are particularly interested in the older population, so we select them for the study. The independent variable in this case is not age but rather participation in the exercise program; the dependent variable is health. In the third study, participation in the exercise program is again the independent variable, looking for the impact it has on physical health. However, the goal of this research is to see if the effects of the exercise program are the same for people of all ages. In this case, age is treated as a **control variable,** a variable that might influence the findings of the study and thus should be included in the design.

The role that age will play in any study—as an independent variable, a control variable, or a selection variable—is an important conceptual decision that has implications for the way age will be measured in the research. This might seem like quite a simple matter; we can just ask people how old they are or when they were born. In fact, much research on aging does just that. However, it is important to consider whether we want to know about the impact of every single year of age or whether the age group of the person is most important (for example, old vs. not old; middle age vs. old age; member of the baby boom generation or generation X).

It is essential to go through the formal process of **conceptualization** in research on aging. Conceptualization is a general term that refers to the process of generalizing or grouping ideas into a category. In research, this term refers to specifying exactly what is meant by an abstract concept. The conceptualization of age for research refers back to the issue of why we think age matters for the topic we want to study. Depending on the particular research question, age may be referring to the passage of time, as in the case of the first study above, which focused on the impact of age on health. In this situation, we might indeed want to track changes by single years of age. Age may also be used to define membership in a group—a generation, a target population for a service or program such as Medicare—or to mark the boundaries of a life stage such as retirement. In these cases, a person's exact age does not matter, and the research will not focus on the impact of every passing year. Conceptualization thus has implications for how age should be measured in research.

Sorting Out Age, Period, and Cohort Effects

Thinking through what we mean by "age" as a variable in research is the first important step in designing a study. Once we have achieved some clarity about why and how we think age matters in our work, it is necessary to pay attention to one of the most challenging issues in research on aging—the age–period–cohort problem. When a researcher studying political participation finds that the percentage of the population that votes is higher in upper age groups (see Exhibit 2.2), what exactly does that tell us? Does it mean that advancing years or changes resulting from aging make us more politically active or involved?

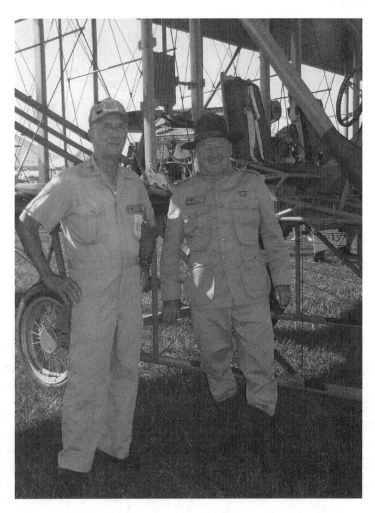

Although age is often a significant factor in social research,
many older persons soar above
and beyond stereotypes based on
their years. (Credit: E. J. Hanna)

Not necessarily. There are, in fact, three related influences that shape changes across age groups and over time: aging, period, and cohort effects. Understanding these three forces is central to understanding the complexity of aging in a social context.

Many researchers are interested in learning about the effects of **human aging**— that is, the changes that occur as individuals accumulate years and move through the life cycle. When most people think of the effects of aging, they think first of the physical effects, such as wrinkling of skin or graying of hair. Yet there is clearly a social side to aging as well. As discussed earlier, chronological age can be a proxy for life stages and can also be an indicator of social and psychological maturation. So questions may arise about the effects of aging on our social as well as physical lives. For example, we may want to know whether and how aging influences individuals' productivity at work, happiness in marriage, choices in saving or spending money, or religious participation. But answering these questions is not as simple as it first appears. The initial inclination would be to observe, for example, workers of various ages to learn how productive they are at a specific task and then draw comparisons by age. But would any differences that appear be *only* the result of aging?

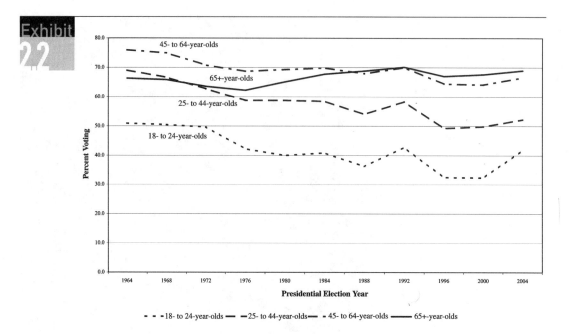

Exhibit 2.2

Percentage Voting in Presidential Elections by Age: 1964–2004
Source: U.S. Bureau of the Census, Current Population Reports 1968 to 2004.

It is very difficult to isolate the effects of aging in research, because human aging or maturation does not occur in a vacuum. Instead, the process of aging is surrounded by social, economic, and historical events that influence the lives of individuals and groups as they age. Beyond aging, a second force that is sometimes responsible for differences between age groups derives from the historical period. **Period effects** emerge from the major events that occur during a study of aging. For example, if we studied a cross-section of adults 25 years ago and again today and saw that the same people knew much more about AIDS now than they did before, should we conclude that their increased knowledge is a result of aging? Of course not. The period effect of growing public awareness of AIDS has influenced individuals of all ages over that same time period—at the same time that the adults were aging 25 years. Because individual aging and period effects are tied together by time, it is important to attempt to separate period effects from those of aging. The time at which we measure knowledge of AIDS, not the fact that the respondents are older, is the real issue with period effects. Major wars, economic booms or busts, and dramatic modifications in the norms and values of society alter people's experiences as they age (Schuman & Scott, 1989). It is important to recognize, however, that more "everyday" period effects—for example, the introduction of new technologies such as personal computers and cellular phones—can also have profound effects.

Finally, **birth cohorts**—groups of individuals born at approximately the same time in history and sharing a collection of historical life experiences—often differ from each other in important ways. These **cohort effects**—differences between groups sharing major life events (such as birth, marriage, college entry) at different points in historical time—are the third piece of this puzzle. For example, if a research study found that appreciation of the music of bandleader Lawrence Welk was higher among older birth cohorts, would it mean that people would come to like this music as they aged? Again, this difference is not an aging effect. Instead, the older cohorts today, who came of age during the era when Lawrence Welk's music was popular, have continued to like it as they have aged. Their preference is a cohort effect. It has moved with them as they aged; the preference was not caused by aging.

A breakthrough article by Ryder (1965) identified the critical nature of the cohort in understanding processes of aging in society. Paralleling some of Mannheim's ideas about "generation" discussed in chapter 1, Ryder identified the flow of birth cohorts through society as both creating and institutionalizing change in society over time. "Each cohort has a distinctive composition and character reflecting the circumstances of its unique origination and history" (p. 845). Members of a cohort share a slice of history and the social and cultural influences of their time, differentiating them from cohorts who preceded them or those that follow. Thus, each cohort has a life of its own. Cohort traits, such as its size or its race or gender composition, influence outcomes for the larger society and shape the life chances of individuals within the cohort (Easterlin, 1987).

The diagram in Exhibit 2.3 is a graphic representation by Riley and her colleagues (1987, 1994) of the triple forces of aging, period, and cohort. In this diagram, time is

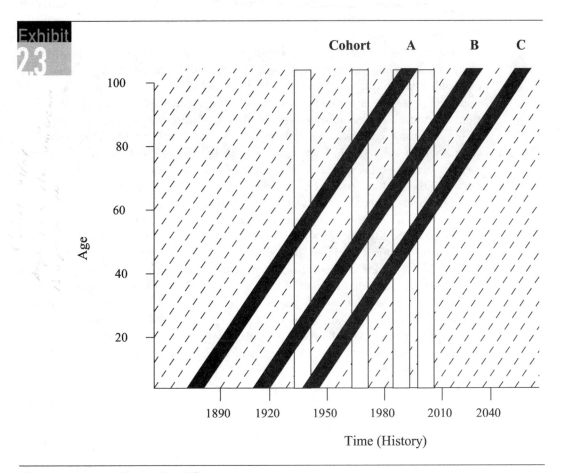

Exhibit 2.3

Changing Lives and Sociocultural Change
Source: Riley, 1987.

represented by the horizontal axis, and age is represented on the vertical axis. The diagram shows three birth cohorts (A, B, and C), each born at a different point in history. For each cohort, we can move from the year of birth on the horizontal axis diagonally upward as time passes and each group ages. Thus, the diagonal black bars represent the aging component. The white vertical bars represent period effects, the first clearly being World War II, the second perhaps the Vietnam War, and the third (potentially) the widespread integration of computers into everyday life. (The fourth is a hypothetical event yet to happen.)

Most of the cohorts intersect each of these period events, but they do so at different ages and stages of their lives. For members of the oldest cohort, World War II occurred when they were in their 50s, the age to be parents of soldiers. Members of the next cohort, born in 1920, were young adults, likely to be heavily involved in actual fighting or war work on the home front. The 1950 cohort did not experience that war directly but was undoubtedly influenced by its aftermath. For them the second event, the Vietnam War, fell at about the same time in their lives (their early 20s) as World War II did for the 1920 cohort. In contrast, the Vietnam War was too late to have much effect on the surviving members of the cohort born in 1890, who were by then about 80. Thus, different cohorts face the same historical events (period effects) at different stages of the life course, and therefore relate to them differently. Such period effects may influence these cohorts as a collectivity in ways that will persist throughout their lifetimes (Riley, 1987).

Any large-scale event, such as a lengthy war or a significant economic downturn, is likely to have an impact on everyone in the society, but the effects are differential based on membership in different birth cohorts. Young adult cohorts, those most likely to be called upon to fight in the event of war, are likely to experience a life-changing effect from the war. At the same time, the birth cohorts who are parents or grandparents of these fighting-age adults, while doubtless affected by the war (worry over the outcome, shortages of goods and services), are unlikely to feel the same magnitude of effect on their lives from the same historical event (Pavalko & Elder, 1990). More mundane examples also apply. Certainly being a teenager in the 2000s is different from being one in the 1940s, even though many of the issues of aging and maturation faced by teenagers remain the same. These sorts of accumulated differences throughout life may make the two cohorts very different when they reach their third or eighth decade of life.

Because they are so closely interrelated, these three factors (aging, period, and cohort effects) are extremely difficult to disentangle in research. In fact, age, period, and cohort are "exact linear functions of each other because Age = Period − Cohort" (Winship & Harding, 2004). In other words, an individual's age can be known by subtracting his or her year of birth (cohort) from the year of the study (period). Because it is so important to sort out the empirical and conceptual distinctions among these three factors, scholars continue to search for research designs and statistical models to sort out their influences. More complicated research designs, such as some described later in this chapter, can assist in separating one type of effect (for example, a cohort effect) from the other two, but no currently available statistical technique enables researchers to routinely distinguish the relative inputs from each of these three factors (Schaie & Herzog, 1982). A great deal of progress is yet to be made in systematically addressing this puzzle.

To return to the example presented in Exhibit 2.2, when we see variations by age in voting behavior, it is not apparent from a comparison across age group whether aging, period, or cohort effects, or some combination of them, is at work. If we make the assumption that the behavior variation is all due to aging, we commit what is called a **life course fallacy**—interpreting age differences in data collected at one time across birth cohorts as if the differences were *caused by* the process of aging, without ruling out other possibilities (Riley, 1987). Although it may be the case that adults do become more politically aware with the accumulation of experience (aging), and therefore act upon that awareness in the voting booth, this interpretation is not the only possibility. A second explanation for this difference by age may relate to cohorts and their experience. Older cohorts, raised at a time when patriotism was more emphasized, may feel a greater duty to vote, and may have voted at higher rates all of their lives when compared with younger cohorts. The age difference in voting, therefore, could be a **cohort effect**. A third possibility is a **period effect**, where a political event, issue, or candidate could increase or decrease the voter turnout or voter registration rates (Firebaugh & Chen, 1995). Finally, it is possible that the pattern of voting behavior is a result of some combination of aging, cohort, and period effects. Despite the research difficulties in disentangling these three forces in the complexities of social life, some research has succeeded in doing so. By way of illustration, we describe three specific research studies in which one of the three factors was successfully separated from the other two.

Aging Effects: Criminal Behavior by Age

Research has clearly established that not all citizens are equally likely to commit crimes. As Exhibit 2.4 shows, many of the crimes of concern to society are committed by adolescents and young adults. Further, peak ages for commission of these crimes have remained consistent or declined since 1940 (Blumstein, 2001; Steffensmeier, Allan, Harer, & Streifel, 1989). Teenagers and young adults commit (and are arrested for) substantially more crime than are children or more mature adults. Why do we think this is an aging effect? In large measure the answer rests on the fact that similar age-related patterns of criminal behavior have been reported in many different societies and in different historical periods, diminishing the potency of explanations based on period or cohort. Although the amount of age difference in criminal behavior and the size of the decline with advancing age vary, many crimes show similar patterns of variation by age (Steffensmeier et al., 1989). When a pattern as apparently consistent as this appears, then we cautiously conclude that there is an aging effect.

But how is aging implicated in crime? Certainly criminal activity may be somewhat related to physical aging, in that some crimes require strength, speed, or agility to execute. More plausible, however, are the social explanations for crime: "Society at large is faced perennially with an invasion of barbarians ... [and] every adult generation is faced with the task of civilizing those barbarians" (Ryder, 1965, p. 845). The barbarians to whom Ryder refers are, of course, the youthful cohorts being socialized to the ways of society and their roles as adults. With limited integration into the social world (few links or responsibilities toward work or family) and with incomplete socialization and maturation, teenagers and young adults face fewer constraints against committing crimes than do their older counterparts. The explanation suggests that as individuals mature and gather more responsibilities and linkages to the social order (that is, increase their **social integration**), the costs of crime rapidly grow to outweigh its benefits, discouraging participation in illegal activities (Laub, Nagin, & Sampson, 1998; Steffensmeier et al., 1989).

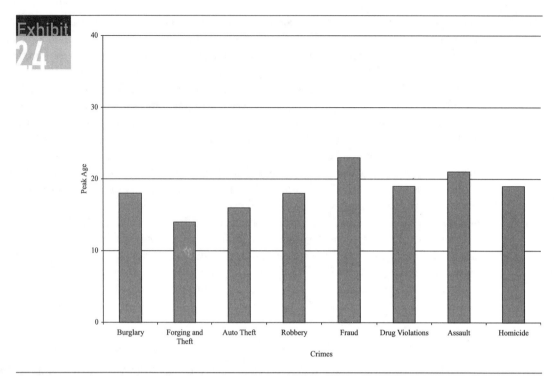

Peak Ages for Arrests for Various Crimes
Source: U.S. Department of Justice, 2006

Cohort Effects: The Nineteenth Amendment and Voting Among Women

Although it is typically very difficult to sort out age, period, and cohort effects, sometimes social life provides a "natural experiment" enabling researchers to clearly identify the consequences of cohort membership. In one such study, Firebaugh and Chen (1995) examined the changes in voting behavior of women in conjunction with passage of the Nineteenth Amendment to the Constitution, giving women the right to vote. The researchers noted that the voting rates of women just after passage of the amendment were much lower than those for men, but that this gap gradually narrowed over the years and then disappeared. Why?

To examine the issue, the researchers compared the voting behavior of three 10-year birth cohorts of White women: those born before 1896, who were denied the vote in young adulthood; those born between 1896 and 1905, who spent their childhoods before women could vote but could vote when they came of age; and those born between 1906 and 1915, who were raised after the enactment of the amendment. Firebaugh and Chen hypothesized that the experience of lacking the right to vote would have a lasting cohort effect on the first group and that each of the later two cohorts would be more likely to vote than the first cohort, because the oldest group had been socialized to think that women should not vote and had been prohibited from voting in their youth.

To make the test more stringent, the voting behavior examined was from much later: national elections between 1952 and 1988. The analysis revealed a true and enduring cohort effect from the passage of the Nineteenth Amendment. Women from the earliest cohort, who had been kept from voting as young women, were less likely than either of the subsequent cohorts to vote throughout their lives. Even though they did get to vote as soon as they reached adulthood, the women in the second cohort, who were socialized during the era when women could not vote, were still less likely to do so 30 years later than their younger counterparts, who were raised when women had the vote. Thus, the critical experience of youth lasted throughout life and differentiated these three cohorts of women in their voting behavior.

Finally, the authors offered an explanation as to why the gender gap in voting rates shrank over time. This reduction was the result of changes in the composition of the voting population. As the older cohorts of women, who were less likely to vote, died and were replaced by women of later cohorts more likely to vote, the gap systematically disappeared. Thus, this change probably did not reflect changes in the voting behavior of individuals or even of cohorts. Rather, the explanation derives from the so-called **cohort composition effect**. As cohorts age and their members die, they are replaced in the population (here, the voting-age population) by younger cohorts whose behaviors and attitudes may differ. This gradual shift in the composition of the voting population, then, accounts for the disappearance of the voting gap between women and men.

Period Effects: Consumer Spending Over the Life Course

As businesses anticipate the needs and desires of aging baby boomers, they might want to track consumer expenditures, looking for changes in the way people spend their money as they age. Hypothetical Company T conducts some research on this topic, wanting to know how these patterns might change with age. Remember, age effects are not just physical; we can be interested in physical, psychological, or social maturation. Company T is assuming that consumer expenditures may change because of life stage, hypothesizing that middle and later life will be marked by greater availability of discretionary income and discretionary time. To test this question, they conducted a longitudinal study, tracking the same people over time as they age. Exhibit 2.5 shows the hypothetical data resulting from this study.

As anticipated, the participants were gradually increasing the amount of money they were spending on travel as they moved into and through middle age. The increase continued until a precipitous drop when they turned 66. Was this an aging effect? Did these study participants suddenly reduce the money they spent on travel when they retired or began receiving Medicare? Unlikely. A major historical event occurred during the time of this study—the September 11 terrorist attacks on the World Trade Center and the Pentagon. It is much more likely that the rapid drop in consumer spending on travel was due to this period effect, not the effects of physical aging or life stage. In fact, we know that the travel industry suffered tremendous losses following the events of 9/11. This example of a **period effect** illustrates how a significant historical event or social change can influence the results of a study that might be designed to help us understand aging.

Designs and Methods Targeted to Research on Aging

Research on aging includes many unique challenges, including the conceptualization and measurement of age and aging and sorting out age, period, and cohort effects. Some research designs are especially suited to these special concerns. These designs focus on

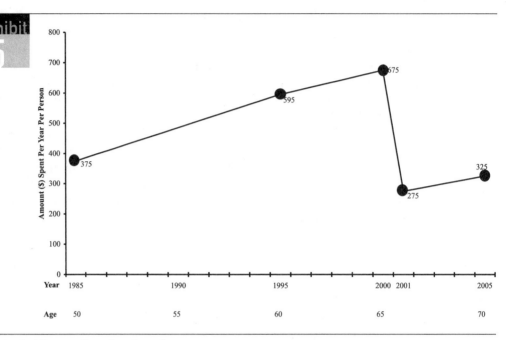

Hypothetical Data on Traveling Spending

who is studied, how data are collected, and how the influences of age, period, and cohort can be analyzed.

Longitudinal/Panel Studies

Longitudinal studies, sometimes also called panel studies, attempt to isolate aging from cohort or period effects by following a sample of units of analysis (cells, individuals, states, corporations, or societies) over time to observe how they change (or remain unchanged). The most often used type of longitudinal study is one in which individuals in a sample are repeatedly surveyed about their lives over a period of years or even decades. Longitudinal designs are contrasted with **cross-sectional studies,** in which data are collected at one point in time, generating a snapshot of differences between age cohorts. Cross-sectional studies can show how age groups may be different from each other, but they cannot reveal the extent to which those differences are attributable to the effects of aging. Cross-sectional studies often entangle aging effects with cohort or generational effects. To illustrate, consider a question about whether people become more religious as they grow older. A cross-sectional study would compare the religiosity of today's 80-year-olds with today's 60-, 40-, and 20-year-olds. If we see that the older groups are more religious (e.g., go to church more often), we cannot be sure how much of that difference is due to aging processes and how much might be due to different cohorts growing up with different emphasis on many aspects of religiosity, such as church attendance. Longitudinal designs help to sort aging effects from cohort effects; because a cohort is followed over time, as it ages, we are not confusing age effects with cohort effects.

Although it is not a panacea for all of the analytical problems we have been discussing (Campbell, 1988), the use of longitudinal data drawn from the study of a sample over time is generally touted as a necessity in the study of social processes of aging. However, the design has drawbacks. Because the commitment in time, financial resources, and effort involved in collecting significant longitudinal data can be staggering, the benefits sometimes are not seen for years (Campbell & O'Rand, 1985). In addition, researchers face challenges in conducting longitudinal studies that are not characteristic of cross-sectional work.

> Despite the researcher's efforts, some respondents will be lost, requiring extensive tracking, and may possibly never be found. The investigator must deal with thorny measurement issues. Should questions be repeated, even if the early data from the study show them to be flawed? And even if questions are repeated in exactly the same form, the structure and meaning of concepts they indicate may have changed over time. What if new concepts emerge that seem germane to the original research objectives? (Lawton & Herzog, 1989, p. vi)

Yet longitudinal data are critical to disentangling the effects of age, cohort, and period on processes of individual aging and social change over time. Especially useful are longitudinal studies that follow more than one cohort as it ages—a cohort sequential design. Exhibit 2.6 shows a hypothetical sequential design, following three cohorts over four time periods. Each group is reinterviewed at 5-year intervals. This design makes it possible to compare cohorts as they age. For example, we can compare the age changes that cohort 1 and cohort 2 go through as they move from ages 40 to 50; even though they will go through these ages at different historical times, knowing whether an age change observed for one cohort holds true for another gives us greater confidence in our conclusions about the effect of age. Following more than one cohort longitudinally enables some separation of the effects of aging, period, and cohort. One study, for example, included 15 birth cohorts (every 3 years between 1916 and 1958) and collected data annually for 11 years, providing a substantial amount of information to sort out age and cohort effects for disease and disability (Reynolds, Crimmins, & Saito, 1998). In the earlier example of women's voting patterns following ratification of the Nineteenth Amendment, by focusing on a span of behavior (voting patterns from 1952 to 1988) with three distinct cohorts, the researchers used a sequential design to clearly isolate cohort effects.

Secondary Analysis

One way around the time constraints and costs of longitudinal studies is to use existing data. **Secondary analysis** "refers to the study of existing data initially collected for another purpose" (Liang & Lawrence, 1989, p. 31). Although secondary analyses need not use longitudinal data or even survey data (for example, secondary analysis of medical records), many of the most valuable contributions to our knowledge of aging have involved longitudinal surveys of aging samples.

A growing number of large, national longitudinal secondary analyses of studies originally designed to examine very specific issues (such as economic status, employment, utilization of health services, and family relationships) have been employed by other researchers in secondary analyses to answer questions about aging beyond those envisioned by their original designers. Many such data sets are available from computerized archives, making them readily accessible to researchers for secondary analyses. The Inter-University

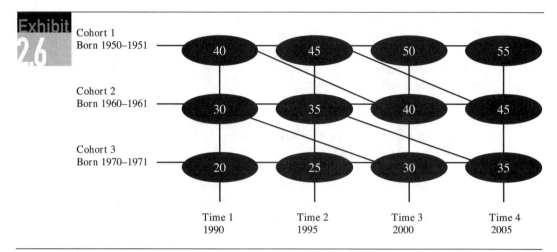

Exhibit 2.6

Cohort Sequential Design

Consortium for Political and Social Research and the National Archive of Computerized Data on Aging are two excellent resources for secondary data. Examples of this type of data can be located through Web sites listed at the end of this and some other chapters. These studies have been used to dramatically expand knowledge in a number of areas about aging, despite having been designed with other goals in mind. Newer longitudinal studies, including the Health and Retirement Study initiated in 1992 with large samples of women and men, updates the information provided by panels initiated in the 1960s and 1970s (Health and Retirement Study, 2006). These longitudinal studies used in secondary analysis have added considerably to our store of knowledge about aging.

The growth in these large, national data sources available to researchers for secondary analysis is a mixed blessing. As Kasl (1995) points out, although these studies provide both a longitudinal design and a large, national sample, which would probably otherwise be unavailable to most researchers on aging, they offer information on a limited number of variables. Researchers may not be able to measure concepts of interest (such as health status, family cohesiveness, or political involvement) in ways that are ideal; essentially they must work within constraints of what the data provide. If a key variable is missing, then the researcher must choose between not using the data at all or attempting to work around this limitation.

Qualitative, Quantitative, Combined Methods

Most of the techniques drawn from other social science traditions that have been applied to the study of aging are quantitative approaches. These approaches include experiments, surveys, and much of the evaluation research discussed earlier in this chapter. Even though these specific designs are different from each other, they share one central feature: they examine numerical data using statistical techniques. The numerical data may derive from medical records, the census, an experiment, or from a survey of individuals, states, or companies; the data are then analyzed in such a way as to suggest that the numbers are meaningful reflections of reality. For example, a person reporting limitations in five activities of daily living (ADLs)—a common measure of functional health status—is assumed in a quantitative approach to be more disabled than a person reporting only two such limitations. Although widely used, quantitative approaches have limitations. Because of the focus on numerically valid data that can be used to make general statements about the larger population, or about the causal connections between variables of interest, quantitative research does not attend to subjective interpretations by respondents. Quantitative research is also criticized for inhibiting theorizing by reducing complex social life into a set of numbers (Cole, 1995).

Complementing quantitative approaches are numerous **qualitative analysis** techniques, designed to deal with the issues that quantitative research cannot address. "Qualitative research starts from the assumption that one can obtain a profound understanding about persons and their worlds from ordinary conversations and observations" (Sankar & Gubrium, 1994, p. vii). Qualitative research is thus based not on numbers, but on words, meanings, and symbols. Key to the qualitative approach are the acknowledgment of (1) people's inherent ability to know and communicate things about their own lives, one another, and their respective worlds; (2) the researcher's role in obtaining the facts of experience; and (3) the importance of seeking to understand the multifaceted and complex nature of human experience from the perspective of subjects (Sankar & Gubrium, 1994). Thus, instead of using questions with multiple-choice answers, which construct the meaning of the social situation for the respondent in advance (e.g., your health is either excellent, good, fair, or poor), qualitative researchers tend to focus their research efforts on in-depth interviewing, life-history collection, and observation, sometimes as a participant, in a social setting. The goal is to represent the participants' reality as faithfully as possible from their points of view (e.g., my overall health is good, except for severe arthritis) (Sankar & Gubrium, 1994). The researcher, rather than being only minimally present for the administration of a questionnaire asking yes/no questions or for numerical ratings of the subject's health, is an active participant in eliciting meanings from the informants, whose reality is often recorded on audio- or videotape for later analysis.

For example, Gay Becker (1993) analyzed the aftermath of stroke in a sample of 100 victims. Her analysis was based on repeated interviews with the sample, participant observation in a stroke rehabilitation ward of a hospital, and observation of patient-practitioner interactions over a 5-year period. The interviews, once transcribed, were used to identify central themes that appeared throughout the data. Those themes became the basis of theoretical explanations and hypotheses for further consideration. Among her key conclusions was that victims viewed stroke as a major life-course disruption, requiring victims to reconstruct their lives with new expectations and patterns of behavior.

In this case, Becker examined the event (stroke) from the perspective of those living through it to learn how they, not physicians or researchers, socially constructed the major issues. As an observant outsider, the qualitative researcher may see aspects of the situation that are missed or taken for granted by those in the situation. The hallmark of qualitative research is looking at the meanings central to social actors, not those that may be imposed by the perspective and goals of the researcher.

When exploring topics about which we have very little information, qualitative research is usually the most appropriate design. It is important to point out that these two approaches—qualitative and quantitative—represent two different, not necessarily opposing, frames of reference for examining the social world and are sometimes combined in research studies. Many studies can be enhanced by the inclusion of both approaches. For example, if we want to develop a new measure that will eventually be used in a large-scale survey, it would be wise to begin with a qualitative phase. In this phase, we can ask people to describe their experiences in depth so that the measure we develop will capture what is meaningful to those eventually surveyed.

At the beginning of any research project, we should consider whether qualitative, quantitative, or a combined approach will be best suited for what we want to understand. This research decision is part of some of the challenging but essential work that must take place before data collection or analysis. Some of these important initial decisions are summarized in Exhibit 2.7.

Event History Analysis

One of the newer tools in the study of aging is called **event history analysis.** In aging research we are often interested in when a particular life event happens or in the social forces that shape its occurrence. Event history analysis attempts to address these issues. This frame of reference draws attention to a particular event of interest, such as retirement, enactment of a new social policy, entry into a nursing home, or divorce.

As its name suggests, event history analysis focuses on when and how particular events happen to the person or group of interest. Based on longitudinal data, this technique explores how much time passes before the event of interest occurs, the rates of occurrence of particular events (for example, widowhood within a population), and how these rates change with the passage of time (Does the rate of widowhood increase as women age?) (Campbell & O'Rand, 1985). This type of analysis allows us to answer questions related not only to when something occurs, but also to the relationships, if any, between events—for example, marriage and childbirth, or passage of a new retirement policy and changes in the behavior of retirees.

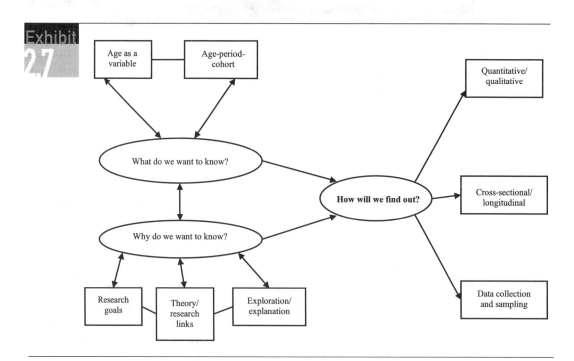

Exhibit 2.7

Designing a Study: Critical Starting Questions

Although event history analysis is most frequently used on the individual level, examining the impact of specific life events, it can also be applied to large-scale (macro) events. It would be equally valid, however, to look cross-nationally at how changes in eligibility age for retirement influence when workers retire in various countries, using the country as the unit of analysis. Regardless of the unit of analysis, it is essential that the unit under study have the potential to undergo a particular change that may have identifiable consequences of interest.

A key to analyses of this type is being able to pinpoint the timing of the event of interest (Campbell & O'Rand, 1985). Current studies often enable us to know only that retirement or marriage or death took place between the third and fourth round of interviews in a longitudinal panel, but not the specific month or year of the event in question. A second complication in this type of analysis is known as censoring. If we are following a large sample to examine the timing and rate of a particular event—say the onset of dementia, which occurs at widely different ages in a population above age 70—this event would already have occurred for some people, not yet have occurred for others, and never occur for still others. In the cases in which the event does not occur and in the cases in which we don't know its timing, the event is considered "censored" and not available for analysis. Therefore, unless we can wait 30 or 40 years to ensure that everyone in the sample has either shown signs of dementia or died without doing so, event history analyses are always dealing with censoring. Censoring simply means that we lack knowledge of when those remaining people will experience the event of interest, if ever. Fortunately, techniques are available to assist in dealing with the problems of censoring.

As a specific example of event history analysis, Moen, Dempster-McClain, and Williams (1989) conducted a study of women's role involvement and longevity. They used a sample of married mothers (originally ages 25–50) who had been interviewed in both 1956 and 1986. The event of interest was mortality. Most women in the sample (76%) had survived the 30-year period and were therefore censored as to the timing of their eventual demise. Another 5% could not be located and were also considered censored as to time of mortality. Only 19% of the sample had died during the interval between interviews. Knowing the dates of death for the women who died, however, enabled the researchers to utilize complex statistical techniques to evaluate the relationship between longevity and the number of social roles held earlier in life.

The researchers were interested in whether the number of social roles (aside from being a wife and mother) was related to longevity. They found, after controlling for social class and age in 1956, that the number of social roles did help to predict longevity. Women who were more involved earlier in their lives, especially those who belonged to clubs or organizations, had greater longevity than those who were not. The authors concluded that social integration of mid-life women has beneficial effects that translate into greater life expectancy. The event history approach enables researchers to examine a variety of life-course events that are of considerable interest. Rather than focusing on "the aged," this technique emphasizes the dynamic nature of aging over time.

Life History and Reminiscence

Some researchers address questions of time, aging, and social change at a more individual level, asking older persons to look back over their lives, emphasizing the transitions and events that were turning points. This life history or reminiscence approach is not only used for research purposes, but is also considered by many to be therapeutic for older persons (Borglin, Edberg, & Hallberg, 2005). Review of past life events may occur spontaneously by an older person alone or in conversation, through a structured interview process, or in a group workshop. It is these latter two settings that have been involved in research and therapeutic activities. As a research tool, life history interviewing is somewhat controversial. Many methodologists argue that retrospection (looking back) involves a mental reconstruction of the past that is subject to bias (Hagburg, 1995). This reconstruction, however, may be what is of interest, rather than a factual accounting of the events as they happened. For example, what is of interest to a researcher today may not be the exact realities of the Great Depression of the 1930s or World War II, but rather how those events and times are recalled over the course of many years and how they influence today those who experienced them.

Bo Hagburg, in a life history study focusing on close personal relationships throughout the life cycle, examined satisfaction with events surrounding retirement. Hagburg (1995) found that positive recollections of relationships in childhood and adolescence were associated with a positive reaction to the experience of retirement. Retirees remembering earlier life stages and the significant people in them most positively were most likely to be satisfied in retirement. Neither the current mental status nor the cognitive ability of the retiree explained this relationship. Instead, satisfaction with retirement was linked to a positive report of relationships to significant others during childhood and adolescence. Was this positive tie to significant others the way these relationships were viewed in childhood and teen years? It is hard to say, but the findings suggest that how they are recalled now is influential.

Much of the life history or reminiscence work is qualitative in nature, focusing on descriptions of past events and how they are interpreted through the passing years. This qualitative approach is not necessarily always the case, however. The Hagburg study, for example, used statistical means to correlate aspects of recalled life history with current events and characteristics.

Other Special Issues in Studying Aging

Separating "Normal" from "Pathological" Aging

Chapter 1 mentions the difficulty in separating out the "normal" aging of the body from diseases that are age-related but not age-caused. Similar problems arise in studying the social phenomena associated with aging. If people typically experience a decline in response time at the wheel of a car or in purchasing power in the marketplace as they age, can we say that these factors are part of the normal process of aging? Often we cannot. Although some social phenomena are clearly age-related (for example, the probability of widowhood for women is clearly related to the ages of their husbands), many times the chain of causation is indirect at best. The decline in response time may result from illness rather than age. A decline in income at higher ages, though common, is a consequence of the manner in which society constructs the systems for income maintenance for older people who have retired and the fact that women, with fewer economic resources in current older cohorts, outlive men. Because we have institutionalized retirement and developed income-replacement strategies that derive from employment and do not always keep up with inflation, many people see their purchasing power erode. A majority of these survivors are older women. So just as physical pathology is hard to separate from the biological components of aging, social effects are intertwined with the individual processes of growing older.

There is nothing natural or inevitable about providing retirement income this way in the social world—age systems are socially constructed. In agricultural economies, where the ownership of land often remains in the hands of the oldest generation, their power and economic security may endure until death. We must remain vigilant to avoid assumptions that because something is common or typical, it is somehow socially "normal." This critical eye enables us to identify and address, through policies and programs, problems of older persons that are not inevitable parts of the aging process but that could in some instances be thought of as social pathologies in need of "treatment" through policy intervention.

Increasing Variability With Age

Dale Dannefer (1988) points out another difficulty related to the study of aging. He argues that there is now an ample body of both psychological and sociological research demonstrating that individuals in a cohort become more differentiated (or, in sociological terms, **heterogeneous**) as age increases.

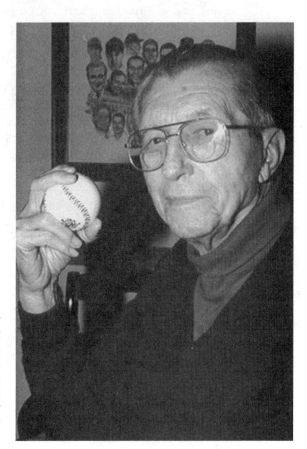

The late Mel Harder, a former All-Star pitcher with the Cleveland Indians, knew a thing or two about life's curveballs and longevity on and off the mound, living to the age of 93. He pitched in the major leagues for 19 years and stayed in the game for 21 more seasons as a coach with the Indians and other major league teams. (Credit: Mike Payne, courtesy of the Ohio Department of Aging)

> Older people have been thought to be more dissimilar from one another than are younger people in terms of physical health status, intellectual capacity, and psychological functioning, material resource availability and life-style. Although such comparisons are often used to contrast different age groups or strata at one point in time, they also implicitly connote a life-course pattern toward greater heterogeneity among age peers. (p. 360)

The processes involved in creating this increased variability are complex, and the growing differentiation with advancing age creates challenges for research. Dannefer argues that neither current theories nor research methods are well equipped to deal with this pattern. Adequate study of variability with aging would require both very large samples and longitudinal data (data collected on the same individuals over long periods of time), which are costly types of research in terms of both time and money required.

Many current approaches to describing age-related changes focus on **measures of central tendency,** such as averages (means) that define how a typical person is doing. We then compare across ages to find any differences associated with age. If a difference is found, we may think we have identified an effect arising from aging, period, or cohort. In fact, on some items older people differ more from one another than they do from younger age groups. Measures of central tendency ignore the variability within each cohort, making such measures less adequate to describe older than younger groups. It is this "mean" that Quinn warns of in the quote that began this chapter. Alternative measures are available, and Dannefer urges their use in the study of aging populations.

Sampling Adequately

In most research, it is not possible to study every person who is a member of the population of interest. So we use **samples.** As Nesselroade (1988) so simply put it, "A sample is a small part of anything (or a few of a larger number of somethings) that is (are) used to show the nature of the whole" (p. 13). In most social science research, a sample is a few units of analysis (people, families, businesses, city governments, or countries) out of all of the possible pertinent units of analysis (the population) that one wishes to study. The units in the sample reflect the location along the macro–micro continuum that has been selected as appropriate for the question at hand, with the number of units in any given sample being highly variable and the number of samples potentially to be drawn from any large population infinite. The goal is to have a sample that represents the entire population (sometimes also called the universe), because it is too costly in time and money to reach every member of that population, and good estimates can be developed from a sample of what would have been found had the entire population been included. This is especially challenging given the diversity among older adults, discussed above.

A study of the entire population of the United States is conducted every decade when the census is taken. The census, by not using a sample, is more the exception than the rule. Since it is impossible to interview every person who is widowed, for example, researchers select a sample believed to represent in most critical ways the larger population from which it was selected (all widowed persons).

A wide variety of sampling techniques can be applied to various types of quantitative and qualitative research (Schutt, 2004). Many of these techniques are directly applicable to studies of aging, where attention is often focused on constructing samples based on age (for example, a survey studying how attitudes toward Social Security vary by age). Sampling by age is a difficult task, because there is no simple way to identify or reach large and representative groups of people across the full range of ages. For example, there is no roster of retirees or persons over age 65 from which we can easily draw samples. Although the Social Security system has information about most older adults, the information is confidential and not available to researchers to use in developing samples for their research.

The study of aging encompasses more than just age in selecting participants for research. Sometimes researchers are interested in locating individuals from more specific groups or "rare populations": daughters providing at-home care for a frail parent; older adults who have maintained high levels of creative productivity in the arts; or African Americans anticipating retirement in the next few years. Efforts to examine specific groups require additional attention to sampling and sometimes the use of special sampling techniques. Not only may these groups be statistically rare, but they may also be resistant to participating in research for a variety of reasons (McAuley, 1987). To develop a high-quality sample in these cases requires considerable resourcefulness.

Studies that focus attention on the oldest individuals in society, who are often frail or cognitively impaired, raise additional concerns. Researchers are ethically bound to use extreme caution in conducting interviews or observations with such samples, given the relatively higher risks of stress, fatigue, and health impacts of upsetting a normal routine. Gatekeepers, such as relatives or health care providers, are often reluctant to give permission for frail persons in their care to participate in research studies. Special protections, including detailed reviews of research methods for risk factors when older subjects are involved, work to minimize problems for such vulnerable samples.

Early research on aging was plagued by samples that were small, local, and unrepresentative of the larger population (Cutler, 1995). Researchers could draw conclusions only in very limited fashion because there was no certainty that their results pertained to the population as a whole. Until fairly recently, most studies underrepresented some groups, making it difficult, for example, to study aging in minority populations (LaViest, 1995; Markides et al., 1990). In fact, many studies were conducted using "convenience" samples that tended to overrepresent White, middle-class individuals. The development in large, nationally representative samples that enable researchers to examine many issues of concern in aging has marked a major advancement in the field (Cutler, 1995; Kasl, 1995).

Ethical Issues in Research on Aging

All researchers have an obligation to do no harm to anyone who participates in their studies. All universities and government agencies, and most agencies or organizations that serve the public, have some mechanism to protect research participants. In many organizations, the group charged with this oversight is called an institutional review board (IRB). This group reviews research before it begins to make sure that any proposed study will not cause undue distress and that people do not feel coerced into participating. The protection of human subjects is of concern to everyone involved in research. Special concerns can arise when studying the older population. In particular, older people who are living in nursing homes or receiving home-care services need to be assured that their participation is voluntary and that they can be honest in their answers. It is understandable that individuals in these situations might worry that they will disappoint the researcher or the agency if they choose not to participate; in addition, they might be concerned about giving any negative feedback, fearing possible repercussions. For example, a home-care recipient might not be willing to say that her worker shows up late sometimes because of worry that the worker might lose her job and not show up at all. These considerations are all part of assuring that human subjects are protected. The integrity of the researcher, and of the research process, are equally essential to the ethical conduct of research.

Cohort-Centrism, Dynamism, and Limits of Current Knowledge

As already noted, the scientific study of aging is a relatively recent development. For example, early research on retirement began in the 1950s and grew dramatically in the decades that followed. Most of what we know about how retirement affects individuals, families, the labor market, and the overall economy is drawn from the 1970s through today. The same could be said about a wide range of topics associated with aging.

Our knowledge of retirement is, therefore, limited to cohorts of workers who were entering or already in retirement at those particular time periods, with all of their related cohort experiences of economic upturns and depressions, education, war, and employment. They represent a truly narrow slice of history upon which to build a knowledge base. Riley (1987) warns against the **fallacy of cohort-centrism,** whereby an erroneous assumption is made that future (or past) cohorts will age (have aged) in the same fashion as current cohorts under study. We should expect research findings to change as new cohorts—with vastly different experiences in health care, the labor market, the family, and in other domains of their lives—approach and enter retirement. These newer groups will retire from a global economy that has changed dramatically in the past 20 to 30 years. Similarly, processes that are influenced by period effects in other areas of aging, even biological aging, should be expected to change as conditions experienced by the individual alter through historical time.

In studying aging, part of the problem is that we attempt to study a moving target. Matilda White Riley (1987) describes this dynamic aspect of the study of aging from her perspective of examining cohort flow through the age structure of society over time. She describes two interrelated dynamisms as underlying this interplay of individual aging and social change. The first process is the *aging of people* in successive cohorts who grow up, grow old, die, and are replaced by people in subsequent cohorts. Because the members of these successive cohorts age in different ways, they contribute to social change. "When many individuals in the same cohort are affected by social change in similar ways, the change in their collective lives can produce changes in social structure" (p. 9).

For example, Riley explains the rising economic well-being of older adults using the "cohort composition" explanation described earlier. The reduction in the poverty level of the older population has been brought about by deaths among the oldest cohorts, who were the least financially secure, and the movement into older ages of their replacement cohorts, more of whom retired with pensions and assets to combine with Social Security benefits. Thus, according to Riley, the fates of particular elderly persons have not improved over the past decades. Instead, the movement of cohorts into and (through death) out of the older population has changed the composition of, and thus society's view of, the economic security of the older population.

Second, there is constant *change in society* as people of different ages pass through the social institutions organized by age. Because society changes, people in different cohorts age in different ways. The economic boom following World War II and the increased availability of pensions has enabled more older persons today to retire at earlier ages. Early retirement, in turn, has created a boom in housing, travel, and leisure pursuits for this economically advantaged group, to which the economy has reacted by providing products and services. "The key to this understanding lies in the *interdependence* of aging and social change, as each transforms the other" (Riley, 1987, p. 2).

The problem, according to Riley, is that we are attempting to study the process of aging within the context of constant change in the social world. Social changes, in turn, modify the process of and the adaptations to aging among successive cohorts, making it more difficult to determine what, if anything, is caused by aging on the macro or micro level. One such dynamic, described below, is change in the size and composition of birth cohorts, which, according to economist Richard Easterlin, may have important influences on the lives of various cohorts.

Sociology of Knowledge and Research Activism

Most of us take the information we get, especially from authoritative sources, for granted. We assume that the information is factual and unbiased. But there are many questions that we can, and perhaps should, ask about it. How do certain ideas come to the forefront in a society? Why do particular theories become popular and taken for granted by researchers or the public? Why do certain discoveries get coverage in popular media whereas others disappear from view? We assume that experts know what they are talking about, use appropriate means to determine and present facts without the influence of political or ideological slants. But these assumptions are not necessarily true. One subfield of sociology, the **sociology of knowledge**, has made knowledge its subject matter, assuming that we need to question how we know what we know and to examine the social influences on sources of information that most of us take for granted. Science is, in fact, a social enterprise and a human activity that is shaped by the setting and the historical context in which it is per-

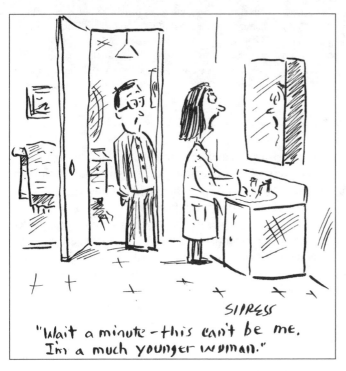

STRESS

"Wait a minute - this can't be me. I'm a much younger woman."

Cohort Size and Life Chances: The Easterlin Hypothesis

Do you believe that your personal fate and your opportunities are entirely in your own hands? Is it only your individual abilities and choices that determine how your life will turn out? Economist Richard Easterlin has formulated an interesting and controversial theoretical argument about the opportunities individuals get in society (what sociologists call **life chances**). His premise is a simple one: The life chances of individuals are influenced to a significant degree by the size of the cohort into which they were born. "For those fortunate enough to be members of a small generation, life is—as a general matter—disproportionately good; the opposite is true for those who are members of a large generation" (1987, p. 3). Prompted by the obvious impact of the baby boom cohorts (which he refers to as a generation), and recognizing an apparently cyclical movement from large to small "generations," Easterlin argues that cohort size affects the well-being and outcomes experienced by a cohort's individual members. Members of large cohorts compete for attention and positions in families, schools, and the labor market; members of smaller cohorts see their fortunes advance relatively easily by comparison. When the members of larger cohorts are unable to achieve their high aspirations, Easterlin argues, they take actions such as having fewer children, and they experience higher rates of unemployment, divorce, suicide, crime, and political alienation (1987).

Although Easterlin has presented a compelling case in his book *Birth and Fortune*, other researchers have demonstrated its limitations as an explanatory scheme. To test one of Easterlin's predicted negative outcomes for large cohorts, Kahn and Mason (1987) analyzed survey data on political alienation from 1952 through 1980. They found that period effects (such as the Vietnam War or Watergate) had more to do with political alienation than did cohort size. Political alienation fluctuated over time in similar patterns for all cohorts, rather than differentially for cohorts of different sizes.

In other studies examining cohort size and crime, findings are mixed. One analysis showed that larger cohort size was related to the commission of homicide (O'Brien, Stockard, & Isaacson, 1999), but others showed, contrary to Easterlin's prediction, that larger cohorts were not especially prone to crime (Steffensmeier, Allen, Harer, & Streifel, 1989). These authors argued that looking only at cohort size is too simplistic and that prediction of criminal behavior needs to take into account the larger social and economic climate as well. Nonetheless, the age structure of society does influence crime in important ways.

As the debate on the validity of Easterlin's hypothesis on cohort size continues, it may be interesting for you to consider the size of your cohort (either your birth cohort or the cohort with which you entered school, the workforce, or marriage) and to contemplate whether the size of that group is likely to shape your opportunities and, as a result, your life chances as you move through your life course.

formed. Researchers bring their personal frames of reference—including ideologies, expectations, interests, and experiences—to the research setting, sometimes unwittingly confounding what they find in their studies with what they wish to find.

These problems of potential bias are much more pertinent in the social sciences than they are in biology or physics, for example, where the topics are more removed from personal interests and goals. When scientists study people and society and how they operate, however, they touch upon topics in which all social scientists have a strong vested interest. It becomes quite difficult to maintain the "objectivity" that scientists are supposed to have regarding their subject matter when the processes under study affect them and all of the people important to them. Because we are all aging and have family and friends who are aging, these issues become very personal.

Not only do forces internal to the scientist shape the kinds of questions being asked and the ways in which answers are sought, external forces, too, can influence the situation. Research, like fashion, has trends that are shaped by a variety of external forces, including political trends, the availability of funding to support research on various topics, and the popularity of particular research methodologies. Conflicts regarding theories or goals among forces external to the research setting, such as changes in the political power of interest groups, may also shape what is studied and how it is studied. A good example of these external forces is the dramatic increase in funding from the mid-1980s to the 1990s for research on both the physical and social aspects of Alzheimer's disease (Adelman, 1995). Although the disease has been identified since 1906, it was "rediscovered" during the 1980s with the assistance of advocacy groups stressing dire projections of the number of the oldest old who would face this disease in the future. Funding for research grew tremendously, resulting in increasing knowledge about the disease, its impact on the health care delivery system, and its effects on family members who provide care and support to its victims (Adelman, 1995). Most diseases receive research funding that reflects their burden on the population, but Alzheimer's disease is an exception, as are AIDS and breast cancer, which receive greater funding than would seem warranted by the number of people affected and their lethality (Gross, Anderson, & Powe, 1999). Obviously many forces are at work in the allocation of research funds. Critiques of the mismatch between research support and burden of the disease are often made in an effort to advocate for a greater allocation of money to the study of another disease. For example, the American Obesity Association argues that "obesity is approaching the level of being the leading cause of preventable death in the U.S. Yet AIDS, another cause of preventable death, receives about 5 times more research funding than obesity" (AOA, 2002). Differential research support to diseases may represent an active social construction (for the benefit of legislators and those funding research) as to the relative seriousness of diseases and their priority for funding. In other social/political contexts, funding might well be allocated in an entirely different fashion.

Thus, rather than being a neutral force, knowledge is both created and shared in a socially constructed context that has overtones of economics, politics, and personal interest of scientists and their sponsors. The sociology of knowledge perspective emphasizes the importance of looking at research on aging with a critical eye for implicit assumptions, potential biases, and alternative conclusions.

A second major critique has to do with the issue of **activism** among researchers versus the objectivity prompted by the scientific method. Because we are all aging, it is difficult for researchers studying aging, as in most other fields focusing on human behavior or society, to separate themselves completely from the topic they study and remain objective. One ongoing dispute about the scientific method has to do with whether science should even attempt to be objective, value-free, or value-neutral, as the scientific method suggests. The opposing viewpoint argues that researchers should be activists, taking a stand on critical social issues of importance and providing applied research findings oriented toward solving these problems. There are compelling arguments on both sides of the debate. Those espousing an objective approach to science suggest that it is critical for researchers to acknowledge and work to overcome any biases or preconceptions they may have. In this way, the research may be more valid, reflecting viewpoints other than those of the researcher, and may have more credibility with any audience. A study finding beneficial effects of nursing home placement, for example, would be more credible if conducted by an independent researcher with no vested interest than if conducted by a group funded by the nursing home industry. Those on the other side argue that it is fundamentally impossible for us to put aside our personal frames of reference in conducting research. Rather, we ought to acknowledge the assumptions and biases that have directed us to select particular topics for study and approaches to studying them. Instead of pretending value neutrality, researchers should acknowledge and work with their biases to achieve applied research that is oriented toward improving the circumstances of some group or solving some problem. They may carry their activism to testifying before legislative bodies or lobbying on behalf of the causes they choose, combining research with individual political activism.

SUMMARY

Researchers studying aging in a social context have a growing number of options. Not only can they draw from traditional techniques from several disciplines, but the field has added some specific methodologies, such as longitudinal and event history analyses, to the methodological arsenal. Increasingly, data are available on selected topics following multiple cohorts over 20 to 25 years, allowing researchers to disentangle some of the changing nature of cohorts as they age. The growing number of nationally representative studies, including lengthy panels on a wide range of topics, has increased researchers' abilities to address important issues without trying to collect their own data in an era of restricted research funding. The recent rise in popularity of qualitative techniques has enriched the information on many subjects in which statistical analyses, though useful, can cause the flavor and meaning of the results to be lost.

The quality of research on aging has improved substantially in recent decades, but numerous challenges remain (Cutler, 1995). Researchers continue to compete for financial support to perform research on aging, and the knowledge builds selectively as research funding for biomedical concerns outstrips that for the social sciences. The need for high-quality applied research on aging escalates as the population ages and we seek solutions to many related social issues. The main challenge for researchers is to clearly identify their research problem, its appropriate unit of analysis, the population from which a sample is to be drawn, the best way in which to collect information (surveys, observations, review of historical records), and specific techniques for analyzing that information to answer the original question. Only then can we be confident that our base of knowledge about aging in a social context is sound. Many studies on aging show failings in one or more of these steps, in part because of the "youth" of the field, and in part because of the practical constraints on research. It is the skill to match methodology to the problem that is the hallmark of important research to advance our knowledge of aging.

WEB WISE

Fedstats

http://www.fedstats.gov

The Fedstats Web site is intended to provide users with easy access to government statistics on a wide range of topics. The site organizes and provides access to information that is collected and made available online or through publications from numerous federal agencies. It is a "one-stop shopping" site and allows searching by topic for information that may be relevant across a range of governmental agencies.

AgeLine

http://research.aarp.org/ageline/home.html

AgeLine is a resource that has been around for a while and is very useful to researchers, including students with paper assignments. It is a searchable database of thousands of articles from journals and magazines screened to be related to aging. AgeLine, supported by the American Association of Retired Persons, has an extensive thesaurus of aging terms that can be used as keywords in a search. Fees are charged for full articles, but this is an effective way to search for references on a topic, even if the full text is received elsewhere.

Health and Retirement Study

http://hrsonline.isr.umich.edu

The University of Michigan Health and Retirement Study surveys more than 22,000 Americans over the age of 50 every 2 years. Supported by the National Institute on Aging, the study paints a portrait of an aging America's physical and mental health, insurance coverage, financial status, family support systems, labor market status, and retirement planning. Data are available at no cost to researchers.

National Archive of Computerized Data on Aging

http://www.icpsr.umich.edu/NACDA

The National Archive of Computerized Data on Aging (NACDA), located at the University of Michigan's Interuniversity Consortium for Political and Social Research (ICPSR) has been a substantial resource for researchers interested in secondary analysis of large databases. NACDA archives and maintains many data sets that can be retrieved by individuals who teach or study at ICPSR member institutions. It also provides a searchable database of publications generated from its databases.

National Institute on Aging

http://www.nih.gov/nia

The National Institute on Aging (NIA), part of the federally funded National Institutes of Health, is involved with both basic and applied research on physical, social, and psychological aspects of health as people age. NIA's Web site provides information on its research agenda, including extramural research (funding to outside groups, such as university-based researchers) on biology of aging, behavioral and social research, neurosciences and neuropsychology, and geriatrics. In addition, NIA funds its own research labs (internal programs) and provides a number of free publications that are available via e-mail requests. To find out what is "hot" in aging research, a good place to look is the NIA Web site.

KEY TERMS

activism	event history analysis	measures of central
aging	fallacy of cohort–centrism	tendency
birth cohorts	heterogeneous	period effects
cohort composition effect	human aging	qualitative analysis
cohort effects	independent variable	quantitative approaches
cohort sequential design	life chances	sample
conceptualization	life course fallacy	secondary analysis
control variable	life history	social integration
cross-sectional studies	longitudinal studies	sociology of knowledge

QUESTIONS FOR THOUGHT AND DISCUSSION

1. The literature on aging is growing by leaps and bounds. Look at one or two published articles, and try to decipher how the authors were using aging as a variable. Were they looking at age as a cause of something or as a marker for group membership? Or were they investigating something about the older population? Were they clear about why they included age as a variable and why they expected age to matter to their topic?

2. Conducting research is always complicated. Taking a question or topic that interests you, go through the questions posed in the final section of this chapter to consider how you might begin to shape a strategy to answer your question.

3. Examining your own life, identify some events or historical transitions that you think might influence your aging to make it different from that of your parents or grandparents.

4. Think about your life and the life of one of your grandparents. What are the commonalities that you expect to find in the childhood and adolescence of these two lives? What differences do you expect in those and later stages? What causes the differences between you and your grandparent?

Will They Play the Rolling Stones at the Nursing Home?

What kind of music do you listen to now? Rock, Rachmaninoff, rap, or reggae? What did you listen to 5 or 10 years ago? Do you like the music of your parents' generation or that of your grandparents'? Can you imagine what the music favored by people of your children's or grandchildren's generation is going to sound like? One thing is for certain—it probably will be very different from what you listen to today.

Analyzing the social aspects of music is in some ways like analyzing the social aspects of age—both are elements of daily life that most of us take for granted (Martin, 1995). Music, like growing older, just seems to "happen" and to be part of everyday existence, rather than some puzzle to be solved. Although age has not been dealt with in a very systematic fashion in connection with music (Martin, 1995), there are some interesting questions that we can pose. Although most attention in the sociology of music has focused on classical music (perhaps because it has been the music of powerful elites in many Western societies), some contemporary analysts also examine class, race, and age as elements of musical preferences (Epstein, 1994; Martin, 1995). Issues such as *how* and *when* musical preferences are formed and change and how the trends in popular music evolve over time have also been addressed in a preliminary fashion by researchers. Here we examine some possible connections of music with the concepts of age, period, and cohort.

Do Popular Music Styles Have a Life Cycle?

Music, like many aspects of our culture, evolves with the passage of time. Every era has its "sound" as well as its sights, smells, and tastes that evoke the ambiance and events of the day. The 1995 50th anniversary celebration of the end of World War II brought back not only the events of the day, but also a nostalgic visit with the music and performers that marked that historical period. In a sense, the music is connected with the events (period effects) that shaped the lives of everyone, but especially of youth most affected by the war. Many younger persons might think of this music as being "old," both by virtue of being out of date compared to contemporary styles and by reflecting a bygone era.

Perhaps musical styles and songs could be described as going through "life stages." Many musical styles make their entries as brash youth, breaking the rules and raising the ire of older generations. Parents in the 1920s were concerned with the moral decay implicit in the fast-paced music behind the dances in vogue, such as the Charleston. The same issues arose with the birth of rock and roll. Chagrin with youthful musical tastes is certainly not new.

With the passage of time, these new musical forms become institutionalized and accepted as part of the musical marketplace. As the musical style matures, we may hear versions of these songs converted into "muzak" for elevators or shopping mall background. By this point in their life cycle, the songs, their performers, and the styles have become an accepted part of the culture. Emphasizing the motivation of youth to separate their music from that of older cohorts, Epstein (1994) claims that,

> As generations of rock fans grow up, and have families of their own, they bring their music with them into adulthood. This makes it necessary for rock music to change, to mutate.... Once a music is co-opted into the mass culture, it can no longer be considered confrontational, as is demonstrated by the Beatles song "Revolution." Revolution was once considered a controversial song about radical political change; now it is used in television commercials to sell shoes. (p. xvii)

The once-shocking Rolling Stones passed this milestone when one of their hits became the anthem for a major software advertising campaign in 1995; their appearance as the halftime entertainment for the 2006 Super Bowl is an even stronger illustration of Epstein's argument.

Artists age along with their audiences. New performers often rocket to stardom, only to fade from the scene after a few years (Martin, 1995). The most innovative, cutting-edge musical artists of today will, if you wait long enough and their music endures, become oldies, both musically and chronologically.

Do Cohorts Have Fixed Musical Preferences?

Especially compelling for each cohort seems to be the music associated with the events of young adulthood and "coming of age." Couples may have a special song to mark their romance and marriage; young adults recall their passage to maturity with the songs they heard as they experienced major milestones toward adulthood. Perhaps Mannheim was right in suggesting that our strongest influences are those we encounter in late adolescence and young adulthood, since they form the standards against which we evaluate whatever comes later. This would mean that each cohort's musical tastes become set in young adulthood. If this hypothesis is true, then no music could have greater impact on us than the music of our youth.

Setting of musical tastes in late adolescence and demographic trends go a long way to explain why many major cities now have at least one "oldies" station, playing the hits of the 1960s and 1970s. Radio station managers have come to believe that each cohort's tastes are fixed in young adulthood, so that baby boomers will continue to listen to the music of that era throughout their lives. The large size of the cohorts of the baby

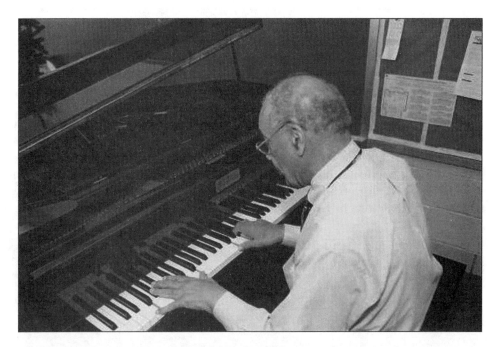

The music we listen to in adolescence will likely be the music we play in our later years. (Credit: Courtesy of the U.S. Administration on Aging)

boom, and their current location in their high-earning middle years, makes them a very valuable market for advertisers. In past years, radio advertisers pushed fast cars and the newest fashions to the boomer market; but now products marketed to this group include insurance, minivans, and relaxed-fit jeans. So what if Mick Jagger is past 60 and the surviving Beatles are becoming grandfathers? The logical outcome of this fixing of musical tastes, of course, is that eventually they will need to play the Rolling Stones in nursing homes.

In contemporary nursing homes, of course, one may hear at least two kinds of music. For afternoon singalongs or performances, the most favored music is comprised of the "old songs," reflecting the youthful period of the residents. (Note: Take the current year and subtract about 65 years for a good estimate of the musical era in question.) Even those residents with cognitive impairment seem to recall the words of and to be buoyed by the old songs that are so familiar. The other music to be heard in nursing homes, however, is that played by the staff, reflecting a younger generation and their tastes in music. Although it may satisfy the workers, the musical tastes of most workers probably would not win many converts among the residents.

But do we all become fixed in our musical tastes in young adulthood? Is musical preference really a cohort-related trait? Probably not completely. There are those who cultivate a taste for other types of music as they mature. A fan of hip-hop may eventually cultivate a taste for jazz or the classics. There once was a maturation hypothesis regarding music, the absolute opposite of the cohort hypothesis derived from Mannheim. The maturation hypothesis argued that musical tastes routinely changed as we matured. Musical preferences, like our bodies, were thought to change in a predictable way. "Easy listening" radio stations once hoped for a major boost, expecting that the baby boomers, once they achieved middle age, would convert from the music of their youth to the style and performers of music that had been favored by their parents in mid-life. Instead of a high decibel level and a heavy beat, they hoped that mature boomers would be more interested in a milder and more settled sound. That change failed to materialize in large enough numbers to maintain the "easy listening" format in many radio markets, and some of these stations converted to talk or "oldies" formats.

To throw the neat musical cohort scheme into chaos, there are occasional aberrations. An example is the mid-1990s embrace of singer Tony Bennett by young adults. Bennett is a star closer to their grandparents' than their parents' generation; he has not altered his pop style to accommodate his youthful fans. Unlike stars of most generations, Bennett, having already become "chronologically advantaged" relative to this new audience, will not have the luxury of growing older with them for too many years in the future.

Aging People in an Aging World: Demographic Perspectives

Population aging may be seen as a human success story. ... But the worldwide phenomenon of aging [brings] many challenges ... concerning the ability of [nations], states and communities to provide for aging population. (Kinsella & Phillips, 2005, p. 5)

The challenges presented by an aging world are only hinted at in the quote above. New reports and articles appear almost weekly that describe the issues facing many aging societies. Work, housing, retirement, transportation, technology, health care, and intergenerational relationships are being transformed by population aging. No doubt, you can see signs of these changes all around. Baby boomer aging is discussed on news programs, reflected in a seemingly endless array of new products, and is the subject of a growing number of Web sites. An aging workforce, with a short supply of younger workers, will cause us to rethink our attitudes about older workers and retirement. Our health care system will need significant overhaul to meet the needs of our burgeoning older population for long-term care and prescription drugs. The debate about privatization of Social Security as a solution to the long-range solvency of the system is directly related to the aging of the population (particularly the ubiquitous baby boomers). The future of Social Security has been widely discussed, from newsmagazine cover stories and debates on the floor of Congress to everyday conversations. Many worry about whether Social Security will be there for the next generation and about how much they will have to pay in taxes to keep it going. The "crisis" in Social Security is defined by and will be resolved as a matter of public policy and public sentiment, as is discussed in chapter 9. The battle lines are drawn by political processes and societal values. However, another influence is at work in framing the Social Security debate: the demography of our aging society. The number of beneficiaries receiving Social Security and the number of workers contributing to the system have a direct impact on the amount of taxes workers will have to pay to keep Social Security viable.

The size of the older population ahead of you in line for Social Security helps to determine how much you will have to pay in taxes during your prime working years. The "crisis" of Social Security, then, is driven by demography. The numbers are the starting point.

The demographics of an aging society and an aging world are an important part of the social context of aging. Many aspects of culture and social life, including those that help shape the experiences of aging, are affected by the size, structure, and composition of a society's population. So, as we begin this discussion of the demography of aging, put aside any preconceived ideas about demography as thinly disguised math that is ultimately irrelevant. As in the case of Social Security, demography is shaping public policy and the future. Even the number and kinds of jobs available when you enter (or re-enter) the job market will be determined in part by demography, especially the size of the generations just ahead of you.

The Aging of Societies

Demographic forces have a great impact on society as a whole, as discussed in chapter 1. One of the most important worldwide trends is **societal aging**. Societal aging refers to the social and demographic processes that result in the aging of a population—the transition to an age structure with increasing numbers and proportions of older people and decreasing proportions at the youngest ages. The specific forces involved in, and measures of, societal aging are discussed later in this chapter. For now, our focus is on the general impact of population aging on a society.

The size and composition of the older population influences the most basic features of social life, from "active adult communities" and so-called lifestyle pharmaceuticals marketed ostensibly to improve the quality of older adults' lives to ethical debates about end-of-life medical treatment. Families, the labor market, education, government, media, and consumer goods are all affected by the "age" of a population. Two brief examples help illustrate this point.

First, consider the number of advertisements and commercials that deal in some way with age and aging. Some of these ads present negative messages about aging and try to sell products that slow down or alter the visible signs of aging. Others use a positive message, such as the Nike Air ad featuring Nolan Ryan; this ad talks about "94-year-old swimmers, 89-year-old weightlifters.... People who forgot to retire ... and never got old." Analyzing the effectiveness and purposes of negative versus positive age-based advertising is interesting. But for our purposes the main point of these ads is their mere existence. Advertisements featuring aging in some way, the appearance of middle-aged and older characters on television, and the design of new products for mid-life are all recent developments, and they are related to the increasing average age of the population. As a large proportion of our population enters mid- and later life, marketers and advertisers are responding to this shift by including a new range of images, messages, and products. The use of 1970s' music in advertisements for financial services is clearly targeted to middle-aged baby boomers. As a result of the aging of the U.S. population, "in one way or another, every social institution in American society has had to accommodate to older people's needs, court their favor, or mobilize their resources and contributions" (Treas, 1995, p. 2).

For another example of the impact of population aging on social life, think about the differences between India and the United States. India is a relatively "young" society: Only 5% of its population is age 65 or over, and average life expectancy is about 64 years. The United States is considered to be an "aging" society, with over 12% of its population in the 65+ category and an average life expectancy of 77 years. As explained in the discussion below of population pyramids, "young" societies have high birth rates (fertility) and high death rates (mortality), whereas "aging" societies have low fertility and low mortality. Many aspects of social life (such as the type and availability of housing, the level of economic development, and the status of women) are related to these patterns of birth and death that produce population aging. For example, health care in India is focused almost exclusively on maternal and child health, family planning, and immunization.

The United States spends its health care dollars very differently; Medicare, government-sponsored health insurance for older people, is the largest and most expensive publicly funded program in the country (Lassey, Lassey, & Jinks, 1997).

The availability of public education, access to safe water and sufficient food, and the demands that compete for limited government resources are very different in the two countries. In the United States, clean water is taken for granted (although there is increasing evidence that perhaps it shouldn't be); education through age 18 is guaranteed as a basic right of all citizens; virtually all people over the age of 65 receive government-sponsored health care; and nearly 90% of the older population is eligible for a public pension (Social Security).

In India, all of the major causes of death in children are directly linked to the lack of clean water and food; two-thirds of older men and more than 90% of older women are illiterate; there is no national policy of health care for older people and virtually no public pension system. Older adults live with and economically depend on kin to meet their needs. Although the different "age" of the two populations does not fully explain these basic and profound differences, the age of a population is a contributing factor. One Indian scholar summarizes the significance of population aging this way: "The aging of society reflects the triumph of civilization over illness, poverty, and misery, and the decline in human fertility" (Goyal, 1989, p. 10).

This chapter presents the aging of societies as an important demographic process that affects our everyday lives, even though it may seem (at a macro level) distant. We discuss how societies age, how we can tell they are "aging," and why it matters. We also present an overview of the demographic characteristics of the older population in the United States, focusing on the uses of such information for policy and planning.

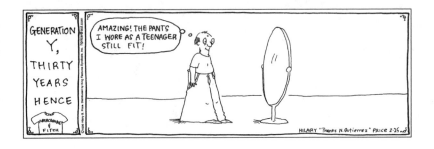

Demographic Transition Theory

The demographic transition is a set of interrelated social and demographic changes that result in rapid growth and aging of the population. The prototypical transition pattern occurred throughout Western Europe in the 19th and early 20th centuries. The first stage of the transition is related to mortality (the rate of death in a society). During the transition, the economies of these countries went through enormous shifts, changing from an agricultural base to an industrial mode of production. At the same time, these countries experienced mortality decline as a by-product of economic development. They gained control over infectious diseases, improved the availability of clean water, and saw the emergence of more advanced medical technology. This shift from high and somewhat variable mortality (variable because of epidemics) to lower mortality is shown in Exhibit 3.1.

As also shown in Exhibit 3.1, fertility remained high longer than did mortality, but then began to decline. In this second transition phase, the lag between mortality decline and fertility decline set the stage for rapid population growth; mortality was not

"removing" nearly as many people from the population as before, and continued high fertility was adding many additional people. Finally, with sustained low mortality and low fertility, population aging occurs. Exhibit 3.1 shows the curves for population growth and for growth in the aged population that result from the demographic transition.

Thus far we have been discussing the demographic transition as a pattern of change in mortality and fertility that accompanied industrialization. Yet we have referred to the demographic transition *theory*. A theory goes beyond description to search for explanations and ultimately to make predictions. *Why* did mortality and fertility decline accompany economic development in Western Europe? Is the pattern of decline consistent? What will happen in nations that are just beginning to enter the transition phase? Data on the consistency of the prototypical pattern suggest that even in Western Europe there were variations in the timing of fertility and mortality declines.

More importantly, *causal* connections between the demographic trends and industrialization are not well established. In Western Europe, the stages of the demographic transition are related to, "and in

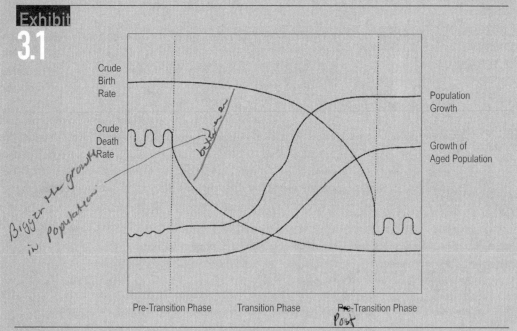

Exhibit
3.1

A Simplified Diagram of the Demographic Transition
Adapted from: Yaukey, 1985 and Myers, 1990.

(continued)

(continued)

part caused by, industrialization, urbanization, and the spread of literacy and education" (Matras, 1990, p. 27). An industrial economy created, for the first time, an economic surplus; all members of a society could be supported by a smaller number of workers. For this reason, it was not necessary for families to have large numbers of children as workers or to ensure that at least some survived. It may seem unusual to imagine that people decide how many children to have based on such a rational calculation. However, there is an extensive literature in demography about the many factors, including the "costs and benefits" of having children, that go into such a personal and emotional decision. Keep in mind as well that the means of birth control were limited and unreliable prior to the past four decades.

We can understand more about the strengths and weaknesses of the demographic transition theory when we consider how well the pattern and predictions are holding for the developing regions of the world that are still "young." The declining mortality rates in these countries are characteristic of the beginning of the second stage of the demographic transition. Whether, when, and how quickly declining birth rates will follow mortality declines remains to be seen. Matras (1990) points out that Mexico, Nicaragua, and Jordan have all experienced dramatic mortality declines, but show little evidence of downward trends in birth rates. Such a decline is necessary for these and other developing nations to move into the third (post-transition) stage, characterized by an older population, a lower rate of population growth, a stable low mortality, and a fluctuating but low fertility.

When and how any country reaches the post-transition stage depends on an array of cultural and social factors that are not thoroughly understood. In developing nations, there is some evidence to suggest that mortality is having a greater impact on population aging than it did in developed nations. This departure from the classic demographic transition model (Coale, 1964), in which fertility has the primary impact on population aging points to the caution we must exercise in applying existing models of change to developing nations. Furthermore, in the United States, Western Europe, and Japan, population aging proceeded along with economic development. In developing nations today, partly because of the rapid import of technology to control fertility and mortality, population aging can occur ahead of economic development. These forces will very likely have an impact on the timing and nature of population aging in the developing regions of the world.

How Do Populations Age?

The simple answer to the question of how populations age is that they grow older when both the fertility and mortality rates are low. In short, population aging occurs when large numbers of people survive into old age and relatively few children are born. In such societies, life expectancies are high, and the proportion of the population age 65 and above is high.. But how does mortality decline? Under what circumstances does a whole society of people decide to have fewer children, lowering the fertility rate? An important framework for understanding these changes is the demographic transition theory.

Measures of Population Aging

The importance of population's age is far-reaching. Kent and Haub (2005) describe the "demographic divide" between countries with low birth rates and high life expectancies (aging/slow or no growth populations) and those with high birth rates and relatively low life expectancies (young/high growth) populations. They point out that the divide is important because of "the disparities associated with the demographic trends—disparities in living standards, personal health, well-being, and future prospects" (pp. 2–3).

How can we show whether a population is aging? The five commonly used indicators of population aging are *population pyramids, proportion aged, median ages, aging index, dependency ratios,* and *life expectancy.* Each of these measures tells part of the story of a society's "age," and each is described and compared below.

Population Pyramids

A **population pyramid** is a graphic illustration of the age and sex structure of a population. It shows the percentage or number of people within a total population who fit into selected age and sex categories. Population pyramids truly are pictures worth a thousand words. They capture and illustrate at a glance many past, present, and future demographic trends. Only three demographic forces directly determine the shape of a pyramid: fertility, mortality, and migration. The numbers of people being born, dying, and moving into or out of a location will affect the relative size of all of the age and sex groupings for that population, whether it is a town or a country. The impact of fertility, mortality, and migration in shaping a population structure can be seen in the examples of population pyramids discussed throughout this section.

Exhibit 3.2a shows the population pyramid for the United States in 2000. The bulge of people in the 35- to 49-year-old range is the infamous baby boom generation (the large number of people born after World War II, between 1946 and 1964). The powerful impact of a past fertility trend is reflected in the shape of the pyramid. The slightly

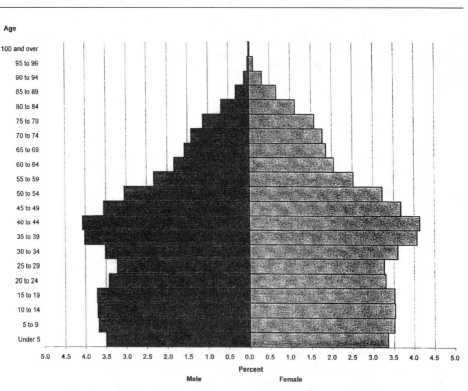

Population Pyramid for the United States, 2000
Source: U.S. Census Bureau International Data Base, Accessed March 2006.

lopsided top of the pyramid shows the greater number of older women than men. This imbalance is a manifestation of past and current trends in mortality. Women live longer than men do. We discuss this phenomenon in greater detail later in this chapter.

Based on the age/sex structure illustrated in the 2000 pyramid, we can make some predictions about the shape of our population pyramid in the future. The most significant feature of that shape will be the movement upward of the baby boom generation. Demographers sometimes refer to this as the "pig-in-the-python," conjuring the image of a whole pig moving slowly through the digestive tract of a large snake. So, too, the baby boom bulge moves slowly upward through the population pyramid of the United States. The mid-life baby boomers of today are the older generations of tomorrow; and young adults today are the middle-aged of the near future. Exhibit 3.2b shows this phenomenon.

The population pyramid for the United Arab Emirates (Exhibit 3.3) has an unusual shape. Working-age men far outnumber women of the same age. Why would this be so? We know that there are only three possible influences on the shape of a pyramid: fertility, mortality, and migration. In this case, the imbalance in the numbers of working-age men and women is due to the immigration of thousands of people from Asia and other parts of the Middle East to work in the oil fields. These workers are nearly always men who migrate into the United Arab Emirates without their families (McFalls, 1998; U.S. Bureau of the Census, 2005b).

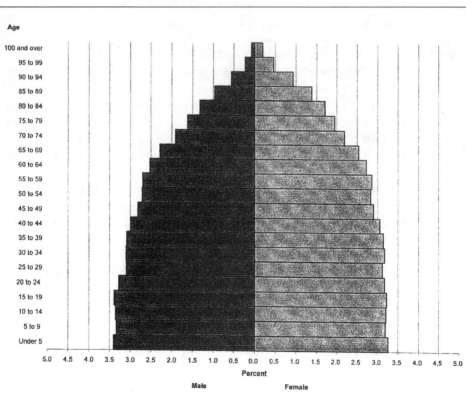

Population Pyramid for the United States, 2050

Source: U.S. Census Bureau International Data Base, accessed March 2006.

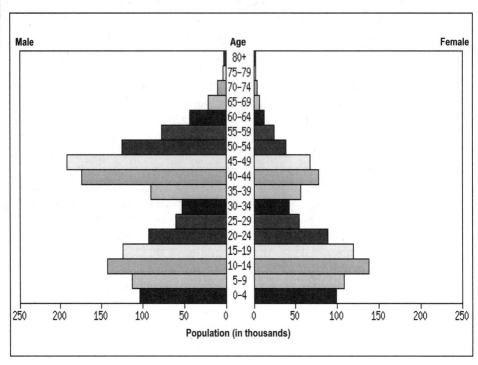

Population Pyramid for the United Arab Emirates, 2000
Source: U.S. Census Bureau International Database, Accessed March 2006.

In most countries, migration does not currently play such a big role in the age and sex structure; fertility and mortality are by far the more powerful influences. However, for smaller geographic units, such as states and counties within the United States, migration can be an important factor. Think about what the population pyramid would look like for a small county that builds a 500-unit, state-of-the-art, low-cost retirement community that can accommodate 1,000 older people. This desirable location would attract people from all around the area, including neighboring counties; the relative size of the older population for the "receiving" county would be affected immediately and significantly. If the receiving county had a small, rural population, a large number of new, older residents could create a T-shaped population pyramid.

The shape of a population pyramid thus tells us something about the past, present, and future of a society—not only the fertility, mortality, and migration trends, but also something about life in that society. Population pyramids often take on one of three basic shapes; each stylized shape distinguishes, in a general way, demographic patterns and other aspects of social life, such as a stage in the demographic transition and level of economic development. Exhibit 3.4 shows two of the three basic shapes. The "true" pyramid, or fast-growth shape, is characteristic of young countries with high fertility and high mortality, such as Kenya. The rectangular, or no-growth, pyramid shows the effects of sustained very low fertility and very low mortality, as in Denmark.

The third classic pyramid shape is a slow-growth, beehive-shaped pyramid; it represents a transition between the "true" pyramid the rectangle. We saw this shape for the United States in Exhibit 3.2b, reflecting a pattern of low mortality and fertility. Some

Exhibit
34

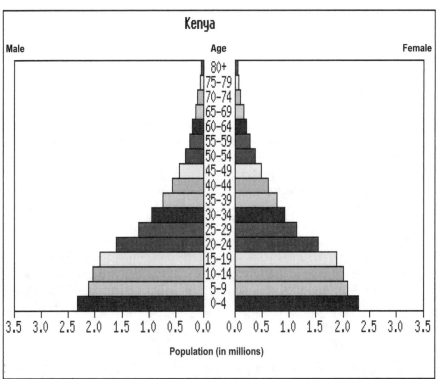

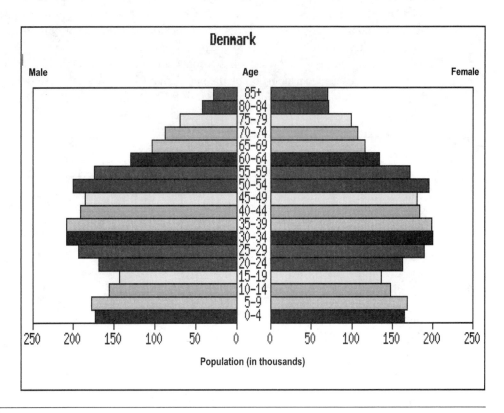

Examples of Classic Population Pyramid Shapes: Kenya and Denmark 2000

Source: U.S. Census Bureau International Database, accessed March 2006.

demographers have suggested a fourth pattern: the collapsing or inverted pyramid, which is narrowest at the base. The bottom half of the pyramid for Denmark (in Exhibit 3.4) has this shape, and it is possible that Denmark will eventually have an inverted pyramid, if current levels of extremely low fertility are maintained.

Students are often curious about which pyramid is most desirable for a society. That question has no simple answer; each of these pyramid shapes represents a different set of challenges. For example, a pyramid with a wide base and narrow apex describes a society with lots of children, large families, and high rates of mortality; in such a society, the major focus of public policy will probably be on maternal and child health, schools, and on family planning. In a society with a rectangular pyramid, it is fairly certain that some public policy and tax resources will be devoted to caring for older people. So, there is no "best" shape for a population pyramid; views on which set of challenge are most acceptable are determined by political and economic development, as well as cultural and social values.

Population pyramids are elegant, informative, intuitively useful representations of the age and sex structure of a society. They give information about how old or young a society is and provide an indication of the level of economic development, the state of advancement in medical technology, and the nature of the resource allocation dilemmas faced by a society.

Proportion Aged

A straightforward measure of population aging is to consider the proportion of a society that is older. "Older than what?" you might ask. Most reports of *proportion aged* use 65 as the marker, but some, especially those comparing countries around the world, use age 60 as a cutoff point. So it is wise to be attentive to the precise definition of "proportion aged." The first column in Exhibit 3.5 shows the proportion of population that is age 65 and over for a broad selection of countries. These proportions range from a low of 2.2% to a high of 17.4%. The average proportion of the population 65 and over for the more developed world is 14.3%; for less developed nations, it is 5.1% (United Nations, 2002).

Exhibit 3.5	% 65+		Median Age		Life Expectancy at Birth		Aging Index	
	2000	2050	2000	2050	2000	2050	2000	2050
Kuwait	2.2	17.8	22.7	39.2	76.5	81.1	14.1	130.4
Nigeria	3.0	6.8	17.2	29.6	52.1	69.3	10.6	41.2
Nepal	3.7	8.3	19.4	31.8	59.8	70.5	14.4	52.7
India	5.0	14.8	23.7	31.3	64.2	75.4	22.7	105.0
China	6.9	22.7	30.0	43.8	71.2	79.0	40.7	183.3
United States	12.3	21.1	35.5	40.7	77.5	82.6	74.4	144.9
Japan	17.2	36.4	41.2	53.0	81.5	88.0	157.9	338.2
Italy	18.1	35.9	40.2	54.0	78.7	82.5	168.5	369.2
Sweden	17.4	30.4	39.7	51.2	80.1	84.6	123.0	270.1

Measures of Population Aging in Selected Countries, 2000 and 2050
Source: United Nations, 2002.

The proportion aged is easily used to make comparisons among nations or across historical time periods within a country, state, or city. Proportions aged are both less complicated and less informative than population pyramids, which give an overall picture of the age structure of the population. Nonetheless, trends in the proportion aged in a society can provide an important indicator of population aging.

Median Ages

Like the proportion aged, median ages are single numbers that are often used in conjunction with other measures of population aging. The **median** is the midpoint of a range of numbers—the point at which half the cases fall above and half below. The second and third columns of Exhibit 3.5 show a wide range of median ages. Sweden, by many measures the "oldest" country in the world, has a median age of almost 40. Nigeria, one of the "youngest" countries in the world, has an exceptionally low median age of 17.2; half of the people in Nigeria are under the age of 17.2. Curiosity about these patterns would lead us to investigate the recent history, fertility patterns, political turmoil, natural disasters, and food shortages that might have befallen a country with an unusual demographic pattern.

Aging Index

The **aging index** is the ratio of older people (60+) to children under the age of 15. It is a straightforward measure of the age structure of a population, telling us how many older people there are for every 100 children under age 15. By 2030, nearly all of the more developed countries of the world will have an aging index of 100 or more (Kinsella & Phillips, 2005), indicating that there will be one older person for every children under age 15. As you might expect, more developed countries have a much higher aging index than less developed countries. In 2000, Europe had an aging index of 116, more than 10 times higher than that of Africa. In Africa, the aging index of 12 per 100 describes a very young population. The fourth section of Exhibit 3.5 further illustrates the differences among nations around the world. Nigeria has less than 11 older people for every 100 children, while Italy has 168 older people for every 100 children. The aging index is an indicator of the pressures that societies may face in allocation of resources.

Dependency Ratios

Dependency ratios are, as the term suggests, measures of the proportion of a population that falls within age categories traditionally thought to be economically dependent: those under age 15 (the youth dependency ratio) and over age 64 (the aged dependency ratio). We can take issue with the definition of anyone under 15 or over 64 as automatically being economically dependent, especially in countries where people work long before age 15 and sometimes long after age 64. In fact, recent discussion of dependency ratios in the United States uses age 18 instead of age 15 (Treas, 1995). Other scholars have challenged the "dependency" assumption by pointing out that some older people fuel economic growth through their taxes and income, and that some working-age people may be unemployed (Kinsella & Phillips, 2005). Despite this limitation, however, dependency ratios are useful as general comparative indicators of the relative proportions of working-age versus non–working-age people. As such, they point to different patterns across states or nations of demand on economic and social resources, such as health care, tax dollars, and the educational system.

The aged dependency ratio is similar to proportion aged, but is calculated in a slightly different way and interpreted in a very different way. The proportion aged in a society is simply the number of older people divided by the total population. The aged dependency ratio is the number of older people divided by the number of people ages 15 to 64. It is interpreted as the number of older people for every working-age person (sometimes stated as the number of older people per 100 working-age people).

Exhibit 3.6 shows the youth, aged, and total dependency ratios for some of the countries in Exhibit 3.5. Of these, the country with the highest total dependency ratio is Nigeria, which has almost 93 younger and older citizens for every 100 working-age citizens. Countries such as the United States, Japan, and Italy have roughly two working-age people for every "dependent" person. If you look at the two components (aged and youth) of the total dependency ratio for countries with very high total dependency ratios and those with relatively low ones, most often the youth dependency ratio con-

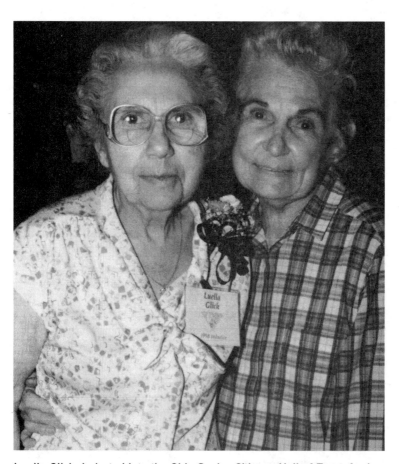

Luella Glick, inducted into the Ohio Senior Citizens Hall of Fame for her volunteerism and commitment to her community, provides a noteworthy exception to the concept of dependency ratios. (Credit: Mike Payne, courtesy of the Ohio Department of Aging)

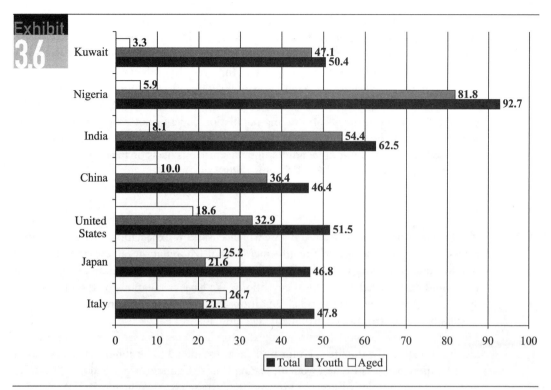

Dependency Ratios for Selected Countries, 2000
Source: United Nations, 2002.

tributes disproportionately to high overall ratios. This pattern would be predicted by the demographic transition theory. Recall that high fertility and high mortality are typical of a country in the pre-transition or early transition phase. Lots of children are being born, and lots of people are dying, producing a low proportion of older people and a high proportion of children relative to the working-age population. The relative sizes of the youth and aged dependency ratios are also demonstrated by the shape of a country's population pyramid.

One final point about dependency ratios is important to keep in mind. Although the numbers and patterns may be interesting in and of themselves, they are most often used to make an argument, defend a position, or influence public policy. In the United States, the increasing proportion of older persons and the accompanying increase in the aged dependency ratio has "prompted concern and even alarm about society's capacity to pay for pensions, to finance health care, and to provide the personal assistance that disabled older adults need in their daily lives" (Treas, 1995, p. 6).

It is certainly reasonable to debate the nation's ability, obligation, and strategies to provide these important programs and services; however, these issues have been used to fuel a political agenda built on the rhetoric of burden. Using "voodoo demographics" (Schulz, 1986), proponents of the burden perspective present data such as the aged dependency ratio to conclude that the number of workers will be insufficient to support age-based entitlement programs for the huge baby boom generation lurking just around the bend. They argue that the economic burden of an aging population will become unfair and unbearable in the near future; their proposed solution is to cut programs and alter eligibility criteria for those programs. Although we may decide to take such action, the demographics of our aging society are not the driving force behind either the problem or the solution. Interestingly, while the aged dependency ratio in the United States is increasing steadily, the youth dependency ratio has been declining, so that the current total dependency ratio is lower than it was in the 1960s and 1970s (Treas, 1995). Our ability to meet the needs of an aging population depends not simply on numbers of old people in relation to working-age people, but on the productivity of the nation, the continued contributions of older adults, and on conscious decision making on the part of politicians and voters (Friedland & Summer, 2005).

Life Expectancy

The final measure of population aging we will discuss is life expectancy. **Life expectancy** refers to the average length of time the members of a population can expect to live. It is not the same as **life span,** which refers to a theoretical biological maximum length of life that could be achieved under ideal conditions. We have calculations of the life span of species that can be raised in optimal conditions, but for humans it is not ethically viable or possible to control the environment. For humans, we gauge the maximum possible life span by using the most recent reliable data on how long a single individual has actually lived. Currently, the life span for humans is estimated to be about 120 years, based on the experience of a French woman, Jeanne Louise Calment, who died in 1997 at the age of 122 (Gerontology Research Group, 2006; Russell & McWhirter, 1987).

Life expectancy, then, is the *average* experience of a population. It is calculated from actual mortality data from a single year and looks at what would happen to a hypothetical group of people if they moved through their lives experiencing the mortality rates observed for the country as a whole during the year in question. The third column in Exhibit 3.5 shows the different life expectancies for the sample of countries we have been discussing. Not surprisingly, countries with the lowest percentages of aged persons, lowest median and **mean ages,** and age/sex structures most resembling pyramids are also those countries with the lowest life expectancies. These various measures of societal aging are related.

Because life expectancy reflects so many biological and social processes, it deserves further consideration. Exhibit 3.7 provides greater detail about average length of life in the United States; it shows the average number of years of life remaining for people of different age, sex, and race categories in the United States in 2002. To use the table, look at the left-hand column to find a target age, then read across to the race and gender category of interest. Find the number of years in the appropriate cell of the table, and add those years to the age in the left-hand column to obtain the life expectancy for someone of that age, gender, and race. For example, the life expectancy for a 40-year-old Black woman in 2002 was 78.1 (40 plus 38.1).

As you calculate life expectancies from this table, you will notice some interesting sources of variation. Average length of life varies depending on age, race, and sex. Life expectancy at birth (all races, both sexes) in 2002 was 77.3; but life expectancy at age 75 is an additional 11.5 years (to about 86). For every year of life a person survives, his or her life expectancy goes up. So, the longer you live, the longer you can expect to live.

The race differential in life expectancy (also termed longevity) is evident in Exhibit 3.7. Black men of all ages have the lowest life expectancies. Black women have life expectancies that are lower than White women but higher than White men. Notice,

	Age	All Races, Both Sexes	White Males	White Females	Black Males	Black Females
	0	77.3	75.1	80.3	66.8	75.6
	5	72.9	70.7	75.8	65.0	71.7
	10	67.9	65.7	70.8	60.1	66.8
	15	63.0	60.8	65.9	55.2	61.8
	20	58.2	56.1	61.0	50.5	57.0
	25	53.5	51.4	56.1	46.0	52.1
	30	48.7	46.7	51.2	41.6	47.4
	35	44.0	42.0	46.4	37.1	42.7
	40	39.3	37.4	41.6	32.8	38.1
	45	34.8	32.9	36.9	28.5	33.7
	50	30.3	28.5	32.4	24.6	29.5
	55	26.1	24.3	27.9	21.0	25.4
	60	22.0	20.3	23.6	17.6	21.6
	65	18.2	16.6	19.5	14.6	18.0
	70	14.7	13.3	15.8	11.8	14.7
	75	11.5	10.3	12.3	9.5	11.7
	80	8.8	7.7	9.3	7.5	9.2
	85	6.1	5.7	6.8	5.8	7.0

Exhibit 3.7

Abridged Life Expectancy Table by Race and Sex: United States 2002
Source: Arias, 2004.

however, that the differences between Blacks and Whites (within gender categories) become smaller and smaller as age increases. The difference in life expectancy at birth for Black and White baby boys is 8.2 years. Black men who make it to age 80, though, have life expectancies almost equal to those of White men (7.5 and 7.7 years, respectively), and Black women at age 85 have life expectancies almost equivalent to those of White women of the same age. This decrease in the Black/White difference in life expectancy is called **convergence**; the eventual reversal (at the oldest ages) of the difference in remaining year of expected life by race is called the **crossover effect**.

These observations suggest two questions: Why is there a race differential in life expectancy at all, and why does it diminish and even reverse itself at the oldest ages? In answer to the first question, most of the race differential in mortality is explained by differences in socioeconomic status (Queen, Pappas, Harden, & Fisher, 1994; Rogers, 1995). Blacks in the United States have historically been economically disadvantaged and continue to have unequal access to educational and occupational opportunity; the numerous health disadvantages that derive from lack of access to important opportunities, such as employer-based health insurance, show up in higher mortality. These racial differences in health status, prevalence of diseases, and causes of death are discussed in greater detail in chapter 10.

The second question—regarding the convergence in the race differential in life expectancy—has received some attention, but no definitive answer. One suggested explanation is that the data are unreliable. Among the current generation of older Blacks, the lack of "official" date-of-birth information may be responsible for some misreporting of age (Preston, Elo, & Rosenvaike, 1996). Another hypothesis for the convergence effect is that Blacks who make it to the oldest ages despite many disadvantages and long odds may be "survivors." In other words, the survivor group may have some complex set of physiological and social psychological advantages that result in greater life expectancy.

A final variation in life expectancy that is readily apparent in Exhibit 3.7 is the gender difference. At every age, for both races, females have higher life expectancies than males. How can we explain this "excess male mortality?" Ideas on the subject are many and varied; some are thoughtful and scientific and others are creative. A colleague offered the hypothesis that the stuff that men cough up and spit out has life-sustaining properties; because women in most cultures don't spit, they live longer (McGrew, 1989).

The most plausible and thoroughly researched explanations for the sex differential fall into two major categories: biological explanations and social/behavioral explanations. Biological explanations are based on the premise that females have a physiological advantage that results in greater longevity, whereas sociobehavioral explanations focus on life-style choices, socialization, risk-taking, stress, and occupational hazards. There is evidence supporting both kinds of explanations.

One example of research support for the biological basis for the sex differential in mortality comes from the sex ratio. About 120 males are conceived for every 100 females conceived, but by the time of birth that ratio is down to about 105 males for every 100 females. Assuming that social and behavioral factors do not play a prenatal role, we conclude that male fetuses are less viable than female fetuses. Another bit of evidence for the physiological basis is heart disease: Prior to menopause, women have significantly lower rates of heart disease than men, but after menopause women's rates increase to approximate those of men. Apparently estrogen (which is high during the childbearing years but low after menopause) provides some protection against at least this one major cause of death.

The "superior biological viability" argument does not tell the whole story, though. Waldron (1993) found that as much as 50% of the sex differential in mortality could be explained by risk-taking and other unhealthy behaviors such as smoking. Men in U.S. culture are socialized to drive fast, drink alcohol, and smoke; they are also less likely to see a physician on a regular basis and less likely to use social support networks to deal with stress. All of these factors help to explain men's shorter life expectancies.

No doubt the life expectancy difference between men and women is explained by some combination of biological, life-style, or environmental influences. Sorting out the explanations has important implications for health promotion and enhancement. The longevity differential had been consistently widening from 1900 until 1972 in the United States but has been narrowing since the late 1970s (Kochanek, Murphy, Anderson, & Scott, 2004), primarily as a result of slower gains in life expectancy for women. For many decades, everyone's life expectancy has been improving, but the rate of improvement varies. AIDS is having a significant dampening effect on the extension of longevity in the United States since deaths at early ages reduce the averages, but life expectancies are still increasing slightly. The recent narrowing of the gender differential in mortality is largely explained by improvements in men's survival.

The same pattern of "excess male mortality" holds true for most other countries around the world, although the difference between men's and women's life expectancies is often not as great in developing nations. For the United States and the European Union, women live on average about 6 years longer than men; in less developed regions, the difference is less than 2 years (United Nations, 2002). In a handful of countries, the difference is in the opposite direction. For example, in Nepal in 2000, life expectancy at birth was 60.1 years for men and 59.6 years for women. The smaller or reversed gender difference in longevity in developing nations is due primarily to maternal mortality—deaths among women during pregnancy and childbearing. This same pattern occurred in the United States in the late 19th century, when knowledge and medical care surrounding childbirth were less advanced and less widely available.

We have seen that life expectancy varies by age, by race, by gender, and by economic development of a nation. Many other factors help to determine how long any individual is likely to live. To get a sense of these other influences and how they can affect an average expectation of life, spend a few minutes taking the life expectancy test in Exhibit 3.8. After you have answered all of the questions, sum up your added and subtracted years of life. Find your total number on the life expectancy table (Exhibit 3.7), and calculate how long you are likely to live. Obviously, this is not a scientific prediction of your life expectancy, but it might be interesting to consider how long your life might be and how you feel about it. Does it seem too long or too short?

The life expectancy test shows the importance of genetics, life-style, social factors, and other social traits such as marital status. For many of these influences on longevity, their impact is intuitively obvious, but the relationship between marriage and life expectancy is perhaps not so obvious. This relationship is well established; it has been observed consistently in the United States and in other nations as well (Hu & Goldman, 1990). Married people live longer than unmarried people. There are two major explanations for this phenomenon (Weeks, 1994). First is the "selectivity" hypothesis that healthy people are more likely to get married and remain married. The second is that marriage is good for your health. Having a stable intimate relationship is argued to be conducive to good health, and the availability of caregiving support is an important health advantage. The numerous influences on life expectancy are relevant to all of us as individuals. They are also part of the complex picture of how, why, and when a population "ages."

Global Aging

Why does the aging of a population matter to individuals or to societies as a whole? In many ways, this entire book is about the effects of population aging—on social institutions such as work, the family, the economy, and the health care system. Chapter 4 explains that the social construction of life stages is partly a result of how long people in a society live. For example, *adolescence* is a fairly "young" life stage in historical terms; in earlier eras, when people married and had children in their early teens and only lived to their thirties, there was no "preparatory" stage of life. Now we take adolescence as an established and essential stage of human development.

Beyond the impact of societal aging on our lives as individuals and as members of a society, one of the most far-reaching consequences of population aging is that the entire world is aging. The world's elderly population is increasing by about 880,000 persons *per month!* (Kinsella & Velkoff, 2001). Exhibit 3.5 shows some of the dramatic change that will be taking place in countries around the world over the next 50 years. For all of the countries in the table, the minimum increase is a near doubling (for the United States,

Exhibit
3.8

Have any of your grandparents lived to age 80 or beyond? If so, add one year for each grandparent living beyond that age. Add one-half year for each grandparent surviving beyond the age of 70. _____

If any parent, grandparent, sister, or brother died of a heart attack, stroke, or arteriosclerosis before the age of 50, subtract four years for each incidence. If any of those close relatives died of the above before the age of 60, subtract two years for each incidence. _____

Do you prefer vegetables, fruits, and simple foods to foods high in fat and sugar, and do you always stop eating before you feel really full? If your honest answer to both questions is yes, add one year. _____

How much do you smoke? If you smoke two or more packs of cigarettes a day, subtract twelve years. If you smoke less than a pack a day, subtract two years. If you have quit smoking, congratulations, you subtract no years at all. _____

How much do you exercise? Add three years if you exercise at least three times a week at one of the following: jogging, bike riding, swimming, taking long, brisk walks, dancing, or skating. Just exercising on weekends does not count. _____

If you enjoy regular sexual activity, having intimate sexual relations once or twice a week, add two years. _____

If you are married and living with your spouse, add one year. _____

If you are a separated or divorced man living alone, subtract nine years, and if you are a widowed man living alone, subtract seven years. If, as a separated, divorced, or widowed man, you live with other people such as family members, subtract only half the years given above. Living with others is beneficial for formerly married men. _____

Women who are separated or divorced should subtract four years, and widowed women should subtract three and a half years. The loss of a spouse through divorce or death is not as life-shortening to a woman, and she lives about as long whether she lives alone or with family, unless she is the head of the household. Divorced or widowed women who live with family as the head of their household should subtract two years for the formerly married status. _____

If you are a woman who has never married, subtract one year for each unmarried decade past the age of 25. If you live with a family or friends as a male single person, you should also subtract one year for each unmarried decade past the age of 25. However, if you are a man who has never married and are living alone, subtract two years for each unmarried decade past the age of 25. _____

Do you generally like people and have at least two close friends in whom you can confide almost all the details of your life? If so, add one year. _____

The Abridged Life Expectancy Test

where the proportion aged will go from 12.3% in 2000 to over 20% in 2050). Other countries will have significantly higher growth. India's proportion aged will nearly triple, and Kuwait will experience a nine-fold increase in the proportion of its population that is 65 or above. Italy and Japan will have median ages of 54 and 53, respectively. The aging index for every country will increase significantly by 2050, signaling a greater number of older people per 100 children than was the case in 2000. China will change dramatically over these 50 years, from 40 older people per 100 children to 183 older persons per 100 children. Japan and Italy will have more than three times as many older people as children under age 15. "This trend may lead to compelling demands for changes in the way society's resources are shared between generations" (United Nations, 2002, p. 16).

Clearly the aging of a society is accompanied by, and is a catalyst for, enormous social change. Some of the greatest impacts of population aging are in the areas of health, economics, and social policy. Developed nations such as the United States are still struggling to adapt health care and economic systems to the challenges presented by the aging of their populations. In developing nations, the aging of a population presents even greater challenges for two primary reasons. First, the infrastructure for planning and providing health care and social services is often not well developed. And, as noted in the case of India, such services are most often aimed at family planning and maternal and child health; it is extremely rare to find a developing nation with a health care system that addresses the needs of growing numbers of adults in later life. Second, the crucial policy debates that take place in the developed nations regarding the distribution of responsibility for care of the elderly among family, government, and individuals have not taken place in most of the less developed nations. In those countries, the number of people surviving to old age has been so small as to obviate the necessity for such discussion but become more urgent as urbanization and technological change alter traditional family-based systems of support.

The issues arising from the aging of the world population, and the growing numbers of older people in developing nations, are receiving increasing attention—for good reason. In 1990, 57% of all older people (60+) lived in developing countries, and this proportion is expected to increase to 69% by the year 2020 (U.S. Bureau of the Census, 1991b). These figures seem surprising, given the relatively low proportion aged, life expectancy, and median age in these countries. But consider that about 80% of the world's total population lived in developing nations in 2000. Take India as an example. Even though only 5% of India's population is aged 65 or above, with a population of more than a billion people, that 5% adds up to a lot of older people. Because so much of the world's population is concentrated in these nations, and because these regions are beginning to experience rapid population aging, a very high proportion of the world's older people will be living in these areas. Another complicating factor is that population aging is occurring much more rapidly in less developed regions than it did in the United States and other already "aging" countries. For example, it took France 115 years for the proportion of population 65 and older to increase from 7% to 14%; in Sweden this change took 85 years; and in the United States this increase will happen in 59 years. For Sri Lanka, this doubling of the proportion of population that is older will take place in only 23 years, and in Singapore it will take only 19 years (Kinsella & Phillips, 2005, p. 15).

In recognition of the many complex and momentous issues, opportunities, and challenges raised by the aging of the globe, the United Nations designated 1999 as the International Year of Older Persons. A sweeping, ambitious, and inspirational International Plan of Action on Ageing was created by representatives from countries around the world. This plan, and some accompanying principles to guide policy development, call for attention to a range of issues: demographic realities; the humanitarian issues related to the situation of older people; the problem of global inequality that will make it difficult for developing nations to meet the basic needs of their populations; and assumptions that old age is inevitably a time of decline, diminished capacity, and alteration of basic human needs. In 2002, the Second World Assembly on Ageing convened in Madrid. This congress developed the **International Plan of Action on Ageing,** which includes specific priorities and action steps to address concerns and contributions of older people around the world. Full participation of older people in society is a major theme of the recommendations.

On a philosophical note, the World Assembly offered that,

> A longer life provides humans with an opportunity to examine their lives in retrospect, to correct some of their mistakes, to get closer to the truth, and to achieve a different understanding of the sense and value of actions. This may well be the most important contribution of older people to the human community. (United Nations, 2003, p. 1)

The demographic facts of global aging indeed have far-reaching consequences.

The trends in population aging have produced a range of responses. At one end of the spectrum is the alarmist call to action and deep concern over the lack of attention given to aging-related policy and planning issues. Driven by the rapidly increasing numbers and by the equivocal success of the United States in planning for our aging population, this

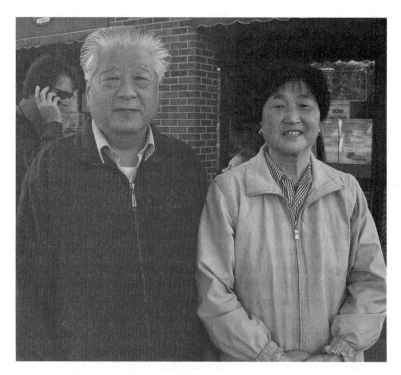

The proportion of older people in the population is expected to increase in several Asian countries as well as in the United States and across most of Europe. (Credit: E. J. Hanna)

position suggests that time is growing short for making decisions about how to handle the older population. At the other end of the continuum are critics who dismiss the alarmist position as ethnocentric: Westerners are defining the problem and calling for a solution by other countries that mirrors their own. In research conducted in Nepal, a number of senior health and planning officials said that aging was not a problem in Nepal and that they were not ready to believe it will be a problem just because Americans said so (Kunkel & Subedi, 1996). They were convinced that older people would be well taken care of by their families, as had been the long-standing tradition, and would impose no significant

Applying Theory

Modernization Theory

As we discovered in our earlier discussion of demographic transition theory, economic development and other sociocultural forces are important in determining the timing, nature, and magnitude of the declines in fertility and mortality that cause a society to age. The importance of explicitly examining ideological and cultural change is borne out by modernization theory as well.

The basic premise of modernization theory is that the status of older people declines as a society modernizes. Changes such as urbanization, technological advancement, health advances, and population growth combine to erode the position of honor, prestige, and respect accorded to older people in simpler societies. Thus, the theory argues that, "with increasing modernization the status of older people declines" (Cowgill, 1972, p. 124). In the least modernized societies, the theory contends that older people supposedly enjoy high status, and family members meet their physical and emotional needs; they require society's assistance only when modernization disrupts the traditional (mostly agrarian) family's economic and social structures. Based on modernization theory, we would expect that in most rural, agrarian developing countries the elderly enjoy high status and their needs are routinely met by families.

Modernization theory has intuitive appeal and some empirical support from cross-cultural research. However, it has also been challenged by other studies and has been criticized for using unclear and inconsistent definitions of social status, oversimplifying the processes of modernization, and ignoring intervening variables such as ideology and value systems.

Perhaps the most significant assumption made by modernization theory is that the extended family

in developing societies typically integrates its older members, eliminating the need for pensions, senior housing, and other older adult services familiar to us. According to Tout (1989), "in some instances, reliance on the traditional extended family may not be the normally acceptable panacea, but may for the old person be a gruesome and cruel experience of dependence, deprivation, and degradation" (p. 300). The traditional situation of widows in India is one clear example of this less-than-idyllic circumstance of family integration. In today's Indian society, most widows do not throw themselves on their husband's funeral pyre as tradition once mandated; instead, the widow is supported with housing and other essentials by her husband's family. However, she holds very low status in his family, is often viewed as a burden, and is sometimes the victim of verbal and physical abuse (Steinmetz, 1988).

In a review of family demography in developing nations, Martin and Kinsella (1994) provide further grounds on which to question the stereotypical model of multigenerational households providing for elders. They found that multigenerational households are declining in many developing countries and that the likelihood of sharing a residence diminishes as age increases—the oldest adults are least likely to occupy them. Multigenerational households are more likely to be based on the needs of sons and daughters than on the needs of older family members. If the needs of elders were the primary motivation, we would expect the prevalence of coresidence to increase with advancing age. Instead older adults sharing a household with descendents are more often supporting others than being supported by others.

Some, though not all, of the developing nations studied by Martin and Kinsella are still characterized by an extended family structure. Nepal is one *(continued)*

(continued)

example. Based on this criterion, we might expect the status of the elderly in Nepal to be high. However, research conducted by Goldstein and Beall (1983) in both rural and urban Nepal found that the equation of membership in an extended family with status, security, and satisfaction for the elderly person is misleading. They found that economic factors (unemployment, low wages, inflation) and social factors (less property as a result of the division of inheritance, migration of eldest sons to urban areas) had affected relationships within the family, often leaving the elderly as relatively powerless dependents on younger family members. Findings from the study indicated

that the status of older people in the family depended on the elders' ability to control property and income. These researchers conclude that, given the socioeconomic conditions of most developing societies and the inability of governments to provide substantial social service programs, there are likely to be increasing numbers of elderly parents with neither property, pensions, nor savings in their old age. This image—older people exchanging promises of economic reward for receipt of care in later years—forces Western scholars to rethink their idealized vision of life in developing nations. Although the premise of modernization theory has much appeal, it is not a uniform pattern of development across societies everywhere.

new burden on the economic, housing, or health care systems. Certainly the enormous pressures of maternal and child health in Nepal take precedence over a longer-range issue that may be adequately handled, at least for a time, by family systems.

What will happen to the growing numbers of older people in the developing nations? An overview of modernization theory will help provide a context for the problems, solutions, and biases involved in the issue of global aging.

The causes, consequences, and measurement of population aging are large-scale issues. Powerful forces, such as fertility and mortality, alarmist warnings about the consequences of global aging, and assumption-laden measures of dependency ratios may seem far distant. However, we hope that you have begun to see that population aging affects us as individuals and our families; on a more macro level it affects our government, public policy, health care system, and economy. A description of our older population will help bring this picture into sharper focus.

Demographic Characteristics of the U.S. Aging Population

This section contains a basic demographic description of the older population in the United States. The purpose of this section is not to provide extensive detail about every possible demographic characteristic, but to provide a general description of the older population. This overview will give you a better idea of the kinds of information available and encourage you to think about how such information is useful. We will also direct attention to the fact that most of these characteristics vary a great deal within the older population. Among the many population characteristics that we could describe are labor force participation, living arrangements, ethnic diversity, geographic distribution, education, and sex ratios. Some of the most important demographic characteristics, such as health, income, and marital status, are discussed in greater detail in later chapters. The major disadvantage of not including them here is that these characteristics provide some of the best illustrations of the great variation among older persons in the population—a point that is important to keep in mind. The major advantage to leaving certain demographic characteristics until later in the book is that we want to convince you that demography provides a fascinating, lively, and useful perspective on the issues of aging. Therefore, we focus on three demographic variables and their interpretations.

Living Arrangements

Information about the *living arrangements* of older people is important for community planners, housing designers, researchers interested in social support networks, and those who are curious about the validity of prevailing societal images. Contrary to a common stereotype, most older people do not live in nursing homes or other "seniors only" housing settings. As shown in Exhibit 3.9, only a very small proportion live in nursing homes—about 5% of all people 65 and over. This percentage does increase considerably by age; almost 25% of the 85+ population lives in nursing homes, but it is still not anywhere near a majority. Exhibit 3.9 shows this age-related increase in the proportion who live in nursing homes for both men and women.

The chart in Exhibit 3.10 shows that living arrangements for noninstitutionalized older people vary by sex, race, and ethnicity. A comparison of older men and women of all races/ethnicities reveals that women are much more likely than men to live alone. Men are more likely to live with a spouse. This pattern reflects differences in marital status. Because women live longer than men, and tend to marry men who are about three years older, women are much more likely than men to become widowed in later life. As shown in Exhibit 3.9, women are more likely than men to live in nursing homes. That

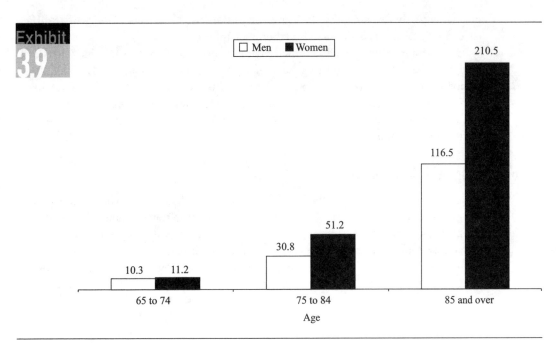

Exhibit 3.9

Nursing Home Residents Among People Aged 65 and Over by Age and Sex, 1999 (Nursing Home Residents per 1,000 Population)

Source: He, Sengupta, Velkoff, and DeBarros, 2005.

Exhibit
3.10

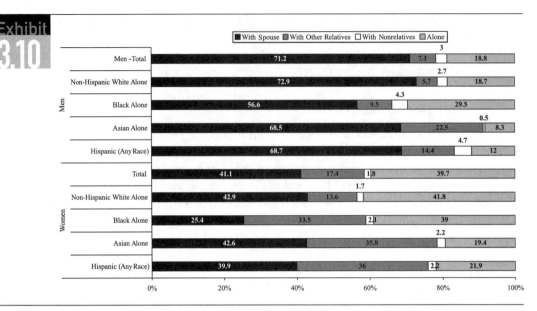

Living Arrangements of the Population Aged 65 and Over by Sex, Race, and Hispanic Origin, 2003 (Percent Distribution) Note: The reference population for these data is the civilian noninstitutionalized population. "With other relatives" indicates no spouse present. "With nonrelatives" indicates no spouse or other relatives present.

Source: He, Sengupta, Velkoff, and DeBarros, 2005.

pattern is partly explained by the availability of spouse caregivers. This gender difference in marital status is discussed further in chapter 6.

Some interesting race and ethnicity patterns are also shown in Exhibit 3.10. Black men are more likely than other groups of older men to live alone (nearly 30% do so compared to about 19% for Whites, and less than 10% for Asian or Hispanic older men). Asian, Hispanic, and Black older women are much more likely than White women 65 and older to live with other relatives (about 35% do so compared to less than 14% of White older women).

Geographic Distribution

How are the households in which older people reside distributed geographically? The **geographic distribution** of the older population (across states, among cities and suburbs, across counties) has far-reaching consequences for a location's tax base, educational system, demand on transportation services, and voting patterns. The numbers of older people, their percentage in a given community or state, and how they got there (by growing older in the same community or by migration)—are all related to outcomes of interest.

It is not surprising to learn that many of the states with large numbers of older people happen to be states with large overall populations. California, New York, Texas, and Pennsylvania are examples of states with large populations and large numbers of older people. The *proportion* of older people in any given location can be a different story; proportion of older people is affected by the three key demographic forces of fertility, mortality, and selective migration, regardless of the location's overall population size. California has a large number of older people, but a lower proportion of older adults than the United States as a whole (10.6% compared to 12.4%), partly because of high rates of international and interstate migration of younger people into the state. In contrast, Florida has the highest proportion of older people in the nation (17% in 2003), largely because of immigration of retirees seeking a sunbelt locale. Although a large proportion of the older people who relocate move to Florida or other warm-climate states, older people are much less likely to move than people under the age of 65. Among older people who did move between 1995 and 2000, only 18.8% moved across state lines (Administration on Aging, 2004). The states, and other locations that receive large numbers of older people, have to factor in increased (and sometimes seasonal) demands for housing, food, retail, and other services and amenities.

A number of other interesting trends and issues relate to the distribution and redistribution of the older population through migration. Longino (1990) has described a model for understanding the causes and consequences of multiple moves by older people. He proposes an initial move motivated by the attractiveness of a particular destination and later moves motivated by the desire to be closer to kin or the need for long-term care. Investigations into seasonal migration are also increasing in number. The presence of "snowbirds" (seasonal migrants to a warmer climate during the winter months) in a given location has important consequences for the economy and daily life; imagine what a seasonal growth of 20% or 30% might mean to retailers, traffic, and housing in a sunbelt community.

In addition to where people live geographically and with whom they live, information about where they are housed is also of interest. Housing availability, affordability, and quality are of major concern. For older people with fixed incomes and increased likelihood of health problems, appropriate housing options are more challenging. Over 60% of older homeowners have lived in their current homes for 20 years or more, speaking to an emotional as well as financial investment in a place and a community. Deciding how and when to make a housing change, and finding desirable and affordable options, are complex and difficult processes. Even though three-quarters of older people own their own homes (a higher proportion than any other age group), reduced income and frailty can place at risk their many years of financial, physical, and emotional investment in home and neighborhood (Callis, 2003). Housing represents a public policy and planning challenge; it is also a matter of personal and family concern, encompassing an array of issues such as independence, autonomy, security, and the meaning of home. While those with ample financial resources have a wide range of choices, those with more moderate incomes may find relatively few attractive choices in the housing market.

Gender Composition

The **sex ratio** is a measure used by demographers to summarize the gender composition of a population. Traditionally, the sex ratio is presented as the number of men for every 100 women; calculated by dividing the number of men by the number of women, it has also been called the "masculinity ratio" (e.g., Yaukey, 1985). In the United States in 2000, the overall ratio of men to women was 96 men for every 100 women. For the older population, however, the sex ratio is less balanced, and it makes more sense to talk about a "femininity ratio"—the number of older women for every 100 older men. For the population 65+ in 2000, the ratio was 143 women for every 100 men; among those 85 and above, it was 244 women for every 100 men (U.S. Bureau of the Census, 2004a). These ratios capture the differential impact of mortality on men and women. The imbalance has implications for remarriage possibilities following widowhood, for the economic well-being of the oldest old, for living arrangements, and patterns of social interaction.

Increasing Diversity

Another important aspect of our demographic future is the increasing racial and ethnic diversity of the United States as a whole, and the older population in particular. Most projections suggest "that there is likely to be a substantive shift in the racial composition of the U.S. resident population" (Kranczer, 1994, p. 21). Exhibit 3.11 shows the numerical and percentage increases in different age and race/ethnicity groups projected to occur in the United States between 1990 and 2020. The highest rates of increase will occur among people 65 and above who are of Asian or Hispanic origin. For example, the number of Asian American elders aged 85 and above will increase tenfold between 1990 and 2020. Since the number of Asian Americans 85 and older in 1990 was small, it takes relatively few additional people to produce a very high percentage increase. Nevertheless, this trend of increasing diversity in the older population is of great importance for everyone trying to understand and describe the experiences of aging in the United States. Because ethnic and racial identities often play a central role in shaping those experiences, we need to be aware of this important aspect of diversity among the older population.

Centenarians

Centenarians—people aged 100 and over—are another important part of our demographic profile. In 1980, there were only about 15,000 centenarians in the United States; that number had almost doubled by 1990, and is projected to grow to around 834,000 by the year 2050 (Velkoff, 2000). These long-lived people have experienced

Percent Changes 1990–2020

	All Races	Non-Hispanic White	Non-Hispanic Black	Non-Hispanic Asian	Hispanic American
All Ages	31.1	22.1	49.0	203.7	129.1
Under 25	19.8	8.7	37.4	179.4	102.8
25–44	3.0	5.4	22.0	145.1	90.5
45–64	75.0	64.0	115.5	312.0	257.0
65–84	64.7	56.9	92.7	402.4	293.6
85+	125.9	121.2	119.7	975.9	553.8

Projected Change in Resident Population by Race/Ethnicity and Age: United States 1990–2020
Source: Metropolitan Life, 1994.

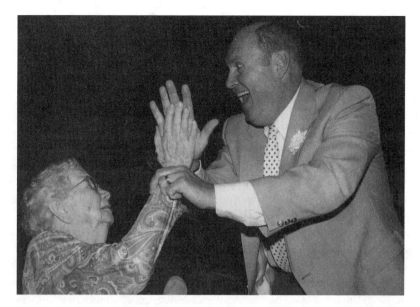

Willard Scott will find no shortage of centenarians to salute in the coming years, with the number of those living to be 100 and beyond expected to soar from approximately 50,000 in the year 2000 to 834,000 by the year 2050. (Credit: Mike Payne, courtesy of the Ohio Department of Aging)

incredible social change and major historical events in a century. There is growing interest in studying centenarians for the many contributions they can make to our understanding of aging, as well as how lives connect to history and social/technological change. In addition, scientists speculate that the study of centenarians may provide clues to factors that influence longevity (Velkoff, 2000).

Interpreting and Using Demographic Data

In describing select demographic characteristics of the older population, we have illustrated some important uses for demographic data. Such information is the foundation for a wide range of professional endeavors, including product design and development, community planning, market research, education about aging, and public policy development. Demographic information can be used to support a position in a term paper, debate, or presentation. We all use such data to help us understand the realities of aging. Throughout this chapter we have been encouraging you to see the importance and usefulness of demographic information. We make those same points in the final section of this chapter.

As we use such data about the older population, it is extremely important not to overgeneralize—not to make blanket statements about all older people or about the "typical" older person. So, while we encourage the use of demographic data as a valuable tool, we caution that such data also uncover the complexities and varieties of aging.

The Fallacy of the Demographic Imperative

One key to avoiding errors in interpretation is to keep in mind that "demography is not destiny." Friedland and Summer (1999, 2005) illustrate various interpretations of commonly accepted demographic wisdom. We hear much about the baby boomers and what their aging will mean to society. Friedland and Summer point out that we can get a different sense of the magnitude of the "baby boom problem" if we consider not just the total number of people in that birth cohort, but rather the additional people born solely because of the higher birth rate. The higher birth rate during the baby boom era added about 12.3 additional children beyond the number that would have been born if the pre–World War II birth rates had continued. If we think about it this way, the baby boom does not seem as large. These authors also clearly demonstrate how economics and policy play roles at least equal to demography in shaping our destiny.

Although the numbers are compelling, we have illustrated several times throughout this chapter that numbers are only part of the picture. In the case of Nepal discussed earlier, it is quite clear that the "demographic imperative"—the aging of Nepali society—is, at this point, anything but an imperative for planning and policy. What any society decides to do about the aging of its population depends not simply on how many older people there are, but on the political, social, and moral values of the society.

The same warning can summarize our discussion of the uses of the dependency ratio to foretell impending economic disaster for U.S. society. The numbers themselves are open to interpretation. Critical choices about which numbers to present are often very ideological decisions, because some "facts" better support a particular policy agenda than others. So, while we encourage you to consider demographic information as a useful resource, we also urge you to be aware of the social and political context that generates the numbers and directs their uses. For example, someone interested in raising the retirement age may choose to present dependency ratios in one way, where the same statistics can also be shaped to support those opposing this change. Keep this warning in mind as you use demographic "facts" and as you critically analyze anything you read that uses such information.

While demographic information provides an essential framework from which to understand the aging of societies, it is equally important to remain aware of the overarching impact of other social institutions (the economy, politics, family systems) as we consider how best to deal with the challenges of aging. "We need not believe ourselves to be at the mercy of blind forces such as demographic and economic imperatives, as if these existed outside the realm of public discussion and debate" (Robertson, 1991, p. 147).

SUMMARY

As discussed throughout this chapter, the increase in the size and proportion of the older population has an impact on every aspect of U.S. social life. In the United States, the number of older people is projected to exceed 70 million by the year 2030, at which time all of the baby boomers will have reached age 65; older people will represent about 20% of the U.S. population by then—one in every five people will be 65 or older.

Around the world, the increase in the size of the older population is equally dramatic and consequential. As discussed earlier in this chapter, a large proportion of all older people will live in developing nations by the year 2020. Those nations will see their older populations grow by an average of 160% between 1991 and 2020. The challenges facing the nations in which rapid population aging will compete with maternal and child health concerns are enormous. Of equal magnitude are the challenges for the global community to define and understand problems and to propose and implement solutions.

When populations age, the labor force is profoundly affected. As large numbers of people retire and come to be supported by company pensions and health insurance, the cost of doing business escalates. Some of this demand can be accommodated by increased productivity from technological improvements. Companies worry that their competitive edge is dulled by the weight of retirees, resulting in recent trends to end private pension systems, converting them to annuities that provide lower benefits than promised.

As we proceed with our look at the social dimensions of aging, the demographic frame of reference will continually direct our attention to the distinct yet diverse characteristics, situations, and needs of the older population; to the aging of our society; and to our connections to the global community in an aging world. Societal aging, patterns of fertility, mortality, and migration, and the demographic composition of the older population may at first glance seem to be remote and irrelevant, but they have a major impact on one's life, family, country, and the planet.

WEB WISE

Following is a list of sites that provide information on demography of the aging population in the United States and in various countries around the world. Not all of the information is free and some of it refers to published (hard copy) materials.

Age Data

http://www.census.gov/population/www/socdemo/age.html

This is a linked Web site maintained by the U.S. Census Bureau. It provides access to national, state, and local sources of information on demography from the Census Bureau. International data are also available. In general, the census provides both statistics on current populations and projections for population change/growth through these sites and its printed publications.

United Nations Statistics Division

http://unstats.un.org/unsd/methods/inter-natlinks/sd_natstat.htm

The UNSD provides a Web page that links to selected national statistics offices. Each of the country statistical information is unique but may be useful for international comparisons on aging issues. Nations are organized alphabetically by continent.

Agingstats

www.agingstats.gov

The Federal Interagency Forum on Aging-Related Statistics (Forum) was initially established in 1986, with the goal of bringing together federal agencies that share a common interest in improving aging-related data. The Forum has played a key role by critically evaluating existing data resources and limitations, stimulating new database development, encouraging cooperation and data sharing among federal agencies, and preparing collaborative statistical reports. In addition to the original three core agencies (National Institute on Aging, National Center for Health Statistics, and Census Bureau), the organizing members of the Forum now include senior officials from the Administration on Aging, Agency for Healthcare Research and Quality, Bureau of Labor Statistics, Centers for Medicare and Medicaid Services, Department of Veterans Affairs, Environmental Protection Agency, Office of Management and Budget, Office of the Assistant Secretary for Planning and Evaluation in Health and Human Services, Social Security Administration, and the Substance Abuse and Mental Health Services Administration.

HelpAge

http://www.helpage.org/Home

HelpAge International is a global network of not-for-profit organizations with a mission to work with, and for, disadvantaged older people worldwide to achieve a lasting improvement in the quality of their lives. The Web site provides information on current projects that HelpAge is working on, research and policy, and news. It also provides an in-depth overview of worldwide emergencies and helpful resources.

International Data Base (IDB) from U.S. Census Bureau

http://www.census.gov/ipc/www/idbnew.html

If you want to know what population pyramids will look like for Albania, Guatemala, or Sierra Leone in 2025, visiting the IDB site provided by the U.S. Census Bureau will enable you to look at projections for population and detailed characteristics of various countries or regions of the world. Choose from a large number of countries and look at the aging rates of the populations (via population pyramids) or at statistics in tables. It is also possible to download IDB data, but review the requirements in advance and be prepared for a large data set.

Population Reference Bureau

http://www.prb.org

The Population Reference Bureau, funded by government agencies, foundations, universities and nonprofit organizations, makes available a range of demographic data, including a page on aging. Articles, reports, and datasheets change over time but focus on the size, diversity, and characteristics of the older population and the baby boomers in the United States and the world.

U.S. Bureau of Census: FactFinder

http://factfinder.census.gov/home/saff/main.html?_lang = enamp;_ts =

The FactFinder is an excellent resource for accessing information that is amassed by the Census Bureau on a wide range of individual characteristics, housing, and business issues. Users of the system can find customized information on a wide array of topics, including many up-to-date statistics regarding aging, family, health, and related topics. Much information on older adults can be found under the People tab.

KEY TERMS

aging index	geographic distribution	mean age
centenarians	International Plan of	median
convergence	Action on Ageing	population pyramid
crossover effect	life expectancy	sex ratio
dependency ratios	life span	societal aging

QUESTIONS FOR THOUGHT AND DISCUSSION

1. How does the age structure of a society affect the kinds of decisions that must be made by national policymakers? Can you think of examples in the United States when the aging of our society has influenced political agendas?
2. Find some examples in newspapers or magazines of the ways in which demographic information about the older population is used to convey messages of alarm or optimism. Is the information being presently in an accurate and balanced way? How might the same information, presented differently, be used to convey a different message?
3. We know that aging is a global phenomenon. Think about some of the ways in which societal aging presents unique challenges in some countries with which you are familiar.
4. How does the life expectancy in a country affect the way life is organized—for example, number of years spent in school, age at marriage, and age at retirement?

The Aging Individual in Social Context

Like gender or height or the presence/absence of ear lobes, age itself is not a cause of anything. Rather, it is ... a socially significant title that covers complex sociocultural formulations, including some which are directly implicated in personal and collective identities. (Hazelrigg, 1997, p. 96)

Aging is a complex social phenomenon because it involves interrelationships among biological, psychological, social, and cultural processes. At another level, aging is also a very personal experience. Most of us care about the issues related to aging because we are aware that it is happening to us and to people around us. All of us, if we are lucky, will grow old and all of us continue to age, regardless of where we are today within the life course. Thus, aging is a more universal experience than any other. Most of us will grow old, but few of us will change our status in other social categories such as gender or race. Even changes in marital status or religion are far less predictable than changes in age status. Since aging is something that happens to everyone at a personal level, it is helpful to discuss what happens to individuals as they grow older, and then to put those insights into a larger context—the social context of aging.

Setting the Stage: Psychology of Aging

The psychology of aging is a well-developed field of study, with a wide range of questions in its scope. The topics covered within the psychology of aging include changes over time in cellular processes in the brain, the relationship between psychology and physical processes of health and illness, changes in cognitive performance, and complex social psychological concepts, such as the self and identity. In all of these diverse domains, the psychology of aging focuses on the stability and change in how humans operate psychologically at various ages and stages of life. To describe the breadth of the research and theory included in the psychology of aging, Salthouse (2006) offered a taxonomy of "what, when, why, where, and how" questions that guide the field. Topics covered by this taxonomy include the psychological ways in which people of different ages vary; the ages at which these changes occur; where they occur (specifically, what structures of the brain might be involved in changes); and why they occur. Because the field is so broad, scholars who study the psychology of aging have different areas of specialization. Some focus on cognitive psychology and neuroscience, which includes the physiology of cognitive impairments; and the impact of aging on memory, intelligence, information processing, and learning; and changes in sensory functioning. Other psychologists of aging are interested in aging and behavior such as problem-solving and decision-making; some focus on the impact of aging on personality and the self; still others look at the intersection of internal psychological processes with social aspects of life. The breadth and depth of theory and research in the psychology of aging are far beyond the scope of this text. Students interested in a fuller picture of the psychology of aging will find a vast array of resources, including the new *Handbook of the Psychology of Aging* (Birren & Schaie, 2006).

One topic with roots in psychology is emerging as an important interdisciplinary focus for gerontology—human development. As a field of study, **human development** examines the progressive changes across the life span. One of the central concepts in the sociology of aging—the life course—also explores the way that individuals' lives change with time. Both concepts refer to the growth and change that people experience over their lives, and both recognize the importance of internal psychological processes as well as external social processes in shaping the way that individual lives unfold over time, creating rich possibilities for connections between sociology and psychology of aging (Settersten, 2005a). The difference between a psychological focus on life span and the sociological focus on life course is the relative amount of attention given to the internal aspects of development compared to the social influences on human development. We briefly review some important ideas related to the more psychological aspects of life span development before focusing on the social context of individual aging.

Human Development and Aging

For many years the focus of human development was on the changes that take place in infancy, childhood, and adolescence; topics such as language acquisition, emergent cognitive abilities, moral development, and problem solving were researched extensively. More recently, attention has been given to questions about the growth and change that take place throughout the human life span, including adulthood and aging. A pioneer in this area was Erik Erikson, who proposed that adults face development tasks, just as children and adolescents do. His initial work on this topic identified two developmental stages for later life. **Generativity**—learning how to look outside oneself and focus on passing on a legacy to future generations—was described as the major developmental task of middle age. For older people, self-reflection and coming to terms with one's life is the developmental challenge Erikson identified; a successful resolution of this stage of life was termed **ego-integrity**. Erikson further refined these stages, offering more detail about the developmental challenges that face us as we age (Erikson, Erikson, & Kivnick, 1986). Erikson's work was vital in drawing attention to the fact that humans continue to grow, develop, and change throughout their lives. His writing set the stage for research on the major questions identified by Salthouse (2006): what developmental changes take place in later life and why do they occur?

Scholars today continue to explore the nature of human development in later life and to understand the unique characteristics of the stage of life. Tornstam (1997, 2005) proposes that later life offers the opportunity for **gerotranscendence**; he describes this transformation as "a shift from materialistic and pragmatic view of the world to a more cosmic and transcendent one, normally accompanied by a contemplative dimension" (1977, p. 143). His ideas are based on interviews with older people who described a gradual change involving self-reflection, refinement of personal qualities they sought to enhance or to modify, and a deeper investment in select important social relationships. Atchley (2004) describes a similar focus on an inner journey of self-reflection but also suggests that service to one's community can be the outcome of this path; "serving from spirit" is the concept he offers to express the unique contributions that can be made by spiritually grounded elders. "Elderhood" is the phase in later life that William Thomas (2004) describes as moving from doing to being; one of the greatest challenges to achieving this state is our fondness for "adult supremacy"—for the phase of life where success is defined in terms of activity and striving. Schachter-Shalomi (1995) sums up many of these ideas in his call for "a new paradigm of aging with emphasis on lifelong learning, brain-mind development, and consecrated service to humanity" (p. 244). Schachter-Shalomi's "sage-ing," Atchley's "serving from spirit," Thomas's "elderhood," and Tornstam's gerotranscendence all build on and expand some of Erikson's early ideas about the unique challenges and opportunities of human development in later life.

Social Context and Individual Aging

As the study of human development suggests, the passage of time signals physiological and psychological development and changes that happen *within* individuals as they age. However, such changes do not happen in a vacuum. For example, the desire and the opportunity to continue to work past the typical age of retirement vary considerably by the kind of jobs that people have, their economic needs, and the policies that their employers have in place (see chapter 8). Working in later life is not simply the result of individual choice; social forces play an essential role. People respond to, and are affected by, the social context and the physical environment in which they live.

Another example of the importance of surroundings comes from what we have learned about the role of social support in later life. Social support can include the network of people we have contact with, the amount of contact we have with them, the support and help that we get from those around us, or the confidence that we can count on others when needed. There is growing evidence that strong social support has a positive effect on health and well-being in later life, and that it is "a key determinant of successful aging" (Antonucci & Akiyama, 1987; Krause, 2001).

Physical environments can also have significant impact on the aging individual, as eloquently described and empirically verified by Lawton and his colleagues. In his influential work on this topic, Lawton suggests that the fit between a person and his or her environment can have an impact on how competently individuals can get by in their everyday lives. Lawton's classic model of the relationship between behavior and the environment visually depicts the optimal fit between environmental pressure that encourages maximum performance by the individual, as well as potential negative outcomes for the person if the environment demands too much or too little (see Lawton, 1986). If the environment demands more of the person than he or she can accomplish, maladaptive behavior and negative affect can result; similarly, if the environment is not challenging enough, an individual may not be motivated to maximize her or his competence.

This work on social support and person-environment fit are good examples of the importance of social contexts for aging individuals. For sociologists who study aging, social context is not just an acknowledged influence on individual change and response—it is the focus of their work. This is the unique contribution sociology makes to the study of aging. Sociology examines the ways in which social life is organized and the ways in which it affects individual actions and behaviors at all ages. As described in chapter 3, demographic forces (fertility, mortality, and migration) help to shape social institutions, and at least indirectly have an influence on individual lives. Recall the discussion of the role of population aging in the challenges facing Social Security and the current high level of competition for jobs that is partially related to the large number of baby boomers in the work force. The demographic perspective within sociology takes the essentially individual events of birth, death, and relocation and sums them up, describes large-scale patterns and trends, and considers the causes and consequences of these events from a macro-level point of view. One of the great values of sociology is to lend a broader perspective—what Mills called the sociological imagination. As discussed in chapter 1, this perspective places personal experiences in a broader social and historical context and provides a frame of reference for understanding individual experiences. This chapter and all subsequent chapters in this text draw upon the sociological imagination to help us analyze the experiences of aging.

There is a tendency in U.S. society to focus on the individual. We are enamored of the concept of free will and autonomy—that individuals can control or shape their futures through their actions. We value independence, and our nation is built on ideas about individual choice and individual responsibility. We are curious about the various circumstances in which people find themselves and often take some comfort in attributing success or failure to a person's choices and actions rather than external forces. Such thinking allows us to believe that good fortune will come to us if we work hard and position ourselves correctly, and that ill fortune will not befall us because we have done the right thing. The sociological imagination makes possible a richer understanding of the power of social structures and contexts that influence individual lives.

One of the most important concepts for understanding the ways in which social factors help to shape the experience of aging is the **life course**. The life course is a road map that influences the individual choices we make about moving into and out of important social roles such as marriage, parenthood, employment, and retirement. This chapter further explores the life course as a fundamental feature of the societal framework within which individual aging takes place.

The Life Course

All societies use age in some way to organize social life—to assign people to roles, to regulate interaction, or as a basis for division of labor. U.S. society has laws about minimum ages for drinking, driving, voting, and holding some public offices. We also have some expectations about what ages are appropriate for people to marry, enter the job market, and retire. Many people thought that the 66-year-old woman who had a baby in 2005 with the aid of in vitro fertilization was definitely too old to have a child. Most of us plan to retire sometime in our 60s. In addition to ideas about appropriate ages for entry into and exit from important social roles, we also share some general expectations about age-appropriate behavior. The dictum to "act your age" is a clear illustration that we have some underlying ideas about what we should be doing at various stages in our lives. "Expectations regarding age-appropriate behavior form an elaborated and pervasive system of norms governing behavior and interaction, a network of expectations that is imbedded throughout the cultural fabric of adult life" (Neugarten, Moore, & Lowe, 1965, pp. 22–23). These expectations are part of our culture; they are taught to us as we grow up and are continually reinforced throughout adulthood. They also sometimes shift, as we have seen over recent decades when ages for having children have extended and ages at which individuals seek higher education have come to include mid-life and older adults.

These expectations are reflected in laws, policies, and organizational rules; they are also part of a general timetable we use for major life events. Neugarten and her colleagues observed that people "are aware not only of the social clocks that operate in various areas of their lives, but they are aware also of their own timing and readily describe themselves as 'early', 'late', or 'on-time' with regard to family and occupational events" (1965, p. 23). This social clock is the life course (Settersten, 1999).

The life course is a sequence of stages people move through as they age; movement out of one stage and into another is typically marked by a significant event or social transition. Some, like adolescence, are marked by chronological age. Other stages of the life course are less defined and may be entered at varying ages. The clearest example is the lengthy stage of adulthood. At what point and by which criteria do we determine that someone is an adult? There are legal definitions of adulthood, and there are social roles that can indicate movement into adulthood (such as, employment, completion of education, marriage, or parenthood). Some of these markers do not occur at a single point in time, and not all of them occur for every person, making many life course transitions fuzzy or gradual. The life course is delineated by the roles we are expected to play in particular sequences or at delineated age ranges. Atchley (1994) defines the life course as "a cultural ideal consisting of an age-related progression or sequence of roles and group memberships that individuals are expected to follow as they mature and move through life" (p. 154). The life course can be applied to many domains of social life, including the family, education, and work. We can talk about the timing of events in the occupational domain and whether they fit well or poorly with the expectations at the same ages for the family domain. For example, career building comes at an age when many are actively involved in parenting small children, and the reduction of time demands at retirement occurs when society demands few other contributions from older adults. Since the life course is subject to social

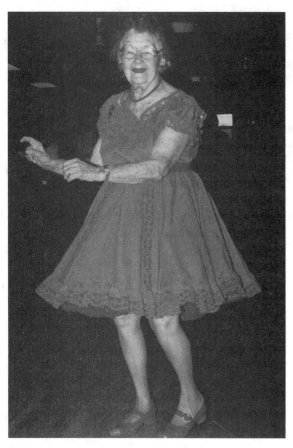

Stages of the life course are not immutable (and you're never too old to dance). (Credit: Mike Payne, courtesy of the Ohio Department of Aging)

change over time, issues of asynchrony (aspects or their timing not fitting together well) regularly appear.

Indeed, many people feel some pressure to achieve milestones at fairly specific ages. Deciding on a college major and finding a job after graduation are two milestones that many college students feel pressured to accomplish within a certain time frame. Think about the following questions, as further evidence of the existence of a life course. Why don't more people work past the age of 65? Why don't people wait until they are in their late 30s to get married? Would you feel comfortable announcing to your family, friends, and professors that you have decided to delay your entry into the job market until you are in your mid-40s and in the meantime you will enjoy your leisure and pick up some odd jobs here and there? Why not plan for a period of middle-aged "retirement" followed by a return to the labor force? The life course carries fairly influential ideas about what we are supposed to do and how we are supposed to behave at various stages of life. It is one of the ways in which society shapes our opportunities, decisions, and behaviors at various ages throughout life. Because it is so thoroughly embedded in our culture, the life course remains largely invisible to us; we do notice, however, when someone does things out of order or at atypical ages.

The concept of **social time** (Neugarten & Datan, 1973) refers to the expectations and definitions that society gives to stages of the life course. These stages, and their timing, are not "natural" or immutable. They are sometimes linked to "natural" processes such as physiological development, most clearly from infancy to adolescence, but the roles accessible to us and their link to age expectations are malleable and are primarily determined by society. For example, childhood did not exist as a distinct stage of life until industrialization made child labor unnecessary (and illegal), and formal education became a social institution in the 17th and 18th centuries (Aries, 1962). Similarly, retirement is a fairly recent life stage; life expectancy had to increase sufficiently for enough people to grow old enough to retire, and income support systems generated by higher productivity were created after industrialization (see chapter 8).

In summary, the life course is a socially constructed, culturally and historically specific sequence of stages, often with connected social roles, that people are expected to move through as they mature and grow older. The life course is closely linked with age-/stage-specific social roles, and the entry to and exit from those roles are influenced by age norms. These two building blocks of the life course require further examination.

Social Roles

The concept of "social role" is one of the fundamental building blocks of the life course (and of sociology). It is the mechanism through which real people are linked to the more nebulous structures of social groups and institutions. There are two aspects to the ways that social roles link people to each other in social structures. First, roles entail socially recognized positions (e.g., father, employee, student) in social networks; second, role occupants behave in certain ways when they are in those positions. A **social role** is a set of expected activities and responsibilities that go along with a position held in a social network. Conveniently, this important concept has an everyday referent; the term "role" conjures up theatrical images of parts to be played. In fact, a social role is essentially that—a part to be played in social life (Goffman, 1969). A role is a set of expectations about how people who occupy a particular position will behave—what they will do, what they should do, and what they should not do. For example, a woman may simultaneously occupy the social roles of sister and employee. Each of these positions is understood to have certain rights and duties, and the woman is expected to behave differently when she is acting as a sister than when she is behaving as an employee. Roles exist in relationship to other roles; that is, each role has a counterpart. Some examples of reciprocal roles are mother/child, teacher/student, friend/friend. Because roles exist in relation to each other, having shared expectations about what each person will do (or will not do) in a given role is essential for social interaction and social order. If we had no idea at all about what to expect when we enter a classroom—that is, no idea what the teacher will do or what the students should do—it would be very difficult to accomplish anything. For our purposes, it is sufficient to understand that "role" implies an organized set of interrelated functions, activities, and behavior associated with a given social position. Remember the theatrical reference; a role is a script.

A central figure in American social psychology, George Herbert Mead, used the idea of a baseball game to explain the reciprocity of social roles and their importance for social interaction. He points out that every player in a baseball game has to learn how to play her own position, but also has to learn what the responsibilities of the other positions are as well. A good player must understand the function of every position on the team in order to effectively play her own position. Similarly, role players in society have to understand how their position relates to other roles in the social structure in order to fully participate in society—as an employee how do you behave relative to your co-workers, your boss, your clients? Role behaviors are structured, but not completely. There is room for variation in how we enact a particular role, such as student, worker, or daughter. Age norms help to define which roles should be undertaken at various stages of life and how they should be played.

Sociologist Irving Rosow (1985) raised the question of whether social roles are always attached to a particular position in a social network, and vice versa. Often clearly defined roles (a well-written script; clear expectations about behavior) are attached to a well-defined position in a social structure, including clear interrelationships with other statuses. "Grandmother" is an example; we have fairly clear (albeit

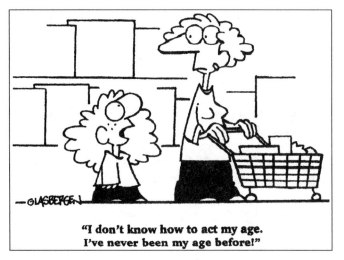

"I don't know how to act my age.
I've never been my age before!"

fairly limited) expectations about how someone should and should not behave in that role, and it is a well-defined position in relation to other social positions (grand-child). However, Rosow suggests that there are situations in which either the role is not clearly defined or the position is not very specific. "Retired worker" is an example of ill-defined expectations about essential activities. The past con-nection to the workplace help define the position rather than any current social position or linked position, but what is one expected to do or not do as a retired worker? Rosow questions whether old age itself, because of the multiple role losses associated with growing older, is a position without substantial role expectations—a "roleless role."

Age Norms

Have you ever seen a small boy dressed in a suit and acting very mature or someone in his or her 70s playing hopscotch? Do these images strike you as inappropriate? If so, it is probably because of age norms. The ideas and expectations shared by members of a culture about how a person of a certain age should behave are **age norms**. Age norms are a subset of all social norms, which tell us how to act in various circumstances or toward particular others (e.g., how to act in a museum versus at a party or toward a peer compared to a police officer). These shared rules guide the behavior of members of a society by specifying what behavior and activities are expected, appropriate, and inap-propriate. **Norms** are broader and more intangible than social roles; they are the deeply learned ideas that are collectively shared by members of a culture and that enable us to predict much of a person's behavior while they are playing a role.

Age norms are "socially governed expectations and sanctions concerning the appro-priateness of role acquisitions and behaviors as a function of chronological age" (Burton, 1996, p. 199). For example, we have age norms about entry into roles (driving, voting, marrying, or working) and exit from roles (retirement, graduation). Sometimes these age norms are formalized into law and policy, but sometimes they remain simply *understood* among people who share a common culture. We also share age-related expectations about behavior, dress, and speech. To explore some age norms about behavior and dress, think about how you would react to an 80-year-old woman wearing a very short skirt, a 70-year-old couple kissing passionately, a 50-year-old man who has never held a full-time job, an 80-year-old woman going to college, or a 17-year-old male who drives very slowly.

There are three important components of age norms: (1) they prescribe and proscribe behavior (i.e., tell us what to do and what not to do); (2) they are shared by some social group (such as society, a work organization, or a subculture); (3) they carry with them some element of social control or sanction (there are consequences of failing to behave according to the social expectations). Some sociologists would add a fourth key feature: the roles must constrain peoples' behavior (see Lawrence, 1996; Settersten & Hagestad, 1996a, 1996b).

These four components of age norms raise conceptually challenging questions. If age norms must meet these four standards, how do we know whether these criteria are met? Who do we ask, and what do we ask them, to find out if a particular age norm exists, and if it constrains behavior? A number of researchers have attempted to answer this question with research on age norms and their operation in society.

A basic dilemma in the study of age norms and the life course is what should be measured: what people typically *do* or what people say they think they (and others) *should do*. Both approaches have been used by researchers. The former strategy—looking at what people typically do—is well illustrated by the work of Paul Glick (1977), who calculated the median age at major life events for women (such as marriage, birth of first child, marriage of last child, and death of spouse), from the 1900s to the 1970s. His findings, summarized in Exhibit 4.1, showed very little change in women's median age at marriage, but dramatic increases in the number of years spent in marriage until the death of a spouse (not surprising given life expectancy improvements), and a substantial decline in the length of time spent in the childbearing stage as family size declined. Similarly, Matras (1990) documented the "compression of employment" into a smaller proportion of the life span (see chapter 7), and Uhlenberg (1996) analyzed the impact of increased life expectancy on opportunity for intergenerational relationships throughout the life course. These demographic patterns speak to "typical" behaviors, relatively predictable

Exhibit 4.1	Birth of Wife	1880s	1890s	1910s	1920s	1930s	1940s	1950s
Family Life Cycle Stage	Approximate Period of First Marriage	1900s	1910s	1930s	1940s	1950s	1960s	1970s
Median age at								
First marriage		21.4	21.2	21.4	20.7	20.0	20.5	21.2
Birth of first child		23.0	22.9	23.5	22.7	21.4	21.8	22.7
Birth of last child		32.9	32.0	32.0	31.5	31.2	30.1	29.6
Marriage of last child		55.4	54.8	53.2	53.2	53.6	52.7	52.3
Death of one spouse		57.0	59.6	63.7	64.4	65.1	65.1	65.2
Difference between								
Ages at birth of first and last children		9.9	9.1	8.5	8.8	9.8	8.3	6.9
Ages at birth of first and marriage of last child		22.5	22.6	21.2	21.7	22.4	22.6	22.7
Ages at marriage of last child and death of spouse (empty nest)		1.6	4.8	10.5	11.2	11.5	12.4	12.9

Demographic Description of the Family Life Cycle in the United States, 1880s–1950s
Adapted from: Glick, 1977; Matras, 1990.

	Age Range Designated as Appropriate or Expected	Percent Who Concur	
		Men (N=50)	Women (N=43)
Best age for a man to marry	20–25	80	90
Best age for a woman to marry	19–24	85	90
When most people should become grandparents	45–50	84	79
Best age for most people to finish school and go to work	20–22	86	82
When most men should be settled on a career	24–26	74	64
When most men should hold their top jobs	45–50	71	58
When most people should be ready to retire	60–65	83	86
A young man	18–22	84	83
A middle-aged man	40–50	86	75
An old man	65–75	75	57
A young woman	18–24	89	88
A middle-aged woman	50–59	87	77
An old woman	60–75	83	87
When a man has the most responsibilities	35–50	86	80
When a man accomplishes most	40–50	82	71
The prime of life for a man	35–50	86	80
When a woman has the most responsibilities	25–40	93	91
When a woman accomplishes most	30–45	94	92
A good-looking woman	20–35	92	92

Consensus in a Middle-Class Middle-Aged Sample Regarding Various Age-Related Characteristics
Source: Neugarten, Moore, and Lowe, 1965.

timetables, and to the evolution of new or altered life stages. They also indicate social changes, as patterns of family and work life shifted during the 20th century.

The second approach to measuring age norms—asking people what they think are appropriate ages for life events—has been adopted in number of studies. Exhibit 4.2 presents results from one of the classic studies on this topic (Neugarten, Moore, & Lowe, 1965). These findings show a high degree of consensus among respondents on appropriate ages for various life stages and events; some of the interesting variations by gender are discussed in the section on modifiers of the life course. Researchers asked respondents about both their own timetables and about what other people expected for timing of life events. There was a difference between personal attitudes and attitudes attributed to others—age norms were consistently acknowledged to exist in other peoples' minds, but were not always accepted as personally valid or constraining (Neugarten, Moore, & Lowe, 1965). At a later time and in a different culture (New Zealand), other researchers concluded that the degree of consensus and overall pattern of age norms had remained fairly consistent since the Neugarten study (Byrd & Breuss, 1992) .

Settersten and Hagestad (1996a) found that age norms are still perceived to be relevant for most major life events for both men and women. Exhibit 4.3 shows the percentages of people who perceived deadlines for major family transitions and the average deadlines for those transitions. A strong majority perceived deadlines for all family transitions except for grown children returning home, a non-normative event until recent years. The average ages for these deadlines varied for women and for men. Women are expected to marry and complete childbearing earlier than men. While the averages were

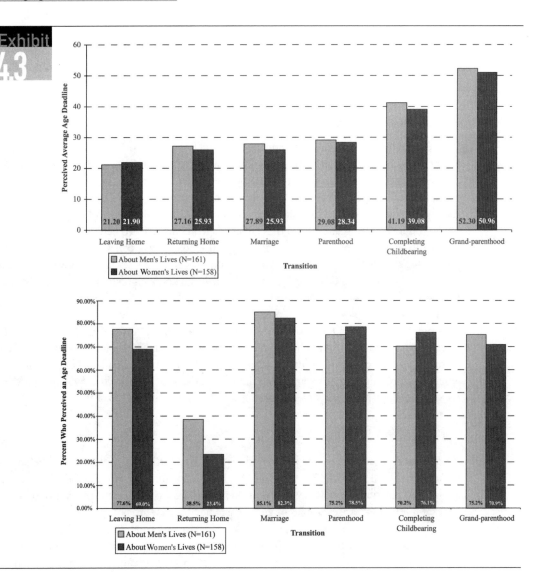

Perceived Age Deadlines for Major Family Transitions
Source: Settersten and Hagestad, 1996a.

interesting, the variations are also important. There was a lot of variation in the ages given for completion of childbearing for men (over 7 years), and for grandparenthood (more than 7 years), but less diversity for the acceptable age for young adults leaving home. This important study suggests that there is a perceived timetable, but that there is some flexibility in the timing of some family events.

Settersten and Hagestad also found that, although most respondents perceive age norms, they did not perceive any negative outcomes for violating these deadlines. "Being late" did not carry with it significant consequences. Lashbrook's (1996) research revealed fairly consistent age norms for promotions in work organizations, but little relationship between being "off time" (either early or late in relation to the social timetable) and job well-being for middle-aged men. The lack of sanction for being off time, and the flexibility in timing led Settersten and Hagestad to conclude that cultural timetables and age norms "may be an important force shaping the life course, but their influence may instead be secondary ... and may be much more flexible in individuals' minds than researchers have assumed" (1996a, p. 187).

Age Norms and Life Course Flexibility

People seem to subscribe to ideas about ages at which it is appropriate to be at certain stages in one's life, but they do not feel particularly pressured to conform to those expectations. These two facts seem inconsistent. This apparent inconsistency can be explained in several ways. Foner (1996) suggests that perhaps age norms are only part of the age structuring of society, and age norms are flexible across social contexts. Settersten and Hagestad (1996a, 1996b) offer the idea that cultural timetables—age norms that we perceive for everyone—can be different from personal timetables that individuals use to construct their life courses. This latter explanation reminds us that age structures and other social forces are not totally deterministic. Humans take some active role in the structuring of their own lives. In fact, people have an impact on social structures and social forces. Individuals are not merely reactive; they are, to some extent, "proactive architects" of their own life course trajectories (George, 1996, p. 254). One of the interesting questions in the study of the life course is the interplay between individual choice and constraints imposed by society. Settersten (2003) summarizes this reciprocal influence as "agency with structure" and identifies a major challenge for researchers to "conceptualize the life course as *actively created by individuals and groups, but within the confines of the social world in which they exist*" (p. 30).

Age Norms and Ageism

As discussed above, age norms are shared expectations for how a person should behave or what they should do based on their age. Earlier in this discussion we asked you to think about your reactions to how people were dressed and how they acted (playing hopscotch, for example). These are examples of general age norms; they are not specifically related to a role. Our expectations about how people should behave and what kinds of roles they should be engaged in because of their age provide some level of social order and organization.

However, an overapplication of these expectations can lead to ageism. **Ageism,** as discussed in chapter 1, is "a systematic stereotyping of and discrimination against people because they are old, just as racism and sexism accomplish this with skin color and gender" (Butler, 1989). While ageism may be related to society's use of age to organize social life and expectations for behavior, it is not a necessary by-product of age norms. In other cultures and at other times in history, older people are and have been valued differently. Ageism is a product of complicated demographic, political, ideological, and economic forces (see Scrutton, 1996, for a discussion of the foundations of ageism).

Ageism is alive and well in U.S. society. Reflecting on his 30 years of research on this topic, gerontologist Erdman Palmore (2005) expressed optimism that ageism can be overcome in our society, but concluded that, "ageism makes a great difference in our society and culture.... It is a social disease much like racism and sexism" (p. 90). In an intriguing exposé of discrimination against older people, author Patricia Moore used makeup and dress to disguise herself as an older woman. Her book *Disguised* (1985) documents the experiences she had traveling as an old woman and presenting herself in various situations. She encountered both negative and positive forms of ageism; she was ignored, patronized, deferred to, ridiculed, and offered assistance. These were not the reactions she received when she presented herself as a young woman. Even participants at conferences on aging treated Moore differently depending on the age she portrayed, often excluding her from conversation or treating her as if she were invisible when she was dressed as an older woman (Ferraro, 1990).

Structural Lag

Although age norms are important influences, Matilda Riley (1996) eloquently argues against "life-course reductionism," which treats social structures, such as age norms, as simply the context for individual lives. She urges an examination of how changes come about in norms and social structures. "As lives change, new norms develop and become widely accepted and institutionalized in structural transformations" (p. 258). But changes in norms do not always occur at the same time as changes in other aspects of society. **Structural lag** is the term used to describe this mismatch between changing expectations about aging and the inertia of social arrangements. Structural lag is based on Riley's age stratification theory, which pulls together some of the most important concepts (such as cohort flow, age graded opportunity structures, and the aging of society) in the sociology of aging. Because this idea captures so well the power, fluidity, and evolution of the life course, we present it in further detail.

In their discussion of the concept, Riley, Kahn, and Foner (1994) clarify the link between real human lives and the more formal, less tangible structure of social roles. They define structural lag as the tendency for the social structure of roles, norms, and social institutions to change more slowly, and thus lag behind, changes in peoples' lives. For example, the majority of people retire at around age 65 (and often before). Because of increases in life expectancy, most people will live an average of 15 to 20 years in retirement. But what roles or opportunities exist for people after retirement? As Rosow asked decades ago, what exactly do we expect a retired person to do? What links do retirees have to the life of the larger society? Society has not kept up with the increase in life expectancy by building opportunities and responsibilities for the new stage of life. Society has lagged behind the changes in peoples' lives—this is structural lag.

Another example of the mismatch between society and peoples' lives is the persistence of age norms about completion of education at a relatively young age. The notion that education and career training should be complete by age 25 or 30 "lags behind individual need for continual retraining in the workplace over the person's whole life; these norms are not in accord with the capabilities of older people and their motivations" (Foner, 1996, p. 222). These education and work examples illustrate the gaps that have emerged between peoples' longer (and changing) lives and the timing of opportunities, roles, and rewards in the life course.

Structural lag occurs, according to Riley and her colleagues, because human lives, including the timing of life course events, change more rapidly than social structures and institutions. Riley and Riley (1994) argue that social life is currently organized in a very age-segregated way. Young people are involved in education, middle-aged people in work, and older people are immersed in the world of leisure. A more flexible, age-integrated arrangement would open up these three areas of social life for people of all ages. Exhibit 4.4 illustrates these two different arrangements of activity through lifetimes. The Rileys suggest that we should be moving to an age-integrated structure to accommodate

Exhibit
4.4

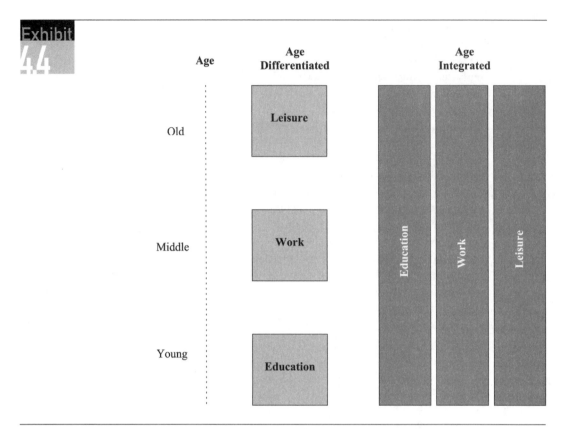

Two Idealized Age Structures
Source: Riley and Riley, 1994.

the needs, interests, abilities, and contributions of people of all ages. These scholars are optimistic that "age will lose its current power to determine when people should enter or leave these basic social structures (work, education, retirement); nor will age any longer constrain expectations as to how people should perform" (p. 110). Whether we reach such a state where age is truly irrelevant in the near future, there are some changes in age structures that reflect the Rileys' position. Elderhostel programs and over-60 audit policies at many institutions of higher education have opened up the opportunity for continued learning for many older people. The integration of "service learning" or community service into the curriculum at many colleges acknowledges the importance of crossing the artificial work/education barrier that is implied by classroom-only curricula. More flexible career trajectories, including protected time off for child or elder care, suggest a loosening of the boundary between work and leisure.

This idea can be used to support a position of advocacy for older adults. One of the clear messages in the discussion of structural lag is the unfulfilled potential of a large proportion of the older population, due to lack of formal outlets and recognized positions in which they can make their contributions. This attention to the costly lack of opportunities for contribution is the backdrop for the growing body of work on **productive aging**—the recognition that older people sometimes want to and often can continue to be involved in volunteer or paid work. This important area of research is discussed more in chapter 7.

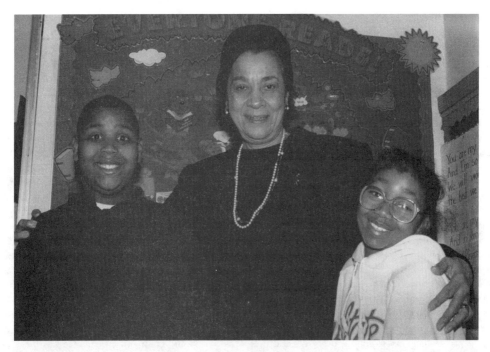

Older persons have much to offer via volunteerism in schools and other areas where others may benefit from the wealth of their accumulated knowledge. Society should work on expanding the ways it taps into the vast resource of the older population's wisdom and experience. (Credit: Mike Payne, courtesy of the Ohio Department of Aging)

Analyzing Theory

The Emergence of Developmental Science

Social theories about aging attempt to explain a wide range of phenomena, from individual adaptation through life to societal changes driven by cohorts. Theories are frameworks that help us to organize information and understand the world. Many of the major social theories about aging are presented in detail in various chapters in this book. This discusses human development in later life, the ways in which social forces shape lives across the life course, and the interplay between individual agency and social structure. To adequately conceptualize and investigate the complex questions related to the many dimensions of aging calls for interdisciplinary theory and methods. Settersten has termed this emerging perspective "developmental science" (2005a), and makes the case for "a new social studies of old people and old age" (2005b). This approach is taking shape in

conceptual and empirical work on the life course in the areas of leisure (Hendricks & Cutler, 2003), work (Henretta, 2003), health (George, 2003), and families (Hagestad, 2003). This emerging scientific framework represents a new stage for gerontology.

Where do new theories come from and how are they developed? How can we understand how new questions and new frameworks develop in the field? Theories reflect historically grounded views of what the appropriate questions are to ask about age or aging and what should be the focal subject matter (Ferraro, 1990). For example, questions about how people adapt to retirement received a lot of attention in the 1970s and 1980s; during this era, the attention of researchers, policymakers, and the general public was turned to the experiences of aging individuals, partly because we were beginning to recognize the tremendous growth of the older population. In this era, more people were retired than ever before.

(continued)

(continued)

Today the research on retirement tends to focus more on larger-scale political and economic questions, including how to finance retirement and regulate employer pensions.

Theories "furnish the boundaries for what we know.... A theoretical orientation becomes a habit of the mind ... and does not easily recognize contradictory evidence" (Hendricks, 1992, pp. 32–33). Theories create competing explanations, or even raise different kinds of questions that might be asked about a particular subject such as retirement or housing or lengthy marriages. To understand how a given theory reflects the historical period during which it evolved, Hendricks discusses "generations of theory." He suggests that there are three generations of theory on the social dimensions of aging. The first generation of theory focused on individual adaptation and adjustment—how individuals react to (or don't react to) changes and continuities in their lives over time. In the next generation, theories began to focus on structural processes and the social organization that surround cohorts of aging individuals, directing attention to such questions as how the labor force responds to retirement or how groups such as the family adapt to more long-lived members. In the third generation, theories of aging synthesized the individual and structural emphases of the earlier generations, examining questions relating multiple levels from micro to macro (along a continuum from individual to societal, as discussed in chapter 1). In this phase, theories became more "dynamic and political ... recognizing the important of structure ... but also seeing people as intentional actors involved in creating social situation and their lives" (Hendricks, 1992, p. 37). In turning our attention to the ways in which theory development is a product of a particular historical and social context, Hendricks (1992) and Ferraro (1990) point out that knowledge itself is a social construction—a product of dominant ideas and assumptions. The emerging "developmental science" of the life course is a well-articulated example of a new generation of theory, full of promise. "This cluster of ideas, old and new, will bring opportunities to reflect on what the field of gerontology now is, reclaim some of what it once was, and dream about what it might one day become" (Settersten, 2005b, p. S179).

As you encounter more detailed presentations of many sociological theories of aging in this text, you can deepen your understanding of those theories by comparing and contrasting them. Does it focus on individual actions and adaptations, the social structure, or both? To what "generation" does the theory belong? What assumptions about the appropriate subject matter are implicit in the theory? What exactly does the theory try to explain and where does it look for answers? These questions can help you analyze and categorize the variety of social gerontological theories of aging.

SUMMARY

This chapter has explored the mechanisms through which society shapes life stages and individual experiences of aging. Americans place high value on a sense of individual achievement and responsibility, and so it is often difficult to embrace the notion that our destinies are not completely the product of our individual actions. Using a sociological imagination helps us to better understand our own and others' experiences. We can see that personal circumstances arise, at least in part, from a particular social and historical context. The ways in which experiences in later life are patterned by gender, race, and social class provide examples of the impact and constraints of social location.

Some sociologists take a purely deterministic view and argue that there is no such thing as personal choice; they suggest that all action and experience are the result of social location and social influences. Others argue that social influences do indeed have an impact, but that humans retain free will are never truly completely "socialized." While this debate is ongoing, many scholars are more interested in the interplay between social constraints and individual actions. This idea of reciprocal influence is presented a few times in this chapter; people are influenced by social forces such as age norms, but they also, collectively, can have an impact on age norms and social structures. "People's lives can only be fully understood as they influence, and are influenced by, the surrounding social structure of roles, groups, nation states, and other social and cultural institutions" (Riley, 1996, p. 256).

In our society is it very popular to focus on individual attitudes, the power of positive thinking, and individual responsibility. Comments such as, "aging is all in your mind" and "you're only as old as you feel" reflect those values. Now that you have been thinking about the ways in which society shapes our lives, we ask you to reconsider such statements. Is it really so simple? Is personal attitude all that matters? Or are there age-related social forces that do have an impact on whether we can find a job, and how "young" we can possibly feel?

WEB WISE

Sociology and the Aging Revolution

http://www.trinity.edu/~mkearl/geron.html#in

Sociologist Mike Kearl of Trinity University has invested considerable time in developing a Web site with numerous interesting links and great visuals. Aside from general information about the discipline of sociology and links relevant to that discipline, he includes a section entitled "Old Age in the Mass Media" and "Old Age Across Cultures and Time."

American Sociological Association—Section on Aging and the Life Course

http://www.asanet.org/sectionaging

Just as psychologists have a specialized division focusing on aging and the life course, the American Sociological Association also has a membership section addressing issues related to aging. This Web site provides access to recent newsletters, membership information, data resources, and a description of sociology's role in the study of aging and life course issues. Included are links to other aging organizations.

American Psychological Association—Division 20: Adult Development and Aging

http://apadiv20.phhp.ufl.edu

Division 20 is the section of the American Psychological Association that is devoted to the study of human development throughout the adult years, including old age. The Web page offers links to recent research on topics such as Alzheimer's disease, depression, behavioral health, and emotional health. A recent visit to this Web site offered links to articles on the genetic components of Alzheimer's disease and the role of social networks in protecting against the effects of Alzheimer's disease.

KEY TERMS

ageism	generativity	norms
age norms	gerotranscendence	productive aging
developmental	human	social role
science	development	social time
ego–integrity	life course	structural lag

QUESTIONS FOR THOUGHT AND DISCUSSION

1. To what extent do you feel constrained by age norms and life course expectations? How aware are you and your friends of these expectations?
2. Informally interview a handful of people and ask them some specific age norm questions, such as the age at which a person should be settled into a career, the age at which they expect to marry (if at all). What do these findings tell you about the power of age norms?
3. Do you think that the stages of human development in later life (such as gerotranscendence and elderhood) are possible to achieve only when we are old? Why or why not?
4. How do societies "use" age? Why does chronological age make any difference whatsoever in our lives? Give some examples of the ways in which social definitions of age, including ageism, have affected your life (or someone you know well).

Love, Sex, and Longevity

As the old song says, "Love and marriage ... go together like a horse and carriage." Perhaps, but which comes first? If you are a well-socialized product of American culture, you probably feel strongly that people should get married after they fall in love. However, in other cultures people assume that love will grow within marriage. Love is not a necessary condition to their decision to marry. Researchers asked college students from 11 countries whether they would marry someone they did not love. Only about 5% of the students in the United States and Australia said they would marry someone with the right qualities even if they did not love him or her. About 50% of the students from India and Pakistan said they would marry without love (Levine, Sato, Hashimoto, & Verma, 1995). The cultural practice of arranged marriages still prevails in countries such as India, helping to explain the acceptability of marrying first, then letting love develop later. In India, people still use the term "love marriages" to describe the small proportion of Indian couples who decide to marry on their own, without parental arrangements, approval, and decision-making.

Although love may not be the basis for the decision to marry in India, it is still highly valued. However, cultural definitions of love vary. In India, love is based on long-term commitment and devotion to the family. In contrast, U.S. culture highly prizes romantic love—an idealized view of partners and relationships—based on passion, erotic attraction, and media images of ever-growing ardor and tenderness.

Where do these different cultural definitions of love come from? There are a lot of factors that contribute to this ephemeral concept. We suggest that one of those factors is a quite "unromantic," somewhat prosaic demographic element: the average life expectancy in a society. In "young" countries, such as India, where life expectancy is relatively low, romance may be a luxury. In such societies, people marry younger and begin childbearing earlier, because life is shorter. "Older" societies, like the United States where people live longer, are more likely to value romance and to favor falling in love before marriage.

We discuss elsewhere the emergence of childhood as a differentiated stage of life. Changes in life expectancy were part of the conditions necessary for that new stage of life to develop. People had to live long enough for there to be time in life devoted to education and learning how to become an adult. Similarly, we can argue intuitively that living long enough is a necessary precondition for having the time to search for a desirable partner and to enjoy courtship and engagement prior to marriage. These stages prior to marriage are devoted to romance—the search for the ideal partner; the excitement, passion, and the anticipation of the new relationship; getting to know each other; and making plans for a life together—all of which fuel a romantic view of love and marriage. When we marry in our 20s and live until our 80s, we have the luxury of time to search for the perfect partner and therefore we have the opportunity to sustain the illusion of romantic love. We are also confronted with the prospect of five or six decades with our marriage partners, so our choices in this matter have quite an impact on our lives. The adage, "marry in haste, repent in leisure," alludes to the care that one should take in this decision and to the potential length of time spent in marriage.

Longer life expectancy can provide the basis for cultural values about romantic love to develop. These two factors together—longevity and preference for romantic love—are also linked to divorce patterns.

> Our culture emphasizes romantic love as a basis for marriage, rendering relationships vulnerable to collapse as sexual passion subsides. There is now widespread support for the notion that one may end a marriage in favor of a new relationship simply to renew excitement and romance. (Macionis, 1997, p. 471)

And, since we live long enough, we have time to pursue, develop, and sustain more than one relationship. Serial monogamy—having more than one spouse sequentially but not simultaneously—is a phenomenon unique to societies with long life expectancies. Just as an extended life course provides opportunities for second careers in the job market, it also provides for second and third chances at love relationships. Having the time to spend in search of new and improved relationships makes it possible to sustain the illusion of an ideal partner, one with the most important elements in romantic love.

Obviously there are factors in addition to longevity that shape a society's values about love and marriage. Other cultural values play important roles. The importance of extended family, the value placed on independence, and the primacy of parental authority are all cultural values that can influence attitudes toward love and marriage. Simmons, Vom Kolke, and Hideko (1986) compared the attitudes of students toward love and marriage. They found that Japanese students, who live in a culture that highly values respect toward parental decisions and the importance of the family, placed a significantly lower value on romantic love than did students in the United States or West Germany. The predominance of arranged marriages in India reflect the very strong familial system (Gupta, 1976), while in the United States the emphasis on independence and autonomy would preclude such a practice.

Countries with higher life expectancies thus have the demographic foundation for romanticized views of love and marriage. The life course in these societies is long enough and differentiated enough for time to be spent in the search for at least one "perfect" partner and in the development of those love relationships. But is there a time in the life course when people lose interest in this vital endeavor? Do people lose interest in love, romance, and sex as they grow older? According to the stereotypes, they do. According to older people, they don't. The Association of Reproductive Health Professionals (2002) has designed a continuing medical education program entitled "Mature Sexuality" to improve the awareness of health care professionals about older people's sexuality. In one of the most extensive studies on sexuality and aging, Wiley and Bortz (1996) found that over two-thirds of the middle-aged and older adults in their study were sexually active. While 60% reported a decrease in frequency of sexual activity over the past decade, 32% reported no change, and 8% reported an increase—and this research predates the availability of prescription drugs for the treatment of impotence, such as sildenafil citrate (Viagra®). About half the women and 70% of the men in this study stated a desire for increased sexual activity. Availability of a partner is, obviously, one significant factor in sexual activity. One study found that over 80% of married people in their 70s were still sexually active (Brecher reported in Hillier & Barrow, 1999). Summarizing findings from a number of studies of sexuality in later life, Hillier and Barrow (1999) report additional findings that challenge stereotypes about sex, love, and aging. Overall, patterns of sexual activity are established in mid-life and remain fairly continuous throughout old age, barring serious illness or disability. But some studies show that nursing home residents often retain their interest in sexuality. Research also reports that three-fourths of older people said their love-making had improved with time; 15% of people aged 60 and over reported increased sexual activity over the course of a 10-year longitudinal study. The rate of masturbation increases for women as they get older, partly related to the lack of available partners. Some people have a first homosexual experience in later life. So sexuality does not cease in later life.

It is not uncommon to respond to the idea of love, romance, and sex among older people in an ageist, stereotypical way. We may find it hard to believe and even distasteful, or we may find it touching and "cute." Both responses discriminate against older people. Both reactions treat older people as different and presume that age brings with it a fundamental change in our interest in and ability to be sexual beings. From older people we know that, for the most part, interest in sexuality and need for intimacy persists throughout the life course.

Current interest is not on whether
groups bonded by kinship persist but
how and why they adapt as effectively
as they do in response to social change.
(Maddox & Lawton, 1993, p. 2)

The Family Institution

E
amilies are the cornerstone
of all human societies; they
have been discovered in every
human culture in history. Family is the social institution that is perhaps closest to us; we
immediately see and feel its influence on our everyday lives. Everyone has a "common
sense" understanding from personal experience and cultural messages regarding what
is meant by the word **family**, yet there is some difficulty in coming to a social consensus on its
definition. Most attention focuses on the concept of the family as the group socially responsible for
bearing and rearing children, rather than on the family relationships that continue as an important
organizing force throughout our lives.

Contemporary Western societies have a wide variety of family forms, contributing to ambiguity
regarding the definition of the family. Our culture in different eras may have different structures
and expectations for family members (Hareven, 1995), and there may be great variation among contemporary cultures in how they structure the institution of the family. Nonetheless, the centrality of
the family as an organizing force in societies cannot be overemphasized. Many of our closest, most
enduring social linkages in life are located in the family, through our social roles as child, sibling,
spouse, and parent.

Research on **later-life families**—those families beyond the child-rearing years (Brubaker,
1990a)—began as a reaction to the emergence (in the mid-20th century) of "nuclear family theory"
(Sussman & Burchinal, 1968). In nuclear family theory the isolated and autonomous nuclear family

unit was the focus of the study, making extended kin relations (such as grandparents and adult siblings) apparently irrelevant (Parsons, 1959; Parsons & Bales, 1955). From this perspective, attention was naturally focused on family formation and kinship relations in the first half of family life, including courtship, marriage, and child-bearing (Cohler & Altergott, 1995). Neither grandparents nor adult siblings were viewed as important to the lives of individuals in nuclear families, who instead were thought to rely entirely on their immediate kin for support.

Family researchers, however, quickly remedied this limited view of kinship by demonstrating the active interchanges of support and the meaningful bonds of affection that exist among extended kin, albeit in different, and sometimes distant, households (Hill, 1965; Litwak, 1965; Shanas, 1967; Sussman & Burchinal, 1968). Families are, in fact, some of the most important age-integrating organizations in society. While many other social contexts segregate people by age, families necessarily bring together individuals of various ages and generations in social groups sharing mutual interests, experiences, cultures, and values. It is through family membership that many of us develop both interest in and knowledge of other stages of the life course. As part of this changing view, a newer family structure has been described: the **modified extended family** (Litwak, 1960).

The modified extended family acknowledges that, although kin may reside in separate households and often at great distance, there remain strong bonds of affection, identity, and support among them. In fact, because the term *family* often connotes the nuclear group, some authors advocate use of the term *kinship* when referring to the wider web of relatives both within and beyond the household, to emphasize these broader intergenerational and interhousehold bonds (Maddox & Lawton, 1993).

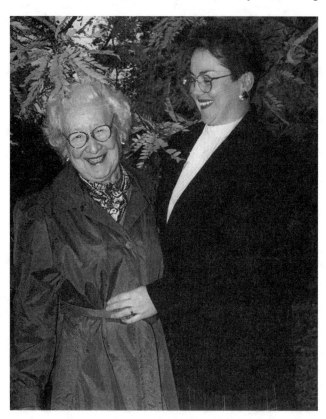

While many other social contexts segregate us by age, families necessarily bring together individuals of various ages and generations. (Credit: Mike Payne, courtesy of the Ohio Department of Aging)

The Meanings of Generation

Linking various ages in the family are the biological **generations** that are key to the family's structure. Although the term *generation* has a wide variety of meanings, its meaning within the family is clear and familiar to most of us. In this context generations are "lineage descent positions within families" (Bengtson, Cutler, Mangen, & Marshall, 1985, p. 305). Grandparent, parent, and child generations in family systems form clearly recognizable social linkages connecting individuals of various ages and cohorts into one of the smallest but most influential social institutions—the family. These generations link the history of the family system through time and provide individual members with connections to both the past and the future. The craze for genealogical research and the development of family trees reflects our interest in better understanding these linkages with our own historical predecessors in past generations. Similarly, grandparents may feel a stake in the future through the younger generations of children and grandchildren in their families.

Another application of the term generation is as a proxy for *cohort*. In studying family relationships, as in other areas, we encounter a great deal of difficulty in distinguishing the effects of cohort membership from those of aging, especially since most of the research on aging and families has been conducted only in the past 30 years, showing the experience of a few cohorts. Generalizing from the experience of historically limited cohorts exhibits **cohort centrism**. This cohort centrism means, for example, that our knowledge of later-life marriage is currently based on the experiences of couples born between approximately 1880 and 1940. Those are the only couples who have entered later life during the recent decades of research on later-life families, showing the limitations of our knowledge. How will future cohorts of married couples differ as they move through their lives? Given the dramatic changes in the overall society, including gender roles within marriage and the increasing experience of divorce and remarriage, it is difficult to project future trends with confidence based on the experiences of earlier cohorts. It is unlikely, however, that future marriage cohorts will be the same as those we have studied to date.

Aspects of Family Variation

Certainly not all families are alike. Not only do they vary by size, composition, and closeness, but researchers have identified several social traits or dimensions of diversity on which families vary. One is the family's stage of development, reflecting the size of the family, the ages of family members, and the types of issues being addressed as central concerns. (See the section on Family Life Cycle Theory later in this chapter). Other differences relate to family form, race/ethnicity, and social class.

In terms of *family form*, a variety of kinship groupings are labeled family. Family form remains a highly controversial area, because society lacks consensus on whether some of these groups constitute "true" family. For example, there seems to be substantial agreement that a married couple or a single parent living in a household with children constitutes a family. But if the couple is childless or if children are being raised by a grandparent, some would withhold the term family to describe that household. Any society's definition of family, as a component of its culture, is subject to redefinition. Although debate continues on this issue, individuals in most of the groups just described, as well as other family forms such as blended/remarried families or same-sex couples (with or without children), consider themselves to be families and act accordingly, even if some religions, laws, and policies do not agree.

A considerable body of research has examined the potential differences by race or ethnicity in how families operate as their members age. Much of the research has focused on Blacks, but recently more attention has been paid to families in other cultures (see Aboderin, 2004; Agree, Biddlecom, Chang, & Perez, 2002). Most research on Black families suggests that relationships demonstrate more interdependence, with members more likely to rely on extended kin and close community (such as church members) for support (Shuey & Hardy, 2003; Sussman, 1985). For example, Black elders are more often cared for at home by relatives, rather than by formal service providers or nursing homes, when their health fails (Miller, McFall, & Campbell, 1994). Such differences may reflect both cultural variations in family norms of mutual assistance (Shuey & Hardy, 2003) and experiences of economic disadvantage or discrimination in access to health care and other services.

Differences between middle-class Whites and Blacks or Hispanics are sometimes attributed to stronger norms of familism in the latter groups, a cultural emphasis on communal sharing of resources directed toward those most in need and a greater emphasis on family bonds and responsibilities. Some researchers have emphasized the apparently greater flexibility in kinship roles among Black families in particular, including a greater likelihood of establishing **fictive kinship** (granting someone who is unrelated the title and rights of a family member, such as "she is like a sister to me") and **surrogate family relationships,** whereby family members or others take on active role responsibility by replacing a parent, child, or caregiver (Burton & DeVries, 1995; Johnson, 1995b).

Most research has shown a higher level of intergenerational exchange and support in Black families than in White families (Mitchell & Register, 1984; Mutran, 1985; Shuey & Hardy, 2003). But efforts to identify the distinct influences of race or ethnicity

Although some research indicates African Americans are more apt to establish fictive kinship roles with nonrelatives, supportive relationships engendering the closeness of family occur among those in all ethnic groups. (Credit: Mike Payne, courtesy of the Ohio Department of Aging)

in families are often obscured by their connection with income and social class. When researchers compare families across race or ethnicity, they have necessarily included effects of class differences as well (Mitchell & Register, 1984; Mutran, 1985). Separating these factors can be difficult, but it is more possible today with growing middle-class Hispanic and Black populations. In an early study, Mitchell and Register (1984) distinguished the effects of race from social class in the family interactions of Black and White elders. Slightly more Black elders shared a residence with a child or a grandchild, but the major finding of the research was that race makes only a very small difference in family relationships and that, in some instances, social class is more important than race in explaining family patterns. In a more recent study (Shuey & Hardy, 2003), Black and Hispanic couples were more likely to provide assistance to parents or parents-in-law even if the effects of resources are taken into account.

Within races, social class differences in family relationships have been the subject of some investigation. The majority of research has focused on middle-class families. The limited research on working-class households shows that they live in closer proximity to extended kin, enabling households in the modified extended family to exchange more face-to-face contact and support (Townsend, 1968). Because working-class spouses maintain more separation in their daily routines and friendship patterns than do middle-class couples (Lopata, 1979), marital relationships are less central to well-being, and widowhood may be less disruptive (Bengtson, Rosenthal, & Burton, 1990).

Core Norms and Expectations of Family Relationships

Family relationships are often thought of simply as bonds based on affection. These critical social linkages are, however, more complex than simply the affection that is characteristic of some, but not all, kinship ties. What keeps family members together when relationships are stressed? Why do adult siblings often assist each other in many ways but seldom help out financially? Why is it often stressful if an adult child moves back in with his or her parents following a divorce? What structures the separations between kin and households in such a way as to promote privacy and autonomy?

Clearly, family relationships are governed by culturally based rules, **social norms** (discussed in chapter 4), regarding how members should act toward one another. These cultural norms for families are specialized in three ways. First, they are specific to particular role relationships. For example, the issue of privacy may be very different between an adolescent and a parent than between a husband and a wife; yet both relationships operate under some social norms regarding privacy. Second, these variations in familial norms may be systematically related to membership in social class, racial, ethnic, religious, or regional groupings. One example, noted previously, is the stronger emphasis on mutual help in Black families reported by many researchers. Third, the norms may vary across individual families, so that particular families, besides sharing a joint history and membership in other social groups, may have their own unique family norms (traditions) to add to the basic cultural rules.

These rules, the social norms governing family life, include two major dynamics, portrayed in Exhibit 5.1. These dimensions include the degree of independence or dependence of bonds and the degree to which relationships are ruled by voluntarism or

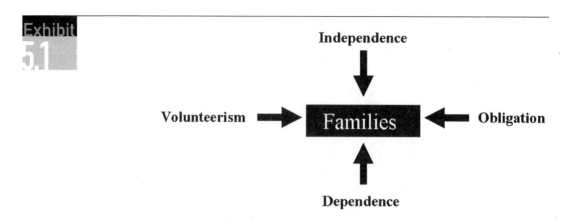

Exhibit
5.1

Dynamics of Family Norms

obligation. Families operate at the focus of these sometimes-contradictory norms. These two underlying themes, though certainly not exhaustive in terms of family norms, are central to an understanding of the social issues faced in families as aging changes them as social units and alters their individual members through aging.

Independence and Dependence

Central to the relationships within the family are issues of **independence** and **dependence**. Young children are physically and emotionally dependent on their parents, and we expect spouses to have dependencies on each other throughout their marriage. Yet we do not expect children to remain dependent on their parents throughout life, nor is a high level of economic, social, or emotional interdependence anticipated between adult siblings (Suitor, Pillemer, Keeton, & Robison, 1994). These norms may be violated, as when unmarried adult children remain in the home of their parents or return there following a divorce or employment disruption (White & Peterson, 1995). Fears of violating norms for independence in adulthood and later life also influence the relationships between older adults and their offspring. The vigor of such norms is indicated by the fact that dependency of an elderly parent, often termed "being a burden" to the children, is a concern often voiced by middle-class Americans (Sussman, 1985).

Living arrangements are indicative of the norm of generational independence in the United States. As Exhibit 5.2 shows, the oldest cohort in a family is more likely to live with relatives other than a spouse (usually adult children or siblings) than are their younger counterparts. However, neither men nor women, except those in cultural groups with norms supporting this behavior, plan to live with relatives other than a spouse. Instead, a majority of older Americans prefer to live independently (Federal Interagency Forum on Aging-Related Statistics, 2004). With adequate financial and housing resources, older adults choose to live independently of their adult children, although some may live in relatively close proximity. This pattern of proximity has been called **intimacy at a distance** (Rosenmayr & Kockeis, 1963), where emotional and social bonds between parents and children are maintained across households. This household autonomy underpins the independence of each of the generations, because neither generation is subject to the rule of the other as household head.

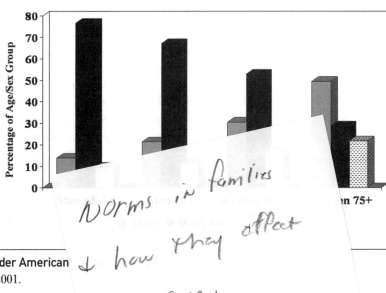

Living Arrangements of Older American
Source: Fields and Casper, 2001.

Norms about interdeper... The
relationships of older relative... hose
of the middle class, have mov... nily
farm to provide for the econon... on
voluntarism among kin (Harev... ...es
of industrial capitalism—self-rel... ...sion of mutual
dependency among two or more g... ...,ying family ties of long duration. Instead, there is pressure to ...... at least the guise of independence between
related adults linked by bonds other than marriage.

The norm of generational independence is also reflected in the **norm of reciprocity.** This norm, which exists generally in social relations, directs repayment of social and
material debts between individuals or among groups; the norm provides an acceptable way
of managing dependency within families to maximize the perception of independence of
adult kin. In family relationships, as in the larger society, the norm of reciprocity dictates
that individuals who are recipients of benefits from others have an unpaid debt or obligation until a comparable favor can be returned to the original helper (Silverstein, 2006). The
common statement "I owe you a favor" is an expression of this norm in everyday life.

Although reciprocity is generally expected between exchange partners—whether
individuals, businesses, or governments—families often exhibit some flexibility in how
the obligation is fulfilled. In some cases, reciprocity may be direct and involve exactly
equivalent goods or services, as when siblings help each other move from one house
to another. In others, reciprocity may involve exchanges of goods or services deemed
equivalent, as when parents loan their adult children money for a down payment on a
home in exchange for assistance with household repairs. Finally, the exchange may be
indirect, with support received from one family member paid back in the form of support to another family member. For example, reciprocity norms may be deemed as fulfilled when parents provide for their children, who, when grown, pay the debt back by
caring well for the grandchildren of the original givers (Antonucci, 1990). In this case,

the norm of reciprocity is satisfied quite indirectly, on the assumption that ultimately all members of the group will benefit through the ongoing assistance passed down through the generations. Even in the absence of direct reciprocity, older kin may subjectively define whatever assistance or advice they give to younger kin as balancing any help they receive, enabling them to maintain their sense of reciprocity (Antonucci, 1990).

Evidence from longitudinal research indicates that reciprocity has an influence on relationships between adults and their aging parents. In a study of multiple generations in 1971, when the youngest generation sampled was between the ages of 16 and 21, questions were asked about the emotional closeness, financial support, and shared time/activity with parents. A follow-up study of these same individuals in 1985 and subsequent years showed that the 1971 teens who received more on these three dimensions were contributing more support back to their surviving parent(s) in later years compared to those who received less—suggesting the influence of reciprocity. Mothers received more support than fathers, and support levels increased over time among those parents who survived to 1997 (Silverstein, Conroy, Wang, Giarrusso, & Bengtson, 2002). Even in families that provided little support to teenagers, however, advancing age generated support from adult children, perhaps from a sense of filial obligation, a social norm discussed below (Silverstein et al., 2002).

The particular form of family reciprocity is based in culture. Akiyama, Antonucci, and Campbell (1990) suggest that Whites have a linear model of exchange, such that older people always give more to younger people within the family; the Japanese culture projects a curvilinear model, in which the middle generation gives more to older and younger; and Black families hold more of a communal model, whereby those with resources share them with all kin on an as-needed basis. Other research, however, suggests that the amounts of support and assistance may vary within a culture and differ from the norms, as described later in the chapter.

Voluntarism and Obligation

Family relationships differ from those of friends in that kinship often carries with it a higher degree of obligation. "Family are supposed to perform in times of need, friends are not so obligated" (Antonucci, 1990, p. 215). Expectations of mutual responsibility and support have been at the heart of most family systems across cultures and throughout history, but the core of obligation and responsibility is thought by some to be diminishing in recent times (Antonucci, 1990; Jarrett, 1985). The degree of **voluntarism** in these relationships (the extent to which individuals have choices regarding whether and when to meet individual versus family needs) has varied widely.

The extent to which **obligation** rules family relationships has also changed. Since the 19th century, families in the United States and many other Western cultures have changed toward a more voluntaristic basis, with families held together more by sentiment compared with past eras when family ties were more strongly based on duty (Hareven, 1994; Hess & Waring, 1978). Johnson (1995b) describes the **opportune family** as a form available to the American middle class. In this family system, individuals can choose the degree to which they invest in themselves (versus the family group), their level of obligation to relatives, and the nature of their significant relationships.

As part of their family roles, individuals clearly have both rights and obligations toward one another, including mutual (although not always equal) responsibility of spouses and sometimes asymmetrical obligations between parent and child (Jarrett, 1985). The specific case most studied is that of the adult child's obligation toward the aging parent.

Filial obligation (or filial duty) refers to the responsibility that children have toward their parents, as mandated by their culture, especially in terms of meeting their needs in later life. As with other norms, filial obligation varies across cultures and historical periods. In some societies and locations, including many U.S. states, filial obligation is mandated by law.

Until World War II, norms for White families dictated that one child, most typically a younger daughter, would forgo or delay marriage in order to provide care for her aged parents until their deaths (Hareven, 1995). Although this practice of having a daughter remain at home as caregiver has waned, contemporary U.S. society still has strong expectations, varying somewhat by social class and ethnicity, that adult children will provide support and assistance for older parents should they require it. Despite a movement toward more voluntaristic family relationships in later life, especially among the middle class, filial obligation demonstrates continued relevance in contemporary families (Finley, Roberts, & Banahan, 1988; Hareven, 1995).

Not all adult children feel these obligations equally (or equally with their parents), creating potential strain in the parent-child and sibling relationships (Jarrett, 1985). Research by Finley and her associates (1988) found that both males and females claimed a high acceptance of responsibility toward aged parents. Factors such as the degree of affection the child felt toward the parent and the proximity of their residences influenced the degree of filial obligation reported toward a mother. For fathers, however, the findings were different. An absence of role conflict predicted a sense of obligation among daughters but not among sons. Agreement or disagreement with questions such as "Adult children should give their parents financial help when it is necessary" and "Every child should be willing to share his/her home with aging parents" are used to evaluate the degree to which these obligations are accepted. Actual behavior often varies from responses to a survey, however, since it is still not socially acceptable to admit conflict, distance, or a lack of a sense of obligation in the family (Jarrett, 1985).

The Cultural Basis of Family Norms: The Chinese Case

Norms, including those for family relationships, are part of every culture and therefore vary across cultural groups and even across time within cultures. The symbolic meanings shared by members of the culture, which direct the manner in which members and groups (including families) relate to one another, vary widely. To illustrate this point, we examine the traditional cultural norms regarding family relationships in China, which are experiencing dramatic challenges today in China's rapidly aging and modernizing society.

According to Charlotte Ikels (1993), China's traditional culture of the early 20th century (pre-Communism) was based on Confucianism "an ethic of familism that not only served as the standard to guide proper family organization for many centuries but was also codified into law" (p. 124). This system emphasized vertical family ties—those between the generations—as more important than horizontal ties, such as those between spouses, which were viewed primarily as a means by which to continue the lineage (or vertical line) through offspring.

Family Life Cycle Theory and Individual Dependency in the Family

Family life cycle theory is one theoretical lens that has been especially pertinent to the study of families as they age. Originated by Evelyn Duvall and her colleagues in the 1950s, when the focus in family research was on the nuclear unit, family life cycle theory focuses attention on the systematic changes that occur in family life over time in conjunction with the maturation of its members. "Families, like individual persons, progress from birth to death in the steps and patterns inherent in the human condition" (Duvall & Miller, 1985, p. 20). According to this developmental approach, family relationships, goals, and routines are differentiated by stages of development. Families with preschool-age children, for example, are quite different in their focus than are families with teenagers moving toward adulthood or **post-parental families,** whose children have left the household via normal "child launching" into jobs, marriage, college, or simply moving out. Thus, it makes sense to recognize these differences and to focus attention on the patterned changes expected as members of the nuclear family mature.

Because the original theory was developed after World War II in a time of high fertility, births clustered fairly closely together, and low divorce rates, it emerged with a set of stages that were driven by the maturation of the oldest child. For example, when the oldest child became an adolescent, according to this formulation, the family moved into a new stage. This emphasis on stages has been criticized for focusing attention on a traditional, idealized, nuclear family in which family events occur on time and without disruption (Cohler & Altergott, 1995). It fails to recognize the variations in family life (for example, families may have both teenagers and preschoolers at the same time) or to account for non-normative patterns, such as childlessness, divorce and remarriage, or single parenthood.

More recently, attention in this theory has turned to understanding the transitions experienced by the family or its members, rather than assigning them to particular stages. This emphasis on family dynamics rather than on stages opens the theory to greater flexibility in examining family careers (Cohler & Altergott, 1995). Regardless of the usefulness of stages, however, family life cycle theory accomplished one vital goal. It focused attention on the fact that family life is dynamic, involving some predictable changes in bonds, closeness, and central concerns of the family based on the changing composition of the household and maturation of its members over time.

Think about family life cycle theory in terms of your own experience. How does the passage of time, paired with the maturation of family members, change the roles, responsibilities, and relationships between you and your kin? One key area of change, mirrored in stages of family development, has to do with the development of children and their dependence on the family. Your own experience is probably one of moving from a high degree of dependence as a baby to greater independence as you moved toward adulthood. Later, others may be reliant on you, if you become a partner or parent, and even later you may have a second phase of dependency, should you experience failing health in advanced old age. Those changes in dependency also shaped your relationships with others in myriad ways. Family life cycle theory separates out one link in the chain of generations—a single nuclear family—to point out that our relationships are not static. Just as individuals grow and change with the passage of time, so too does each nuclear family unit.

In earlier times, parents arranged the marriages of their children, because they had a strong stake in the selection of an appropriate mate to continue the line. Because the system was also strongly patrilineal, and only members of the male line were considered truly related, the word for grandchildren was reserved for only the offspring of a son. Sons remained in residence with their parents following marriage, whereas daughters left to be with their new husbands and parents-in-law, who considered them full members of that kinship group only if they bore children. Thus, sons and their wives provided the support system to aged parents within the same household. Each household was under the control of the senior male until his death, at which time the property was divided among the sons. This continued subdivision of property for each new generation sometimes meant that sons needed to leave home to seek economic support elsewhere, including overseas. Sons who emigrated, however, retained their obligation to provide financial support for aging parents back home.

Daughters-in-law took responsibility for the physical care of aged parents-in-law and continued this care with offerings to the honored ancestors after their deaths. If widowed, a daughter-in-law would be discouraged from remarriage because of her responsibility to the ancestors and her links, through her children, with her husband's kinship group.

Although the advent of the communist regime in the mid-20th century changed numerous aspects of the traditional family system, many components remain. For example, 73% of urban elders and 89% of rural elders still lived in multigenerational households in the late 1980s, a legacy of the traditional Chinese family norms. In addition, the imposition of China's one-child policy to control the size of the country's population initiated in the 1980s, has turned the family tree on its head, with very few children and grandchildren suddenly available to provide support to a growing number of parents and grandparents.

More recent analyses of living arrangements of older adults in numerous countries and cultures throughout the developing world indicate that the Chinese case is one of many variations in how adult children and their aging parents choose to relate. Shared households are common in many places in the world, but solo residence by older adults is more common with higher levels of education and economic development. Modernization prompts concerns that many countries may face crises as traditional systems of care for older adults, such as China's traditional family system, lose favor and no alternatives for housing, financial, or social/emotional support are in place (Bongaarts & Zimmer, 2002).

The Waltons Myth: Coresidence of Grandparents in the United States

The once-popular 1970s television show "The Waltons," now widely syndicated, presented a nostalgic view of family life during the Great Depression of the 1930s. The strong family household of three generations included both paternal grandparents, their son and his wife, and a large number of grandchildren. Did the Waltons present a realistic image of family life in the past for the United States, with grandparents happily co-residing with their children and grandchildren?

Although a myth persists regarding the prevalence of **intergenerational households** (those with three or more generations) in the past, the number of households including an aging grandparent, parents, and grandchildren continues at a low level today (see chapters 3 and 6). Demography offers ample evidence that this type of household was not as common as the cultural myth suggests and certainly not the experience of the majority of families at any given time for several reasons. First, the life expectancy of the time was short. It is probable that either Grandma or Grandpa Walton would have died before all of their children had reached maturity. Second, even if they had both lived, it is even less likely that they would survive the nearly 20 additional years together that would be required to produce grandchildren of the ages shown in the television program. Finally, if the grandparents raised a large number of children, as their depicted son had done, a lot of other adult Walton sons and daughters, married and perhaps raising other grandchildren in households elsewhere, would not be sharing a household with aged parents. Assuming four siblings, for example, only 25% of offspring households would have grandparents for some period of time.

Demography aside, we may question the nature of the warm and emotionally intimate grandparent-grandchild relationships that were portrayed. Research has shown that grandparents in that era were less likely to be warm and companionate than is true in more recent cohorts (Cherlin & Furstenberg, 1986). Grandparents were more often distant authority figures rather than nurturers of younger children. In short, the idyllic picture of happy multigenerational living portrayed in "The Waltons," though not impossible, was not the commonly lived experience of most families of that era.

Social Changes and the Family's Future

Neither the family as a social institution nor individual families are static. They respond to changes in the larger society, and they contribute to, resist, or accelerate societal changes through the decisions and actions of individuals or family units. Changes that take place in the lives of young and mid-life individuals carry forward, creating ripples of change as these cohorts move into later life. Given the important changes that have taken place in the past several decades, we anticipate changes for later-life families, intergenerational relationships, family structures, and much more in the future. As we move ahead in the 21st century, what predictions can we make about how families may age differently?

There has been a major change in attitudes and behaviors related to childbearing in recent decades, involving more non-marital births in younger cohorts. Looking at life-course studies that show greater poverty in later life among women who were single parents for 10 years or more, the question arises as to whether this growth in non-marital births portends greater female poverty in later life. Seldom are changes that simple, however, since most of the current older cohort became single parents through divorce or widowhood, rather than births outside of marriage (Johnson & Favreault, 2004). Therefore, single parenthood that does not result from marital termination may have different results, especially given that many other factors (i.e., women's education and labor force involvement) have also changed for these cohorts.

This exemplifies why cohort centrism becomes a risk is in projecting changes for families of the future based on the experiences of older adults of today. Major social trends, including the growing rate of divorce and remarriage during the 20th century, shrinking numbers of children born to each woman, increased employment of women throughout their lives, and legal changes regarding familial rights, such as the rights of grandparents to visit grandchildren after divorce, all portend major changes in the family experiences that baby boomer cohorts, and their successors, will bring with them to later stages of their lives. Although it is difficult to predict precisely, some major changes have already emerged and will continue to reshape the **later-life family** in future cohorts.

Changes in Marriage

One important area of change involves marriage, including both its timing and its gender-related norms. Significant changes have taken place in age at first marriage for women. This raises the question of whether marriage is simply being delayed or whether there will eventually be growing percentages of adults moving through life outside of marriage—although perhaps not without a partner. Research on the cohorts born in the 1950s and 1960s suggested that most will eventually marry, although the ages of first marriage were substantially higher than those for preceding cohorts (Goldstein & Kenney, 2001). In addition, contrary to earlier cohorts, rates of marriage are now higher for women with college degrees than for women with less education regardless of race. Later marriage, especially when driven by advancing education, also implies later childbearing, potentially smaller families, and economic advantage for these dual-earner couples (Goldstein & Kenney, 2001). Populations in other countries are also seeing de-layed ages at marriage; in some cases cohabitation seems to be replacing legal marriage, a pattern which may spread to the United States in the future.

Some of the change in marriage is gender-specific. There is a long-standing link between male education/earnings and the likelihood of marriage that did not previously exist for women. However, as more women achieve higher levels of education and more are fully engaged in the labor force, their likelihood of marriage is becoming more like that of men. This suggests that the traditional norms differentiating economic roles within the nuclear family (i.e., the breadwinner/homemaker model in which women were more economically dependent) will be less common life experiences as these cohorts reach their later years (Sweeney, 2002). Rather than education and earnings enabling women to skip marriage and remain independent, as some theories had predicted, the opposite is happening—as women and men with college degrees rework the economic bargain in marriage from patterns that had existed for their grandparents' generation to create new marital norms (Sweeney, 2002).

Changes in the Size and Shape of Families

Increased longevity has created the growing potential for four- and even five- or six-generation families. The advent of the four-generation family was first heralded back in the 1960s (Townsend, 1968). In a **five- or six-generation family,** an individual can simultaneously be a grandparent and a grandchild, providing a richer possible set of in-tergenerational family experiences. The possibilities for exchanges of support across so many generations raise many questions, such as whether all generations will have some responsibility toward the oldest or youngest. Will elderly sons and daughters be able to adequately assist their even older parents? What rights and duties do great-grandpar-ents have toward their offspring three generations removed?

Changes in fertility also have long-term implications for family structure. As U.S. fertility rates have stabilized in recent years near replacement rate (just under two children per woman), the family tree has changed its shape in a process sometimes called *family verticalization.* From a narrow base of one couple, fewer children and grandchildren will eventually emerge, leading to a description of this structure not as a tree but as a **beanpole family** (Bengtson et al., 1990). As Exhibit 5.3 shows, the change from a fertility rate of 3 to a fertility rate of 1.5 alters the numbers of siblings,

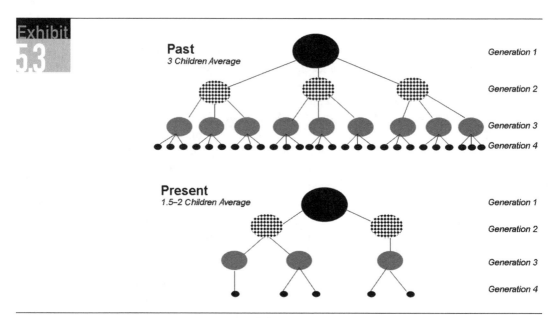

Exhibit 5.3

Family Structure and Size, High Versus Low Fertility

cousins, grandchildren, and great-grandchildren any individual is likely to experience. The beanpole family, resulting from lower fertility, contains fewer siblings, in-laws, nieces, and nephews and relatively more kin located in older or younger generations. We expect, for example, to see more grandparents who attend the marriages of grandchildren and have time to know their great-grandchildren. It is unclear whether this change in structure will be accompanied by a systematic change in filial expectations when fewer adult children are available to be supporters and caregivers.

Future Changes in the Timing of Family Life Events

Major events of family life, such as marriage, birth of children, or child launching, occur at times that are dictated by social norms, cultural traditions, individual decisions, and (sometimes) fate. Ethnic and cultural variations in the expected timing of family events such as marriage and childbirth were discovered in a sample of adolescent girls (East, 1998). Research on social norms described earlier shows that, despite considerable variation in when people achieve particular family milestones, we still share some consensus regarding the appropriate age for many of these events. When asked by what age certain major family events (such as marriage or completion of childbearing) should occur for men and women, most people suggest ages within a 6-year range, with only slight differences in the timetables for men and women (Settersten & Hagestad, 1996a). Less consensus appears for the age of becoming a grandparent, which ranges more widely.

An unanticipated early or late pregnancy or the unexpected cancellation of a wedding (events that throw a person "off time") can shape the timing of events throughout an individual's life in ways that influence later outcomes. Expansion of educational opportunities, for example, means that some delay the establishment of families, so that these events will occur at later ages than was true for their parents. Others, through teenage childbearing, accelerate the ages at which family milestones can be reached. Exhibit 5.4 shows the differences in timing of selected family events for members of female cohorts born between the 1920s and the 1950s. Although time of first marriage was surprisingly consistent for these cohorts, differences are visible in both life expectancy and the time spent parenting. Over time, because of reduced fertility and increased life expectancy, the top period, reflecting the post-parental stage of life, has expanded. We are spending a smaller percentage of our time as parents and more time before and after parenting.

Despite these overall trends, considerable variation is possible within any cohort. Consider the female generations in two hypothetical families: the Hobarts and the Fultons (see Exhibit 5.5). Brenda Hobart was born in the 1930s, married at age 22, and started her family two years later with a daughter, Beth, followed by three other children. Beth grew to adulthood and continued her education through a master's degree. Having waited for marriage, Beth had her first child, Brenda's first grandchild, at age 32. This granddaughter plans to be a physician and also to have children late. Brenda became a mother at 24 and a grandmother at 56; her daughter Beth became a mother at 32 and expects to become a grandmother at age 65. Generations of this family are clearly farther apart in age than dictated by age norms, a pattern referred to as **age-gapped** (Bengtson et al., 1990).

Sarah Fulton married early, bearing her first child, Susan, at 19. Susan became pregnant at age 16 and gave birth to a daughter who followed her mother's example and had a first child at age 15. In this family, Sarah became a parent at 19, a grandparent at 35, and a great-grandparent at 50. Susan, the daughter, became a mother at 16 and a grandmother

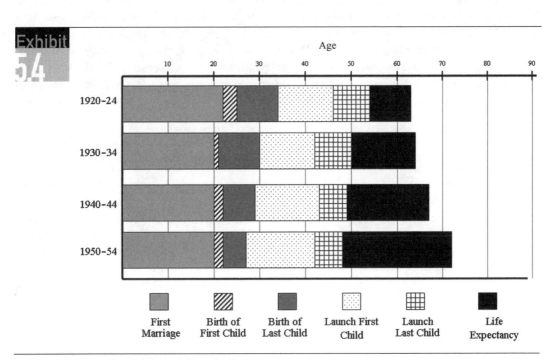

Life Event Timetables of Selected Female Cohorts
Source: Schmittroth, 1991.

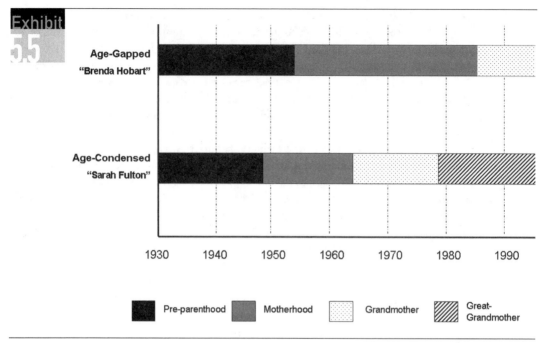

Exhibit 5.5

Timing of Age-Gapped and Age-Compressed Lives

at age 31. In this case, the generations are closer in age (**age-condensed**) in comparison to societal age norms (Bengtson et al., 1990). The potential for an increase in four- and five-generation families rests on two forces: longevity and the number of years between family generations. While individuals are living longer, the choices of family members regarding the age at which to procreate shape the timing of these events. While the Hobarts experienced an expansion of the time between generations, the Fultons encountered an increasingly rapid-fire addition of generations. Since very early childbearing is associated with negative outcomes (poorer income, education, and health) for both mothers and children, the relationships between generations for the Fultons, especially the dependence or independence of generations, may differ significantly from the experience of the Hobarts.

In a study of Canadian women, most women timed the events of their family lives (marriage, births of first and final child) in ways that fit social norms, but 35.7% were classified as following an age-condensed pattern and 9.1% fit the age-gapped pattern. Age-condensed women averaged less than 20 years of age at first marriage, had their first child at about the same age, and completed their three- or four-child average fertility within about 8 years. Age-gapped women, in contrast, first married at age 28, had their first child at age 32, and completed their to- or three-child average fertility in just under 6 years, resulting in very different patterns for the remainder of their lives (Kobayashi, Martin-Matthews, Rosenthal, & Matthews, 2001).

Although a set of age norms establishes when events in the family life cycle are expected to take place, these norms are subject to change. Events happening on time are not problematic, but family events that happen off time, especially early, are more challenging transitions (Cohler & Altergott, 1995). Grandmothers in age-condensed families are often

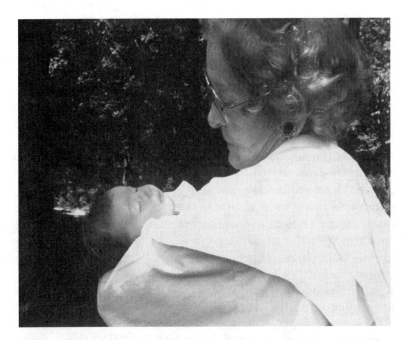

Great-grandparents and even great-great-grandparents are becoming more common as the average life span increases. (Credit: Mike Payne, courtesy of the Ohio Department of Aging)

uncomfortable with the early onset of this role, because it is viewed as occurring "off time" compared with their expectations (see Brubaker, 1990b). Both early childbearing and early widowhood are more stressful than comparable events that are off time by being late.

Divorce also plays a role in timing. People may have children in a first marriage, in a second or third marriage, or have multiple sets of children with different partners. In addition to contributing to the complexities discussed below, divorce and remarriage may mean that a single individual is parent to teenagers and newborns simultaneously with different spouses, presenting challenges not typical of their parents, for whom ordering of events through time typically was much clearer.

Greater Complexity of Family Relations

Although relatively few of the current population of older adults have experienced divorce, the percentage of ever-divorced persons will increase dramatically in future cohorts (Crown, Mutschler, Schulz, & Loew, 1993; Uhlenberg, Cooney, & Boyd, 1990). Unless the divorce rate, which increased dramatically after World War II and leveled off in the early 1980s, declines dramatically, coming cohorts will have a much higher percentage of people having one or more divorces as part of their life course experiences. Because the likelihood of remarriage diminishes rapidly for women as they age and given shorter male life expectancy, more women will enter later life in divorced status (Uhlenberg et al., 1990). Even among current cohorts of older adults, many have experienced the stress, familial dislocation, and relationship complexity resulting from the divorces of their children or grandchildren. Grandparents may lose touch with grandchildren or find themselves providing housing and childcare assistance to a newly divorced child in conjunction with a transition out of marriage (Johnson, 1995a). These responsibilities may tax the resources of aging couples or individuals.

Increasing numbers of older adults in future cohorts will have divorced, sometimes followed by remarriage. Many will have spent a considerable number of years in families with stepchildren (or with stepsiblings). There are probably important but not yet researched differences between older persons who are newly divorced and those who have spent a number of years in divorced status as they aged (Brubaker, 1990b). Given the association between divorced status and poorer economic security in later life (Crown et al., 1993), the coming cohorts of elders with their increased experience of divorce give society cause for concern (Uhlenberg et al., 1990).

Many unanswered questions about family relationships arise from the complex families that emerge in a society with divorce and remarriage. Will adult children feel strong filial obligation toward a biological parent, stepparent, or both? How enduring will relationships become between half- or stepsiblings as they grow older? How are decisions made about the priority of family obligations toward younger and older kin when there is a web of relatives (or former relatives) to whom one may feel some degree of duty? Who will have legal rights in terms of life-and-death health care decisions? Will men who have divorced have a sufficient network of social support as they move through later life (Cherlin, 2004)?

These complex changes in family relationships associated with the increase in divorce and remarriage have only begun to receive attention. Some research has confirmed a decrease in support exchanged or expected between fathers and adult children following divorce but has not confirmed a similar decline for mothers (Amato, Rezac, & Booth, 1995; Cooney & Uhlenberg, 1990). A national sample of adults was examined to see whether relationships were comparable for full siblings and step- or half-siblings (White & Reidmann, 1992). Full siblings had more contact and higher-quality relationships than stepsiblings, but having spent more time together in a household while growing up increased the amount of contact. Some factors that shape interactions between full siblings also influence stepsibling relations: Residential proximity, lower age, being female, and being Black were associated with more contact with siblings of all types. Thus, divorce seems to diminish the strength of relationships that may be critical to well-being in adulthood and later life.

SUMMARY

What conclusions can we draw about aging families? First, family relationships are maintained throughout life, holding deep personal and social significance for most individuals. Second, a set of social norms directs relationships within families, with variation in those norms by class, race, ethnicity, and gender. Not all persons are expected to act the same toward all other persons; structured relationships have their own norms in addition to general norms regarding obligation and reciprocity. The family as a social institution is a dynamic force within the larger society, both contributing to and responding to social changes in politics, the economy, and other social institutions. But families are also internally dynamic, experiencing ongoing change as new generational units are formed, add members, mature, and eventually pass from the scene as they age and die. Throughout this dynamism, however, are threads of continuity connecting the generations and patterns of family norms that are often passed down as part of familial heritage. Family relationships are a force for continuity in the lives of individuals, bridging decades of societal change.

It is difficult to talk about family as though it is a singular phenomenon. Families differ in structure; individual families change in composition and closeness over time; and forces such as class, race, and culture shape the manner in which family life unfolds. The age-integrating family system will undoubtedly continue its pattern of change in the coming decades. Four- and five-generation families will be paired with sequential marriages to create intricate and complex family systems that may be more or less responsive to the needs of older adults of future cohorts. As we age, the families we build and the manner in which we enact family roles will help to shape the norms for this future and the place of the family within it.

WEB WISE

Grandparenting: The Essential Sites

http://www.thirdage.com/guides/family/grandparenting.html

This Web site, operated by Third Age Media, provides advice, information, and support for grandparents raising grandchildren. It also shows links to other sites related to contemporary grandparenting issues.

Profile of Older Americans

http://www.aarp.org/research/reference/statistics/aresearch-import-519.html

AARP collaborates with the Administration on Aging and the U.S. Department of Health and Human Services to develop annual profiles on characteristics of the older population. Each year shows detailed tables on a range of characteristics, and several years' reports are available for comparisons through time on particular issues. Marital status and living arrangements are included.

KEY TERMS

age-condensed	filial obligation	modified extended family
age-gapped	five- or six-generation	norm of reciprocity
beanpole family	family	obligation
cohort centrism	generations	opportune family
dependence	independence	post-parental families
family	intergenerational	social norms
family life cycle	households	surrogate family
theory	intimacy at a distance	relationships
fictive kinship	later-life family	voluntarism

QUESTIONS FOR THOUGHT AND DISCUSSION

1. Do some genealogical sleuthing and map out the structure of your family tree. Examine such things as the number of siblings in various generations and ages at marriage and at death. What larger social changes in the institutions of the family do you see reflected in the history of your family?

2. Thinking about younger adults of today (in their 20s), what changes in the timing of family events, family norms, and individual behaviors are likely to differentiate their cohort experiences of family life from those of individuals in their 70s today?

3. Countries such as China, where family members had a strong tradition of housing and caring for their elders, are seeing pressures on those systems as economies modernize and the population urbanizes. Should countries try to enforce traditional patterns through laws and penalties or let go of old ways and adopt more Western styles of meeting the needs of elders for housing, health care, income support, etc.?

4. Riley, Kahn, and Foner (1994) describe the family as an age-integrating structure, because it links together individuals of different ages and historical eras. What impact might such age integration have on the society as a whole?

Aging Persons and Their Families

6

The myth that old people are alienated from their families and children has guided much of social gerontological research about the elderly for the last 30 years. ... [E]ach time evidence has been presented that old people are not alienated from their families, new adherents of the myth rise up. (Shanas, 1979a, p. 3)

Families as Personal Network Versus Public Institution

E arly gerontological theorists hypothesized that the family's importance to individuals increased as they aged and as other social roles and statuses (such as employment) fell away through disengagement (Cumming & Henry, 1961). These theorists thought that whatever life space remained to the individual was reallocated to remaining roles, including important familial roles (Neugarten, Moore, & Lowe, 1968). We have since learned that families carry importance to individuals throughout their lives; the family's span grows with increasing longevity to permit many shared decades with parents, spouses, siblings, and children.

Because of gendered views of family roles, early gerontologists also believed that women experienced aging with more ease than did men. Women were thought to have two family-based advantages. First, a primary identity with the family, as opposed to employment, guaranteed a strong source of continuity throughout their lives in the kinship system. Second, because family roles involve continual changes with the addition, maturation, and departure of family members, women were thought to be more accustomed to changes than were men, whose continuity of identity (presumed to be in employment, rather than in the family) would be suddenly interrupted for the first

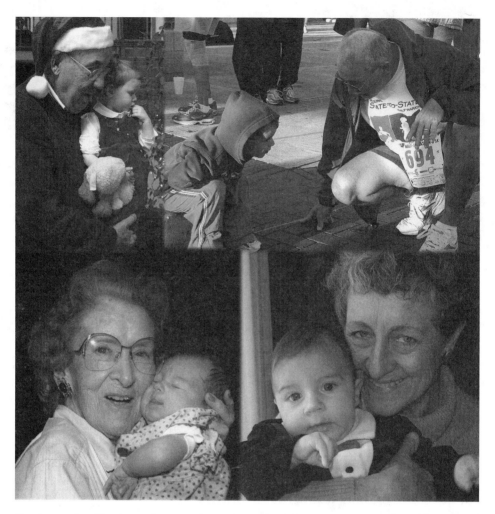

Our increasing life span allows more years to cherish spouses, children, grandchildren, great-grandchildren, and other family members. (Credit: E. J. Hanna and Mike Payne, courtesy of the Ohio Department of Aging)

time at retirement (Maddox, 1968). We now recognize that these ideas are overly simplistic and stereotype both sexes. Today women and men clearly hold core role identities both in families and in employment; nonetheless, these early gender-based assumptions were important in shaping the questions posed by researchers.

Of the aging topics studied from a social perspective, perhaps the largest body of research is associated with family relationships and their impact on the older individual. Most of the research is micro level in its analysis, focusing on small-group or two–person relationships or on individuals' reactions to their families. Few researchers have examined mid-level or macro-level questions relating to the family, although there are many of interest. Because the material in this area is so extensive, the information presented in this chapter is necessarily selective.

Strengths in Later-Life Families

Families are resilient and resourceful groups that connect us to the past and to the future in personally meaningful ways. In addition, families provide a close network of emotional and practical support that shifts over time as their members and their capacities and involvements change over the life course. Family members are usually pivotal in the "convoys of support" that provide continuity over time with individuals as they grow, mature, and age (Antonucci & Akiyama, 1987). Typically individuals consider family roles among their core identities and hold high expectations for the part that the family plays in meeting their emotional, social, and personal needs (Cherlin, 2004).

As discussed in chapter 4, the focus on individualism within the family is relatively new in historical terms and characterizes Westernized cultures rather than family systems everywhere (Cherlin, 2004). Social norms regarding the place of families in the lives of individuals have changed from earlier historical periods in the United States, when families in the largely agricultural economy were units of basic survival for their members (see Giarrusso, Feng, & Bengtson, 2004). No longer do adult sons wait to inherit the farm from an aging father (Hareven, 1993); instead they seek education and employment independent of their families and may move far away to pursue careers, fundamentally changing the role of the family from one of obligation and economic interdependence to one that is more voluntary and supportive (Hess & Waring, 1978). The higher expectations for emotional gratification within the modern family have also been linked to other more negatively viewed changes, such as the growth in the divorce rate (Cherlin, 2004). Nonetheless, for most individuals the family is a source of continuity, meaning, and connection throughout life.

Despite the strengths and positive connotations of family bonds, not all relationships among kin are close and affectionate, including those involving older adults. Just as positive and supportive relationships can have a positive impact on the lives of older adults, negative interactions add to psychological distress and increase risks of chronic illness (Finch & Graziano, 2001; Wolff & Agree, 2004). Some family bonds may be distant or acrimonious over many decades as a result of early-life events. For example, if a father and teenage son have had a difficult relationship, punctuated by serious conflict, it is unlikely that this conflicted history will be forgotten in later decades and that they will develop unambiguously warm and affectionate bonds (Suitor et al., 1994). Negative aspects of family relationships may coexist simultaneously with positive ones in the same relationship, reminding us not to stereotype family relationships of older adults as being either purely positive or purely negative (Pillemer & Suitor, 2004). The normative obligations that exist in family relationships also mean that relatives, even those with some negative feelings or history between them, will most often continue to maintain some type of family ties (Krause & Rook, 2003).

Strengths of families as units and as resources for older adults are also tested by changes that have taken place in family systems in the late 20th century. Fewer adults are marrying and are doing so later, divorce rates continue to be high, and both premarital and post-divorce cohabitation are increasingly common. Stepfamily relationships are everywhere. As described in the last chapter, these changes are gradually moving the family lives of older adults in directions that are sometimes difficult to predict. Regardless of these changes and limitations, the value of the family remains pivotal to the vast majority of people of all ages.

Continuities in Later-Life Families

Brubaker (1990a) defines a **later-life family** as one that is moving through the child-launching phase and into the post-parental phase, in which couples may eventually experience retirement, health limitations, and widowhood. Spousal, parental, and sibling relationships are well established by the time families reach this stage. Typically these relationships exhibit considerable continuity in how they operate over time. One approach to understanding family relationships in later life is to examine these continuities.

Family members are typically involved to some degree with one another's lives, providing advice and emotional support, making demands on time and loyalty, and sometimes giving or seeking assistance both across and within generations. This mutual exchange is so routine that it is hardly noticed as anything special or important by members of the family. It is these regular, ongoing activities and traditions that constitute the bulk of family relationships over the years (Matthews, 2002). On occasion, however, a crisis intervenes to upset the routine operation of established kin relationships. A crisis can be a non-normative event, such as the divorce of an adult child, or the more expected, but no less stressful, illness of an older parent. In these circumstances, family relationships may change, with shifts in living arrangements, increased assistance, or more frequent interaction. Major transition events, either positive or negative, may call for at least a temporary and sometimes a permanent modification of the established patterns that have characterized family relationships. Although the research literature focuses on events of change and crisis, the great majority of time that families share is based in the routine, not the extraordinary, aspects of life.

Key Familial Roles and Relationships

Despite being a group, the family has largely been studied from the perspective of the individual member. Research studies tend to focus on single family members as units of analysis, not **dyads** (two-person relationships) or the complete family network. Most research examines the family through the eyes of only one of its participants, a limited view on such a complex system of roles and linkages. Consequently, the research described in this section focuses on views of the individual about dyadic relationships within the family.

Spouses/Aging Couples

The majority of older men (78% of those 65–74 and 73% of those 75–84) were listed as "currently married" in 2003 (Federal Interagency Forum on Aging-Related Statistics, 2004). For women the picture is quite different, with 56% of women 65–74, but only 36% of women aged 75–84, currently married. Instead, the growing category for women is found among the widowed, reflecting women's higher life expectancy and lower age at marriage . Few women or men in today's older cohorts were divorced or never married, figures that may change in the future (see Exhibit 6.1). These figures on marriage overlook older individuals who are in couples without being married (Huyck, 1995). These

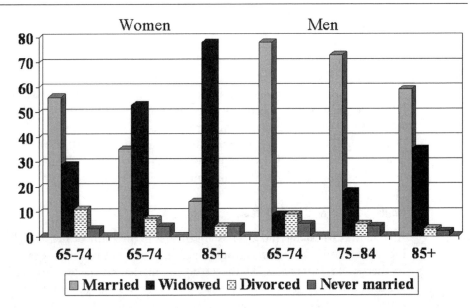

Marital Status by Sex and Age, 2003
Source: Federal Interagency Forum on Aging-Related Statistics, 2004.

uncounted individuals are often erroneously presumed to be without an intimate relationship because they are not legally married.

Marital relationships for persons born in the United States at the turn of the last century were much shorter than today. Given median ages at marriage then of 21.2 for women and 24.6 for men and average life expectancies of about 51 years for White women and 48 years for White men (35 and 32.5 years, respectively, for Black women and men), it is not surprising that many persons were widowed before their children were grown (National Center for Health Statistics, 1989; U.S. Bureau of the Census, 1991a). Today, couples marrying at higher median ages (27 for men, 25 for women) can, because of increased life expectancy, expect to be married 50 or more years. Of course, about half of first marriages don't make it to that landmark, but the reason today is primarily divorce rather than death of a spouse (Cherlin, 2004). This increasing potential duration of marriage has led to suggestions, only half humorous, that growing divorce rates may be one of the outcomes of greater longevity. Couples who might be able to tolerate a problematic marital relationship for 15 or 20 years choose not to endure it for 50 or 60 years, opting instead for divorce. Most divorces occur among younger rather than older adults, but this pattern, too, may differ among older adults in the future.

Marriage does not remain static over the second half of adult life, because the roles and responsibilities of the partners change over time with the launching of children, the deaths of family members, and the addition of grandparental roles (Huyck, 1995). Differences may also exist between marriage cohorts (groups married at different times in history) in the manner in which household labor is divided and gender relations are structured. It is possible to confuse the effects of aging with cohort differences. In many of today's retired middle-class couples, the wives were homemakers and probably continue to do much of the household work in retirement, but baby boomer couples will reach retirement with a two-earner couple having been typical and a more even division of household chores.

Decades ago, deriving her approach from conflict theory, Jesse Bernard (1972) suggested that within each marital relationship were actually two marriages—"her" marriage and "his" marriage—with differing expectations, responsibilities, and pressures. This view seems to have been supported by studies revealing that men benefit more (in terms of greater life expectancy, higher life satisfaction, and better health) than women do from being married. Perhaps this is due to more of the work involved in maintaining family relationships (called **kin-keeping**) and the household falling to women (Bengtson et al., 1990; Rogers, 1995). Marriage thus benefits men more than women.

Marital Satisfaction Over the Life Course

Among the earliest and most persistent themes in the study of marital relations in later life is that of **marital satisfaction**—the degree to which couples are satisfied with their partners and relationships. An early study on marital satisfaction involved a longitudinal comparison of 400 couples married in the early 1930s (Pineo, 1961). In this study couples were evaluated soon after marriage and again 20 years later. Results showed lower marital satisfaction at the 20-year mark, a change that Pineo dubbed "marital disenchantment." Other studies have confirmed a similar decline in satisfaction over the first years of marriage (Lee, 1988).

Later cross-sectional analyses of satisfaction among couples of different marital cohorts and ages suggest that marital satisfaction follows a curvilinear path—from a peak during the honeymoon to a valley during the rearing of children, followed by an improvement as couples move through child launching and into later life. This research has been criticized for concluding that individual couples go through this curvilinear pattern because the researchers (1) compared across cohorts with very different marital experiences; (2) relied on the average marital satisfaction score to describe a highly variable trait of marriages; and (3) ignored the survivorship effect (as time passes, many of the unhappiest couples get divorced, leaving behind a pool of marital survivors who were probably happiest all along) (see Vaillant & Vaillant, 1993; Weishaus & Field, 1988).

Recent research has not resolved the confusion by revealing any uniform pattern of change with aging. One analysis found no "typical" pattern of change in marital satisfaction in conjunction with aging (Weishaus & Field, 1988). Gary Lee (1988) contends that role overload might be responsible for declining marital satisfaction in mid-life and its subsequent improvement in later life. His cross-sectional research suggests that reduction of parental roles (as children become adults) is associated with improvements in marital satisfaction, but that loss of or exit from other roles has no similar effect. In another study, golden-wedding-anniversary couples, true marital survivors, were asked to describe retrospectively their levels of marital satisfaction at various times during the family life cycle. The results, interestingly, showed the curvilinear pattern for both men and women, but with wives reporting a deeper decline in marital happiness during the middle-age and early old-age periods (mirroring Bernard's concept of "his" and "hers" marital experiences). Wives experienced more distress during child launching than did husbands, whose satisfaction improved during that period (Condie, 1989). Other studies have confirmed that the "empty nest," created by the launching of children into

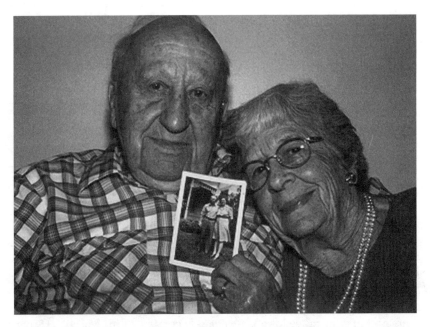

Many married couples observe that their love grows stronger in the later years.
(Credit: Mike Payne, courtesy of the Ohio Department of Aging)

adulthood, results in improved marital happiness of partners (White & Edwards, 1990), rather than the distress described by popular culture. Again, we must be cautious not to generalize too quickly beyond these cohorts, where marital experiences differ from couples in subsequent cohorts or to universal reactions among highly varied couples.

Termination of Marriage: Widows and Widowers

The differential in average life expectancy dictates that more women than men will survive their spouses (Kinsella & Taeuber, 1993). Past the age of 65, widows outnumbered widowers 4.7 to 1 in the United States in 2000 (U.S. Bureau of the Census, 2005a). As Exhibit 6.2 shows, the incidence of widowhood increases overall with age, but the gender gap remains. Added to the life-expectancy differential are the facts that: (1) women tend to marry men older than themselves and (2) widowers have ample opportunity to remarry, should they wish to do so (Bengtson et al., 1990). Both because of their larger numbers and more pressing problems (e.g., higher rates of poverty), most widowhood research has been conducted on women rather than men.

The transition from married to widowed is one of the most stressful, removing a central role identity as wife or husband and the relationship to the late spouse, changing social relationships with friends, collapsing the division of labor in the household, modifying relationships with kin and friends, and often diminishing economic well-being. Marital roles are highly salient to individuals of all ages, structuring much of their identity and social activities. Even an unhappy marriage influences self-concept and activities. The loss of this relationship has both expected and unexpected consequences. Widowed women, for example, experience a disruption in their friendship networks, which are (at least for the middle class) based on couples that interact socially with other

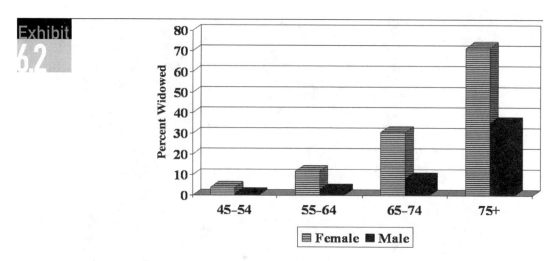

Exhibit
6.2

Percentage of Men and Women Widowed by Age, 2000
Source: U.S. Bureau of the Census, 2003a.

couples. Upon being widowed, a woman becomes a "fifth wheel," creating social dis-comfort if she continues to socialize with her former friendship group (Lopata, 1979). Gradually, most widows modify their friendship and social patterns, spending less time with married friends and more time with other widows.

In earlier cohorts, a gender-based division was more strictly maintained. This meant that many women and men who were widowed were unfamiliar with (and thus unable to perform) the tasks assigned to the spouse. Among the oldest cohorts of women, these un-familiar tasks often included driving, managing finances, and overseeing household repairs (Lund, Caserta, Dimond, & Shaffer, 1989). Among men, who often went from the home of their parents to marriage, many never learned how to cook, manage family or social networks, or clean house. The strict division of labor meant that the surviving spouse was vulnerable in terms of the other spouse's tasks; widowers might not eat properly and wid-ows might manage their money poorly. In more recent cohorts of couples, this strictness of the division of labor attenuates, and the young cohorts of today typically spend some time living on their own and learn most of the basic survival skills once divided into strict male or female duties. While tasks still may be divided between the couple while they are married, fewer should enter widowhood completely without knowledge of these tasks.

Among the most important changes in family relationships following widowhood are those relating to children. Relationships with adult children are intensified, as sons and daughters assist the surviving parent (Lopata, 1979). Long-term modifications in these relationships, however, tend to be specific by gender. The amount of interaction with adult children increases and persists at the higher level for widows, but widow-ers' levels of contact with adult children remain similar to those during their married lives (Morgan, 1984). Why this difference? One possible explanation is the emotionally closer relationships felt toward mothers (Finley et al., 1988) or the concern that widows are more vulnerable following the loss of their spouses (Morgan, 1984). In either case, widowed persons in the United States, conforming to norms of independence and intimacy at a distance, seldom move in with adult children if they are healthy and have adequate income, unless their culture dictates otherwise.

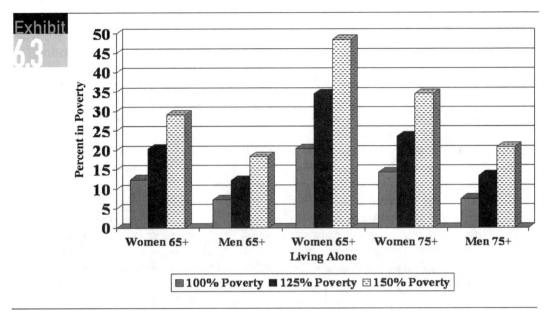

Risks of Being Poor/Near Poor by Household Status and Sex, 2003
Source: U.S. Census Bureau, 2003a.

Economic security is especially tenuous for widows, in part because of the rules for Social Security and private pensions (see chapters 8 and 9 for further details). As Exhibit 6.3 shows, rates of poverty are significantly higher for widowed women living alone than for other women or for men over age 65. Both Social Security and private pension systems were developed when wives in the middle class were economic dependents of their husbands, so rules presume him to be the primary breadwinner. Both systems were established primarily to protect workers (men/husbands) and secondarily to protect their dependents (wives and growing children). Social Security, upon the death of the beneficiary, reduces the benefits to a widowed woman who was a traditional homemaker to 66% of the couple's amount, although research suggests that the survivor needs 80% of the couple's previous income to maintain her standard of living (Burkhauser & Smeeding, 1994). In addition, until 1985 many retiring employees received pensions with no survivor protection. Thus, many widows were forced to adjust economically from sharing a Social Security benefit *plus* private pension to having only two-thirds of the prior Social Security benefit. In addition, movement over recent decades to greater reliance on 401(k)-type pension programs (see chapter 9) increases widowed persons' risk of becoming poor, since many exclude spouse protection (Johnson, Uccello, & Goldwyn, 2005). Widowers, in contrast to widows, also see their benefits from Social Security reduced after the death of a wife, but more typically maintained their private pensions. Under these conditions, it is predictable that poverty among older, widowed women has been among the most persistent problems (Burkhauser & Smeeding, 1994).

Parents and Children

We discussed a number of issues that are central to understanding the nature of parent-child relationships in chapter 5. As both parents and their children mature, the dependencies between them shift, reciprocity becomes a long-term pattern, and there is continuity in the contact between generations and its quality (positive, negative, or mixed). For most of the adult years, these relationships are governed by the norm of independence. Parenting varies across cohorts, simply because the numbers of children born to cohorts differ, sometimes substantially. As Exhibit 6.4 shows, cohorts of women born between 1906 and 1910 had significantly lower fertility than did their successors born between 1931 and 1935. Thinking about the time frames during which these cohorts of women were having their families, how might you use historical events (period effects) to partially explain these differences? Today, fertility is much lower, hovering around replacement level (2.1 births per woman) nationally but varying across class, race, and educational groupings.

Beyond these central characteristics, two contrasting themes have characterized discussions of relationships between older parents and adult children over the years. The first, and perhaps most persistent, mythical theme regarding later-life families is that adult children neglect and abandon their older parents, indicative of the poor relationships between them (Shanas, 1979a, 1979b). This theme of abandonment was described in the quotation opening the chapter. The second theme is that of family solidarity, support, and affection as universally descriptive of parent–child bonds in later life. Although these themes have traded places in terms of prominence over time, both probably reflect unrealistic stereotyping of parent–child relationships. As is often the case, the truth lies somewhere in between.

A good deal of research has been conducted on the levels and types of interactions between adult generations in a family. According to research in this area, older persons are not isolated from their families, and a majority of interactions across the generations are positive (Bengtson et al., 1985). Interestingly, it is often assumed that *more* interaction is *better* for the elderly family members, ignoring the possibility of prior conflict in

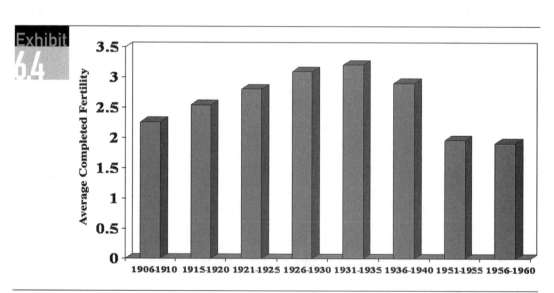

Variations in Completed Fertility for Birth Cohorts of Women
Source: Bachu, 1997; U.S. Bureau of the Census, 2001.

familial relationships (Antonucci, 1990). This oversimplifies relationships between parents and children, where majorities recognize some conflicts in their relationship along with prominent positive aspects (Antonucci, 1990; Clarke, Preston, Raksin, & Bengtson, 1999; Lueschler & Pillemer, 1998).

In an effort to overcome the myth of family abandonment of the elderly, researchers may have gone too far in emphasizing support and consensus within the family. It would clearly be a mistake to assume that family relationships are untroubled, and that more is always better in terms of family interaction. At the other extreme is **neglect and abuse** of older persons by family members, often those providing care for them (Steinmetz, 1988). Relationships with older family members, either within or between generations of a kinship group, may have a lengthy history of stress and violence. As discussed earlier, growing older does not cure troubled family relationships or reduce tension and violence.

There is more than one potential explanation for elder abuse. First, some researchers argue that abuse and neglect result from violations of the norm of independence. When an older person becomes dependent, it violates this norm and places an unexpected stress on the relationship with a caregiver, especially a child (Gelles & Cavanaugh, 2005). A second hypothesis, not yet thoroughly tested with regard to elder abuse, is that violence is a product of reciprocity; that is, adult children who are violent toward a frail parent are returning violence that they received as children. Indirect support for this argument comes from studies showing that children from violent families are more likely to be violent toward kin (Wallace, 1996). Some researchers suggest that elder abuse is related to pathology and dependency (Steinmetz, 2005).

Finally, research has examined the fact that many of those committing abuse and neglect are *spouses*, not adult children. What remains unclear is whether this abuse began when the person reached later life (or physical dependency), or whether this pattern of violence is a long-standing characteristic of the marital relationship (Vinton, 1991). Since not all couples experiencing violence get divorced, especially in today's older cohorts where divorce was less acceptable, one component of elder abuse may be "spousal violence grown old" (Harris, 1995).

Parent-child relationships are influenced by a variety of factors. Increasing life expectancy means that often the child caring for an aging parent is old—for example, a 65-year-old "child" caring for a 90-year-old parent. Second, smaller family size means a changing ratio of younger to older family members, lessening the availability of kin for support and kin-keeping functions. Third, mobility has meant that adult children are less geographically proximate to their parents, modifying the numbers and types of interactions possible between them. Not all researchers are convinced that the changes in intergenerational relations will be as dramatic or occur as quickly as some anticipate. Demographer Peter Uhlenberg (1993) contends that the changes over the next several decades will be slow and gradual, enabling ample time for societal and individual adaptations to changes in the family structure.

Research has consistently suggested that parent and child gender influence the relationship between them. Mother-daughter dyads are typically closer than any other combination, with more daughters acting as confidantes and fewer likely to disappoint their mothers (see Suitor, Pillemer, Keeton, & Robison, 1994). The relationship most likely to experience conflict is that between a father and son, with cross-gender dyads (mother-son, father-daughter) falling somewhere in between.

Siblings

A majority of older adults have one or more siblings with whom they continue to interact in later life (Brubaker, 1990b). Sibling relationships have some unique characteristics that differentiate them from other familial ties. First, sibling relationships are likely to be the longest-enduring kinship bonds (Brubaker, 1990a). Whereas a marriage typically starts after 20 or more years of life have elapsed, siblings are often born only a few years apart. Because they live their early lives in physical proximity, siblings essentially share a childhood in the family (Cicirelli, 1991). In addition, siblings often share a cohort and its experiences at similar points in their lifetimes, encountering the same major innovations, historical events, and societal value shifts. Since kin, unlike friends, are not chosen, there are no guarantees of closeness or affection in their relationships. Indeed, the aftermath of sibling rivalry or violence can exact a toll on these relationships throughout adulthood (Scott, 1990).

Changes in Contact and Intimacy Through Life

Until recently, most of the research on bonds between siblings presumed that, after adolescence, siblings were unimportant (Bedford, 1995). More recently, limited studies of siblings have suggested a continuing salience of these relationships throughout adulthood (Bedford, 1995; Cicirelli, 1991; Scott, 1990). Although their energies may be absorbed by their spouses and children in early to middle adulthood, siblings maintain emotional bonds and tend to reactivate their bonds (if they have become dormant) as they mature and their children depart (Bedford, 1995).

Siblings can and do provide friendship and support to one another as adults (Wellman & Wortley, 1989), often maintaining relationships even when they are not geographically proximate. Exchanges among siblings seldom include financial aid or substantial assistance with health care, probably because of norms of independence (Suitor & Pillemer, 1993; Wellman & Wortley, 1989). There is some evidence that the amount of intersibling support and assistance declines in old age (Bedford, 1989), but this research is rather limited by small, unrepresentative samples.

Variations in Sibling Linkages

Not all sibling relationships are created equal. A range of social factors shapes how a sibling relationship will be enacted through adulthood and later life. As with other family relationships, research shows that sibling bonds vary across racial and ethnic groups. Two major studies have confirmed that older Blacks rely more on siblings for assistance than do their White or Hispanic counterparts; these results are especially compelling because income differences were not a factor—all groups studied had low family incomes (Bedford, 1995). The norm of independence from siblings may be weaker and expectations of reciprocity stronger in the culture of Black and Hispanic families.

The number of siblings is also important, because the amount of support given by any single brother or sister may be limited. Not surprisingly, the more siblings a person has, the more likely it is that she or he relies on one as a confidante or provider of support (Connidis & Davies, 1992). But older adults who have other family relationships, such as adult children, may turn to them rather than to a sibling for some types of support. Marital status also influences the interdependence of siblings. Individuals who have never married or those whose marriages have ended appear to turn more to siblings for assistance (see Bedford, 1995). Being married and having one's own children are thought to provide more compelling role involvements, pushing sibling relationships to a somewhat lower priority.

Finally, what is the role of gender in shaping the closeness of sibling bonds? Some early research has suggested that relationships with a sister are closer; other studies suggest that same-sex dyads are closer than those consisting of a brother and sister (Bedford, 1995; Scott, 1990). Same-sex pairs, especially sisters, are noted for the stronger emotional bonds throughout their lives (Cicirelli, 1991).

Grandparents

What pictures come to mind in thinking about grandparents? Typically we carry mental images of grandparents that feature advanced age, gray hair, leisure, kindness, and celebration of family rituals and holiday traditions fostered by advertisers. Do grandparents really fit this image? What exactly do grandparents do?

Most persons now over age 65 are parents, and most have also become grandparents, often well before reaching old age. Although being a grandparent is a familial role that most people associate with later life, most individuals enter grandparenthood while still in mid-life, married, employed, and with one or more surviving parents and a child still living at home (Bengtson et al., 1990). For women this means spending nearly half their lives as grandparents. As we saw in chapter 5, the timing of grandparenthood is highly variable, depending in large measure on the age at which an individual bears his or her own children.

Although entry into grandparenthood is variable, once entered it is an enduring role, lasting until the grandparent's death. By that time the grandchildren are often grown parents themselves and surviving grandparents have aged decades. Neither partner nor the relationship remains static. Grandparents report that they enjoy their roles best when grandchildren (and grandparents) are young (Cherlin & Furstenberg, 1986).

Voluntary Nature of Grandparenting in Middle-Class Families

What are the duties and rights of a grandparent? As a social role, being a grandparent is not well structured. Early research, mostly on White middle-class grandparents, has attempted to identify the roles played by grandparents within the family system and toward the grandchildren (Roberto, 1990). Relatively few clear-cut duties are mandated for grandparents, because their roles, unlike those of parents, typically are not critical to the survival of children. Given that only recently have large numbers of people lived long enough to spend much time as grandparents, the lack of behavioral norms is understandable. This cultural void gives grandparents the chance to structure the role in any way they see fit, but it also provides them with few guidelines on how they should act as grandparents (Kennedy, 1990). Probably as a result, much of the early work on grandparenting has focused on how adults view and structure their relationships with grandchildren. Several studies have identified styles of grandparenting, showing a wide variation in how the relationships are viewed by their partners (Roberto, 1990).

Less research has examined the relationship from the perspective of the grandchild. One study (Kennedy, 1990) asked more than 700 college students about their grand-

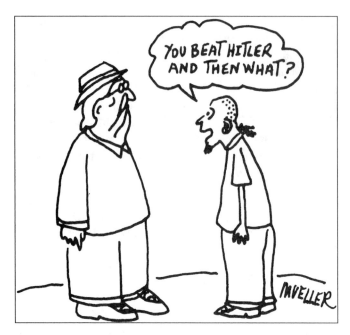

parents' roles. "Students tended to agree most strongly with items that described grandparents as being loving, helping and comforting, as providing role models, and sharing family history, as being persons who are important in the lives of young people and persons with whom they have fun." The responsibilities of grandchildren were to "express love and provide help to their grandparents, that they are a part of their grandparents' sense of the future" (Kennedy, 1990, pp. 45–46). Within the sample, female students emphasized the closeness of the relationships, and Black students described grandparenting as a more active role. Even with these expectations, however, there is a wide range of ways in which grandparents could fulfill this role.

Relationships between grandparents and grandchildren are built within a larger context of family relationships. The middle generation plays a critical role, linking the older and younger generations. This role has been described as the **lineage bridge**—the span connecting two generations (Thompson & Walker, 1987). The quality of the relationships between the grandparents and parents, acting as lineage bridges, will inevitably shape the closeness, geographic proximity, and frequency and types of interaction between grandparents and grandchildren. This linkage becomes especially important in the case of divorce, where paternal grandparents may lose contact with grandchildren unless they maintain ties to their former daughter-in-law or exercise legal rights to visitation (Roberto, 1990).

Variations in Grandparenting Roles

Beyond differences based on the respective ages of grandparents and grandchildren, other factors that influence the bonds between grandparents and grandchildren include economic status, race/ethnicity, and gender. Overall 3.9 million American grandchildren (5.5% of children under age 18) lived in the same household with their grandparents in 1997 (Bryson & Casper, 1999); most often the head of household is the grandparent, so that dependencies involve middle and younger generations rather than grandparents, many of whom are relatively young (Bryson & Casper, 1999). The percentages sharing a home are higher for Black than for White children. Almost 13% of Black children live with grandparents, and 36% of those children have neither of their parents living with them, creating a skipped-generation household. Nearly 6% of Black adults over age 45 are caring for a grandchild, with more women than men, more disadvantaged than well-off, and more physically challenged individuals likely to have a grandchild in their care—including those who share a residence (Minkler & Fuller-Thompson,

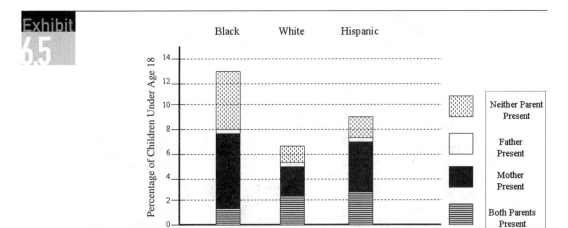

Children Under Age 18 Living in Grandparents' Households by Race/Ethnicity
Source: U.S. Bureau of the Census, 2003a.

2005). Smaller but significant percentages of White (6.2%) and Hispanic grandchildren (9.4%) share a household with at least one grandparent (U.S. Bureau of the Census, 2003a). Exhibit 6.5 shows significant differences by race in the percentages of grandchildren who reside with their grandparents. Within each group, most children live with their mother and one or more grandparents, but a substantial number live with grandparents only, without either parent in the household (Saluter, 1996; U.S. Bureau of the Census, 2003a).

In these and other instances, grandparents take on active roles in lieu of parents, acting as **surrogate parents.** Grandparents acting as surrogate parents take on short- or long-term responsibility for care of grandchildren because of the problems of their adult children (including illness, job loss, drug abuse, homelessness, and incarceration) and because policy changes in the 1980s and 1990s supported "kinship care" when children needed to be placed in foster homes (Cherlin & Furstenberg, 1986; Hogan, Eggebeen, & Clogg, 1993; Minkler & Fuller-Thompson, 2005; U.S. Bureau of the Census, 1991a, 2003a). This unexpected resumption of parenting responsibilities can be stressful for the grandparents, who may be facing challenges associated with health or income (Burton & DeVries, 1995).

Families as Caregivers

Considerable attention has been given to family caregiving, both in research and in the media, as the number of very old adults in the population has swelled. In fact, examining some of the literature, one might come to the conclusion that caregiving is the major factor in most family relationships involving adults over age 65. But let's stop for a minute and consider this issue. Even if many individuals now live into their 80s and 90s or beyond, typically they do not require care and support from the day they turn 65. Instead, the need for care is typically delayed to more advanced ages, and for some individuals, death is unexpected and preceded by little or no period of illness or dependency. In

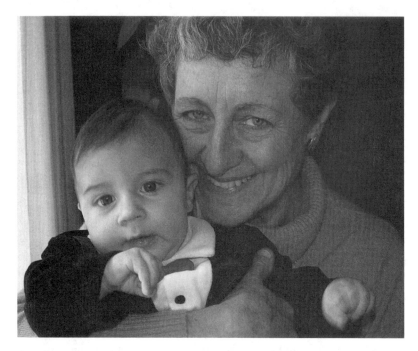

Age, income, gender, and other variables are tied to the closeness of relationships between grandparents and grandchildren. (Credit: E. J. Hanna)

recent decades typical families have experienced many years after retirement age where
older kin and their adult, middle-aged children enjoy a time when neither generation has
been dependent on the other. So, although caregiving is a challenge for many families
and an issue in the larger society, it is not a long and inevitable "sentence" for every
family relationship involving someone over 64. And, more importantly, when caregiving
needs arise, it is not a purely negative experience, as we explore in more detail below.

Applying Theory

Exchange Theory and Family Caregiving

What is really happening when individuals, groups,
or societies interact with one another? What is the
essence of the interactions that occur every day on
any level from person to person or corporation to
corporation or nation to nation? One framework
for answering these questions derives from **social
exchange theory**. This theory views social life as
consisting of exchanges among social actors (individuals or groups) of a variety of valuable resources,
including material goods, financial resources, and
intangible social goods (humor, respect, information) (Dowd, 1975). In a traditional middle-class
marriage of the 1950s, for example, it was expected
that the husband provided income for which the
wife exchanged household work and child care. In a
friendship, friends exchange emotional support, information, respect, and help of various types in an
ongoing fashion. Social exchange may also happen
across a range of levels; individuals may exchange
with organizations (such as exchanging work effort
for a paycheck); companies may exchange with countries (taxes for services).

(continued)

(continued)

Exchange theorists argue that social life is based on these exchanges, in which the parties desire to maximize their exchanges by getting as much back relative to what they give in exchange. If one party to the exchange is not receiving an equitable return, that party will withdraw and seek other exchanges. But social life is not quite that simple. In exchange theory it is essential to consider whether those making exchanges hold equal power (equal resources), because power influences how the exchange will occur. More powerful exchange partners—whether individuals, corporations, community groups, or nations—have a larger reserve of valued resources to give. Being privileged in this way, they have a wide range of potential partners eagerly awaiting an exchange opportunity. Because they can pick and choose among exchange partners, they can control the terms of the exchange to their own benefit.

In applying the concepts of exchange theory to aging, Dowd (1975) proposed that individuals in Western societies systematically gain power throughout mid-life and lose power and resources as they age, putting them at a disadvantage in exchanges. This loss of power may lead to unequal exchange relationships and force older people to behave in ways that are not of their choosing. Dowd defines the process of retirement as one of exchanging the prestige and higher wages of employment for the security of a fixed income and health benefits (pension, Social Security, and Medicare). In an unequal power situation with an employer, employees may be prompted to "choose" to retire either by improvements in the exchange rate if they comply (a "golden parachute" benefits package) or by the prospect of a much less profitable exchange should they stay.

In terms of "acting one's age," Dowd argues, "The older person who restricts his social life for fear of what his acquaintances would think is actually exchanging his compliance to their standards of acceptable conduct for their social approval" (p. 591). Because older persons may lack high incomes and powerful social positions and are, as a group, socially devalued, they must give more to maintain their exchanges, further depleting their limited resources.

Applying exchange theory to the family, we could examine the relative power of participants in the exchange—which may be shaped by age, gender, family roles, or other social factors—as well as the various types of exchanges that are ongoing in family life and those undertaken under special, crisis conditions. Principles of exchange and reciprocity are sometimes visible in the support of various types that occurs in later-life families, including caregiving for elderly kin. How does exchange play a role? Some people argue that caregiving by adult children is essentially delayed reciprocity—a repayment on a deferred debt for caregiving received while they were children. In this sense, the norm of reciprocity is a special case of exchange theory operating between the generations.

Some research suggests that keeping the exchange at least somewhat even is important to the well-being of participants. Older relatives who are recipients of support often value the opportunity to help their children or grandchildren in return, even if that support involves simply being a good listener or giving advice (Pearlin, Aneshensel, Mullan, & Whitlach, 1996). Support provided to others—whether emotional, financial, health care or other types—enables feelings of independence important to well-being (Stansfield, 1999). Both giving and receiving support remains important to older adults as a continuous aspect of family ties over time (Liang, Krause, & Bennett, 2001). People with health impairments requiring a lot of physical care can, by broadly defining support that is exchanged to include being a good listener and advisor, understand that they are still making a contribution (Walker, Martin, & Jones, 1992).

Context of Ongoing Norms of Mutual Assistance

Families have always served both their members and the larger society by providing various types of support and assistance to their members (Cherlin, 2004). This support has received considerable research attention, because of the needs of various dependent members, including children, disabled, or frail elders. These supports vary across the life course; across class, culture, and ethnic groups; and historically within a given culture. Within families, support flows both within and across generational boundaries.

Our understanding of caregiving toward older adults should be nested within the long histories of mutual support that typically exist in families, rather than as something new or distinct (Davey, Savla, & Janke, 2004). Wives and husbands continue to care for one another. Children and parents exchange support of various types over time, providing a template for how assistance comes to older adults as needs arise. Sarah Matthews (2002) examined patterns of assistance toward parents over 75 and found that the gender of the participants and the long history of family relationships provide a key to understanding who provides care, how it is shared or specialized among relatives, and ways in which the older adult participates in the care. In other words, support is a natural, ongoing aspect of family relationships that shifts over time as needs and capacities of members change; intensive caregiving is a subset of this larger pattern.

Intergenerational Support

Despite ideas in the mid-1900s that nuclear family units were independent of outside assistance, a 50-year research tradition reveals ongoing patterns of exchange both within and among related households. Among the pioneering work was that of Reuben Hill (1970), who examined the exchanges among three-generation families in the 1950s. That study showed that family members in all generations were typically involved in giving and receiving assistance of several types, including assistance during illness, child care, financial aid, emotional support, and household management. Hill's research found the middle generation to be net givers of support—that is, they provided more types of help to other generations (their elderly parents and their adult children) than they received. As Exhibit 6.6 shows, the young adult generation more commonly received assistance and gave less. The grandparent generation gave the least and received the most help with household tasks, illness, and emotional support, but (for obvious reasons) received no child care support. Hill's analysis, though path-breaking, was rather unsophisticated. It did not take into account issues such as the frequency with which each type of assistance might be given—for example, child care might be daily, whereas assistance during illness might occur only a few times each year—or the amount of time and energy each task demanded. In addition, the sample was not highly diverse, being primarily White and working to middle class.

Amato and his colleagues (1995) replicated this work 40 years later, including four types of assistance studied by Hill and his colleagues, sampling exchanges of assistance between just two generations, young adults (19+ years of age, still living at home) and their parents (see Exhibit 6.6). In Amato's study, adult children were much more likely to provide assistance with household tasks (understandable for a shared residence with parents), and many more said they both gave and received advice. The fact that fewer received child care help than in the Hill study may have to do with the fact that fewer in the second sample were themselves parents. Finally, fewer reported providing financial gifts or loans to parents than was true in the earlier study. Differences in the studies' samples or cohort and period effects might explain the differences in the results. Both studies confirm that active exchange patterns are normal in families.

Another study with a different sample (Hogan, Eggebeen, & Clogg, 1993) examined intergenerational support in a large national sample of more than 5,000 adults who had both surviving parents and one or more children under 18 living at home. Four types of support were examined: financial, caregiving (to a child or parent), assistance with household tasks, and emotional support or advice. Analyses of exchanges between the older two generations indicated that more than half (53%) of middle-generation adults

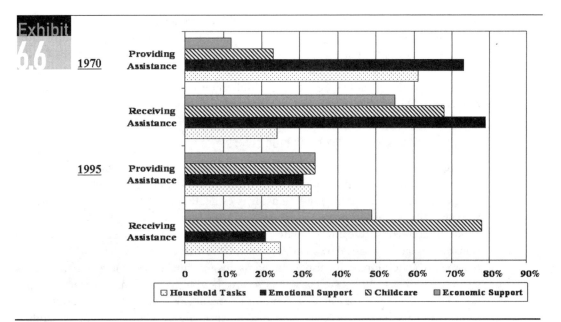

Percentage of Young Adults Receiving or Giving Intergenerational Support
Source: Amato et al., 1995; Hill, 1970.

were low exchangers, giving or receiving very little; another 17% mostly gave advice to their parents; 19% received support from their older parents; and 11% were high exchangers, typically both giving and receiving a variety of support with their aging parents. Many aspects of family relationships and family structures influenced the likelihood of an active exchange. Women were more active exchangers than were men, and co-resident parents both received and gave high levels of support. Black families were, contrary to the findings of previous research, *less* likely to be involved in intergenerational exchanges, a result explained by a shortage of resources within their families.

Finally, the study by Hogan and his associates revealed that family structure influences the exchange of support. When adults had several siblings, each was less likely to receive support from their older parents, who had to divide resources among several offspring. Older parents, on the other hand, improved the odds of being recipients of support with each additional adult child. This analysis was, of course, a snapshot cross-sectional view of support and did not convey the lifetime experience of giving or receiving support, which would be much higher. In fact, Riley (1983) suggests that low levels of assistance at any given time may mask a **latent kin matrix,** "a web of continually shifting linkages that provide the potential for activating and intensifying close kin relationships" when and if they are needed (p. 441). Thus, current exchange and support may be much more limited than the potential for exchange and support should greater need arise.

More recent research has focused on families as providers of routine support to elders rather than on the reciprocity of exchanges (Hogan, Eggebeen, & Clogg, 1993). In addition, research has expanded to examine cultural influences and the effects of migration on the support exchanged across the generations (see Silverstein, 2004). Although this research continues to show that older adults receive considerable assistance from adult children, especially in crises, it would be erroneous to conclude that they are only the recipients of support. Numerous studies also reveal the ongoing support of many types that older adults provide to their grown children and grandchildren (Walker et al., 1992). Most multigenerational households are created in response to the needs (economic, housing, child care) of adult children rather than the needs of older adults, as was once believed (Ward, Logan, & Spitze, 1992).

Family Members as Caregivers to Frail Elders

In times of illness or disability, most older adults receive both emotional and practical assistance from kin. Turning to others for this support can be thought of as a means of compensating for functional limitations. It is estimated that 80% of informal care for frail and disabled elders is provided by **family caregivers** (Dwyer, 1995). Although adult children constitute approximately one-third of family caregivers, their contributions are actually surpassed by spouses (Stone, Cafferata, & Sangl, 1987). Other relatives (siblings, grandchildren) are also included in this informal caregiving group. Estimates suggest that 5% to 10% of older adults receive help from non-kin, voluntary caregivers who are neighbors, friends, or community members. These other caregivers, who sometimes have lengthy personal relationships, provide significant support, including some cases where fictive kinship is established (Barker, 2002). Although family and other informal caregivers are sometimes limited in their skills in providing health care, there are pressures toward placing more of the responsibility for skilled procedures in their hands to control health care costs (Glazer, 1993). Older adults who lack supportive ties are at greatest risk for institutionalization when they can no longer care for themselves (see review by Antonucci & Akiyama, 1995).

Who Are Family Caregivers?

Nearly two decades of research on informal caregiving have established that most adults receive much of the help they need from a single caregiver. The person most responsible for the care of an impaired person is referred to as the **primary caregiver**. Others who provide assistance both to the primary caregiver and to the impaired older adult are referred to as secondary caregivers (see review by Gatz, Bengtson, & Blum, 1990). The provision of care to older adults often follows a hierarchical pattern (Cantor, 1983; Horowitz, 1985a). Caregivers are selected from available kin, with the role often, but not always, falling first to a physically able spouse (Allen, Goldscheider, & Ciambrone, 1999). Because male partners are generally older, more wives than husbands face the duties of caregiving (Chappell, 1990). If the older person is widowed with multiple children, a decision must be made about who takes primary responsibility; studies consistently show that one primary caregiver (often with assistance from other kin, neighbors, or friends) takes the major responsibility for care (Matthews, 2002; Stone, Cafferata, & Sangl, 1987).

Gender, marital status, and relationship quality influence the selection of a caregiver and the way support is provided. The percentage of male caregivers is slowly increasing (36% in 1999), but hours of care provided per week vary significantly by relationship and gender. Wives provided a median of 28 hours, husbands 15; daughters and sons differed less, with 13 hours for daughters and 10 for sons (Center on an Aging Society,

2004). Daily contact for care requires proximity, ruling out adult children who live far away. In some cases, an unmarried child or one without children will be tapped as caregiver on the assumption that this child will have fewer role conflicts (Brody, 1985). It is unlikely that an adult child with a distant or conflicted relationship with the parent will undertake caregiving unless there is no other alternative.

Researchers (Horowitz, 1985b; Matthews, 2002) have found notable differences in how sons and daughters performed the caregiver role. Although both groups were highly involved in providing care (27% shared a household with their older parent in the Horowitz study), they differed in the types of care they provided and their motivations. Aside from the emotional support commonly provided by both sons and daughters, more of the hands-on care of transportation, household chores, meal preparation, and personal care fell to daughters. Perhaps not surprisingly, daughters experienced more stress in association with their caregiving duties, largely because of their greater commitment in time and task responsibility.

Sons involved themselves in typical male gender-specific tasks (financial management, dealing with bureaucracies) or gender-neutral tasks, spending less time and doing a smaller number of tasks overall than daughters. Most married sons also involved their spouses in the caregiving, whereas fewer than half of daughters did. Sons appear to be more motivated by norms of obligation, whereas daughters are more often motivated by the affection of the relationship, confirming the kin-keeping role of women in the family system (Silverstein, Parrott, & Bengtson, 1995). Sons frequently were interested in attempting to restore the parent to independence, rather than accepting their dependence (Matthews, 2002).

Women in the Middle

It is well established that female kin provide the bulk of caregiving, while providing ongoing care for members of their households (Center on an Aging Society, 2004). Early research by Brody (1981) identified the risk of being a **woman in the middle** (also known as being in the **sandwich generation**). These women are caught between the responsibilities of providing care to their own dependent children at home and assisting frail parents or parents-in-law. Both increased longevity and decreased fertility (providing fewer potential caregivers) are thought to accentuate the problem (Rosenthal, Matthews, & Marshall, 1991). Although this structural problem of being in the middle may be a serious one for those upon whose shoulders it falls (Brody, 2004), research has revealed that the problem is not as common as once believed. First, the peak for adult-child caregivers occurs between the ages of 45 and 54 (17% of this age group has a disabled older parent) (Cantor, 1995). By this age, most women have raised children beyond early childhood and into adolescence or young adulthood, times when parental duties may be waning. Second, as longevity increases and disability is delayed, the onset of caregiving responsibilities should occur at later ages for adult children, further reducing the potential for being "in the middle" (Cantor, 1995). One study, for example, has demonstrated that only 50% of women are at risk of this dual responsibility, with fewer actually facing demands from both generations. By the time older parents reach ages at which disability becomes prevalent, their grandchildren are typically grown, leaving women with caregiving responsibility toward only one generation (Rosenthal et al., 1991). A recent study showed that only 10% of informal caregivers to older adults were also caring for children under the age of 18 in their homes (Center for an Aging Society, 2004).

What the "women in the middle" approach originally did not address was the other major role conflict, being caught between the conflicting responsibilities of employment and caring for an aged parent (Brody, 2004). Recent data suggest that nearly one caregiver in three is employed; they often need to reorganize their schedules or cut work hours to provide care. The low percentage of workers who are also caregivers reflects the fact that nearly half of care-providing kin are themselves over 65 (Center for an Aging Society, 2004). When the work–caregiver role conflict does occur (Matthews & Rosenthal, 1993), it may detract from effectiveness at work, and sometimes results in quitting. Although family leave (without pay) is now available for limited time periods, the ongoing demands of care for a parent with chronic health problems often forces choices between reducing or stopping work (with the attendant loss of income and reduction in pension benefits) and purchasing care or services. Although the retirement of adult children may enable them to have more time to attend to caregiving duties, such duties may intensify the caregiver's own issues of aging, such as economic security and health problems. So the dilemma, especially for adult daughters, remains fraught with the potential for role conflict (Brody, 2004).

Caregiver Burden and Rewards

Families provide many types of assistance to kin with health limitations, most of it for routine tasks of everyday living (Chappell, 1990; National Alliance for Caregiving, 1997). Despite the obvious benefits to older adults' functioning and independence, the stress experienced in providing such care may decrease the physical and psychological health of the caregiver (Center on an Aging Society, 2004; Schultz, Visintainer, & Williamson, 1990). Caregivers often experience stress and **caregiver burden** in conjunction with their duties. The experience of burden—a degree of strain reflecting lower life satisfaction, depression, and a decline in health—is highly variable, depending on the level and type of impairment of the care recipient and several aspects of the relationship between the care provider and recipient (Chappell, 1990). For example, adult children seem to be more prone to stress than spouses acting as caregivers, perhaps because the high intensity of responsibility for an aged parent violates the norms of generational independence, as well as presenting the potential for role conflicts with mid-life marriage and employment responsibilities. Caregivers to those with dementia and its associated behavioral problems (e.g., night wandering, agitation, or dangerous and embarrassing behaviors characteristic with Alzheimer's disease) also report greater caregiver burdens (Chappell, 1990).

Despite the burdens, research also reveals that caregivers report rewards and gains from their efforts (Kramer, 1997; Seltzer & Greenberg, 1999). In fact, it is quite possible for both strain/burden and rewards/gains to simultaneously characterize a caregiving experience (Lawton, Moss, Kleban, Glicksman, & Rovine, 1991). There have been both ethnicity and gender variations in the relative weight of rewards to burdens, but the literature on the positive aspects of reward/gain from caregiving are much less developed than they are for burden (Long-Foley, Tung, & Mutran, 2002). This growing literature reinforces that caregiving, while often demanding, is not without benefit to individuals who undertake these responsibilities.

House hold

Involvement of Older Adults in Their Care

Research on caregiving often characterizes older adults as passive objects toward whom care is directed. The study by Sarah Matthews (2002) of siblings and their age 75+ parents suggests that this is far from the case. Examining the dynamics of care within these families, Matthews found that older adults were active participants in arranging care and services for themselves, directing children regarding who should do what tasks, and resisting or rejecting services that appeared to violate norms of independence between the generations.

Matthews (2002) provides rich examples of instances where parents fought their children's well-intentioned efforts to assist them by rejecting home-delivered meals, resisting moves from their houses to live with children or in specialized housing settings, or dismissing offers to manage their finances. Her research clearly shows that, except for the subset of parents who were extremely ill or cognitively impaired, the efforts of children were often effectively mediated and shaped by older parents' wishes. Additional research that focuses on medical care or housing services reflects the concern that services may ignore the older adult, dealing instead with the adult child as the primary client for services, ignoring the capacity and interest of older individuals in participating in decisions regarding their lives (Frank, 2002; Schumacher, Eckert, Zimmerman, Carder, & Wright 2005).

SUMMARY

Family relationships are among the most enduring that people experience during increasingly long lives in most societies. Families provide considerable assistance and support to their members, with most of that assistance being viewed as routine or normal across the decades. Families take mutual assistance as a given in many of the relationships among individuals. Finally, families are not static, either through their own life cycle or historically. Structural changes with the maturation of members and social changes both modify the tasks faced by kinship groups and their expectations of how to meet these challenges. While families are a durable social institution, we can expect them to continue to change as the society does.

We have seen throughout this chapter, for example, that Black families differ in some important ways from White families, including more mutual assistance, closer sibling relationships, and a more active role for grandparents in rearing their grandchildren. Such differences are the products both of culture and of socioeconomic difference, creating a tradition encouraging greater reliance on kin networks.

Nor should we overgeneralize the positive nature of family relationships. For most of us family ties are close, and many of those ties are positive. Assuming that reliance on family caregivers is better than using formal health care services in all instances, however, ignores the realities of negative relationships, abuse, and neglect that characterize some dyads. For many individuals as they age, however, the continuity and support of familial roles, both as responsibilities and as resources, forge the key linkages that connect them to the social world of the past, present, and future.

WEB WISE

Caregiver Survival Resources

http://www.caregiver911.com

Caregiving is a major issue for elderly people, children, and disabled people of all ages. This Web site provides information and support to caregivers in various situations, including but not limited to caring for older relatives. A variety of resources are offered, including books, an "ask Dr. Caregiver" option, and links to a variety of other resources and more specialized organizations. This is a good first stop for assistance for someone seeking information or assistance with caregiving problems. This is a very friendly site for caregivers or professionals interested in support or information.

National Center on Elder Abuse

http://www.elderabusecenter.org

This site focuses on the issue of elder abuse. It provides basic information, legal and reporting aspects of elder abuse, a clearinghouse of information and statistics on elder abuse, and discussion of interventions.

KEY TERMS

caregiver burden	later-life family	sandwich generation
dyad	lineage bridge	social exchange
family caregivers	marital satisfaction	theory
kin-keeping	neglect and abuse	surrogate parents
latent kin matrix	primary caregiver	women in the middle

QUESTIONS FOR THOUGHT AND DISCUSSION

1. Identify your major partners in social exchange at this point in your life. Consider friends, family, employers, teachers, your college or university, religious or community groups, etc. among the potential partners. Think about what you give and what you get from your ongoing exchanges with these partners. Is exchange theory correct in proposing that you withdraw from exchanges that are unprofitable (i.e., that cost you more than you get from them)?

2. Research to date suggests that marital satisfaction among older adults is high. Given social changes in marriage, divorce, and expectations, what predictions would you make regarding marital satisfaction and divorce among older adults in future cohorts?

3. Kin-keeping tasks are important to maintaining relationships in the modified extended family over distance and busy schedules. Think about your own family experience—who hosts the holiday dinners, organizes the weddings

and reunions and memorials? Is this work now being shared more equally since more women are employed?

4. Providing care to an ailing or frail older relative provides both burdens and rewards to families. What new supports can you imagine that would promote caregiving to shift the balance toward greater rewards?

Ironies of Crime: Silver-Haired Victims and Criminals

The conventional wisdom is that older people are frequently victims of crime, including violent confrontations. This notion permeates our culture, but is it realistic? Are older people more likely to be victims of crime than younger people? Data from the Bureau of Justice Statistics (Klaus, 2005) suggest that this image of widespread victimization is far from accurate. Persons over age 65 are substantially less likely than younger people to be victims of violent offenses, and this low rate has been true for many years. In contrast, teens experience 25 times the risk of people over 65 of being victims of violent crime. While 9 of 10 crimes that do occur against older adults involve property (burglary, auto theft, or other property theft), the age 65+ group has the lowest rates of property crime of any age category as well (Klaus, 2005).

Because older persons are more likely than younger victims to report crimes to the police, the difference in the statistics is not an artifact of under-reporting by those over 65. Furthermore, both of these areas of crime have shown declines in the past 20 years, suggesting that our images of worsening crime do not apply, at least to those over age 65. This conclusion carries some important caveats. One has to do with the specific crime of purse snatching, of which older persons are equally (but not more) likely to be victims as those in younger age groups. Thus, our image regarding this specific crime has some basis in fact. Older adults are more likely to be victims of purse snatchers/pickpockets than of many other crimes. A second caution has to do with the circumstances and implications of crime against the elderly. Elderly victims of crime are more likely to suffer a serious injury than are younger victims, are more often victimized at or near their homes, more frequently face an assailant who is a stranger, and are (slightly) more likely to face an armed offender. Although smaller in number, the crimes perpetrated on older persons may be somewhat more dangerous than those on younger victims.

Fear of crime among the elderly, on the other hand, is very high and has been so for at least 20 years. This fear has resulted in the so-called victimization/fear paradox, suggesting that older persons' irrational fear of crime leads to overreaction in their behaviors. Most of the studies that have used cross-sectional data to compare fear of crime by age have shown dramatically higher levels of fear among older adults (Ferraro & LaGrange, 1992).

Fear of crime can be paralyzing to older persons and can have significant negative consequences for quality of life (Ferraro & LaGrange, 1992). Fear often leads elderly people to bar their doors and windows, avoid going out after dark, and experience high anxiety during forays outside of their homes. What is responsible for these high levels of fear? No one is certain, but a variety of methodological weaknesses in the research have been noted (Ferraro & LaGrange, 1992). Most of the research has been based on single questions about level of fear. When people were questioned in more detail about fear of specific types of crime (such as being murdered or having a car stolen), it was found that older people were not more fearful than their younger counterparts. Based on this more detailed measurement, younger people, the more likely victims, were more fearful of crime (Ferraro & LaGrange, 1992).

Older Persons as Criminals

The other side of this image, less often seen in the media, involves the age of criminals held in state and federal prisons. When we picture criminals, we generally imagine young or mid-life adults (predominantly male), rather than those in their 70s and 80s, and this image is largely correct. Older persons are underrepresented in prison populations—they make up about 5% of the state prison population nationwide—primarily because they commit less crime; but this proportion is growing (Aday, 1994).

Why are older men and women incarcerated? Many of the older prisoners of today have life histories of crime, punctuated by alternating intervals of incarceration and freedom. Others are serving lengthy or life sentences for a single crime, such as murder (Gewerth, 1988). The number of persons over age 50 arrested for serious or violent crimes has been increasing in recent years (Aday, 1994). Stricter sentencing laws, including "life without the possibility of parole," and "three strikes and you're out," which make imprisonment a permanent status for serious criminals, will dramatically increase the older prisoner population in the future. As crime has increased and public support for extended imprisonment has grown, criminals being sentenced in many jurisdictions today are facing all of their remaining years, including their old age, behind bars.

This older prison population creates some new issues. Crime by older persons without prior criminal records may result from cognitive impairments (such as Alzheimer's disease), a condition that law enforcement and prisons are not well suited to address (Gewerth, 1988). Prison officials are scrambling to accommodate a growing population of older, increasingly physically frail individuals within facilities designed for youthful and mid-life offenders (Aday, 1994). Prisons were typically not built to accommodate wheelchairs, nor are their medical facilities equipped to manage some of the chronic conditions common in later life, such as arthritis and diabetes (Johnson, 1988). Aged prisoners, in fact, pose the risk of dramatically increasing prison costs because of their needs for long-term health care and medications and their limited ability to work in prison industries and agricultural programs that help to defray the costs of prison systems in many states (Shatzkin, 1995; U.S. Department of Justice, 1989).

As society encourages courts to lock up violent offenders and "throw away the key," we are, over the long term, creating a geriatric prison population that has no precedent in U.S. history. This situation raises numerous questions. Does lengthy prison time rehabilitate? How do we assess the relative risk of recidivism (i.e., returning to crime) by a 70-year-old who murdered when he was 25 or a 70-year-old who murdered when he was

65? What will happen to criminals released after 40–50 years behind bars? Where will they go? Who will they know? How will they find a place in society (Gewerth, 1988)? What costs are we as a society willing to incur to maintain our resolve on "life without parole?" Is this a judicious use of society's economic resources? These and many other questions have not yet been addressed by policymakers at the state and federal levels but will be a natural outgrowth of current sentencing policies.

Work and the Life Course

Aside from issues of war and peace and nuclear holocaust, the most important dramatic social, economic, and political issues and developments facing the societies with aging populations are those associated with the reduction of employment in the life span while the life span itself is extended. (Matras, 1990, p. 75)

Employment as an Organizing Force in the Life Course

We may or may not agree with Matras that the changes in employment rank just under the possibility of nuclear holocaust on the list of compelling social issues. It is, however, difficult to argue with the centrality of employment to the structure of the larger economy and of individuals' lives. **Employment**—work for pay or being a worker— is one of the core roles around which we organize life in complex, modern economies.

As societies age and longevity increases, we need to rethink employment and how it fits with the social context of lives and the more macro-level needs of the labor market. For example, one major international trend among men—the **compression of employment** into a smaller proportion of life—has been identified in aging societies worldwide (Guillemard, 1996). Male labor force participants in the United States enter jobs on average at higher ages, after more extended education, than prior cohorts and, in recent cohorts, ended employment earlier through retirement. Compression applies only to men, because the revolution in labor force participation among women shows an opposite trend, increasing from an average of 14 years of labor force activity in the 1950s to about 32 years by the late 1990s (Gendell, 2005). However, trends for both groups are dynamic and subject to change as social norms, economic conditions, and attitudes change over time (Exhibit 7.1).

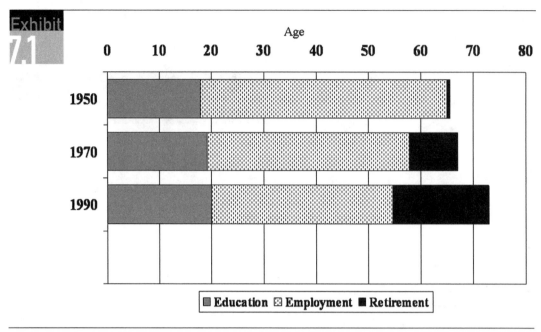

Compression of Male Employment, 1950–1990
Source: U.S. Bureau of the Census, 1977, 1987, 1997.

In this chapter we use the term employment rather than work, because the latter concept also includes household and other unpaid activities of value (Reskin & Padavic, 1994). There are numerous productive activities that are not called "work," although they are necessary to the survival of individuals, families, and the larger society. Child care, household work, community volunteering, and similar activities, while taking time and effort and producing goods and services, are not paid or included in most peoples' definitions of "work." This is paralleled by their unpaid status and the fact that we don't consider this part of our calculations of social and economic productivity—people don't earn credits toward retirement income for rearing children, as an example. The issue of how work is defined frequently arises in conjunction with the topic of productive aging, where ignoring the numerous unpaid contributions of older adults renders them as economically "dependent" in the eyes of some policies and measures (Bass, 1995).

Modern economies organize themselves around employment. We cannot fully understand retirement (see chapter 8) without considering its links to the structure and meaning of employment; in turn, employment and retirement can only be understood within the context of the economic structure of the larger society. Highly developed and developing economies differ dramatically in how employment is managed and whether retirement even exists (Kinsella & Taeuber, 1993). We focus here on issues of employment from the individual level to the societal level and direct our attention to retirement and other aspects of the economies of aging societies in chapters 8 and 9.

One caveat is in order as we begin this examination of employment and the subsequent issues of retirement and the economy. The world is in the midst of tremendous economic change; these changes are having an impact on jobs and job markets, on the meanings of employment and retirement, and on the questions we pose about these institutions.

Such dramatic changes require that we frame our discussion with an eye to the future and to avoiding cohort centrism. Thus, we describe the critical changes in these institutions and provide some educated speculation about the future of employment, although predicting the future in such a dynamic system is risky at best.

Dynamics of the Labor Force

Both the **market for labor** (the demand for employees with specific skills) and the **labor force** (the supply of available employees with their particular skills and experience) in a society, a given locality, or a specific company are highly dynamic. Over the past several decades, both supply and demand have shifted, changing the opportunities for individuals to find appropriate employment and for employers to meet their needs for skilled labor. As anyone experiencing the major shifts arising from the early 21st century economy recognizes, major corporations, industries, and job categories can and do shift dramatically and in unexpected ways. Major changes, such as outsourcing of jobs in the global economy and development of new technologies, continue to reshape the labor market in ways that are increasingly difficult to predict. Economies have always changed, but the pace and the scope of change have expanded in the past 50 years.

In macro terms, labor can be considered like other commodities in the economic marketplace, except that communities or societies cannot suddenly produce a greater supply of labor, because it takes considerable time to produce and prepare new cohorts to enter the labor market (Cooperman & Keast, 1983). When shortages of labor occur, the demand can be met more quickly by bringing less active groups into the labor force (for example, when more women were lured into the labor force during World War II), economizing by making workers more productive with technology, attracting workers from regions or countries with labor surpluses, or keeping current

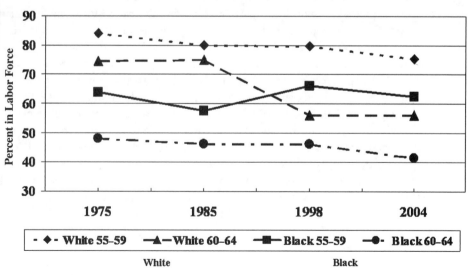

Changes in Labor Force Participation Rates for Men by Race and Age
Source: U.S. Department of Labor, 1975, 1985, 1995, 2005a.

employees on the job longer through wage and benefit incentives or disincentives to retirement. For example, a decade ago there was a "youth squeeze" in the restaurant, grocery, clothing, and retail sales fields, which typically draw their labor from young adults. When small cohorts entered the labor market, these employers scrambled to meet their labor force needs (Doeringer & Terkla, 1990). When labor is more difficult to find and keep, conditions become more advantageous for workers, who can bargain for better wages and benefits. When labor is abundant, however, employers offer lower wages and benefits, because workers are easier to replace (Reskin & Padavic, 1994).

Labor force participation rates describe the percentage of the population that is employed (or seeking employment) at a given time and, by extension, indicate the prevalence of retirement or other forms of nonemployment in various groups. In 2003, 17.8% of men and 10.2% of women over age 65 continued in the labor force (U.S. Bureau of the Census, 2005a). Exhibit 7.2 shows that, while participation was declining slowly for White men aged 55–59, their involvement remained the highest in 2004 of all four groups. Black men aged 60–64, with the lowest rate of participation over three decades, also declined toward 40%. The two other groups demonstrated more movement. Older (ages 60–64) White men dropped their involvement, and relatively younger (55–59 year old) Black men showed an increasing labor force participation rate in 1998, which was declining again by 2004. These trends reinforce an overall decline in participation among men over age 60 and the long-established difference in labor force participation by race.

In mid-life and beyond, Black men more often experience physical disability resulting in labor force exit, a situation that reflects their earlier economic and educational disadvantages (Bound, Scheonbaum, & Waidmann, 1996; Hayward, Friedman, & Chen, 1996). Despite this disability gap, Black men spend a greater percentage of their adult years in the labor force; although their working years are shorter, lower life expectancy more than corrects for this (Hayward et al., 1996).

Trends in labor force participation for mature women show a sharp contrast with those for men. As Exhibit 7.3 shows, during the decades when mature men were departing work in growing numbers via retirement or disability, more women 55–59 remained active in the labor force.

This pattern is largely the result of increasing labor force involvement by sequential cohorts of American women. In each cohort since the 1950s, adult women have had: (1) increasing participation and (2) have spent increasing percentages of their adult years in the labor force. Much of the remaining gender gap in labor force participation is associated with marital status. These gender differences in employment are rapidly diminishing among younger cohorts, as demonstrated by the upward trend lines in most groups of women. Race and age dynamics are also evident in women's labor force involvement, as White women 55–59 catch up to and pass the traditionally higher rates of labor force participation long found among Black women of the same age. Even though the older groups show lower participation, the rates are slowly increasing over the three decades shown here. Although mature men and women differ overall (i.e., note that the scale for the men goes to up 90% and for women only to 65%), there is no gap in labor force participation between unmarried men and women over age 50, after the competing demands of childrearing are diminished (Ruhm, 1996).

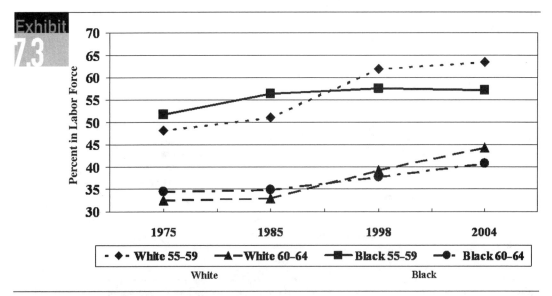

Changes in Labor Force Participation Rates for Women by Race and Age
Sources: U.S. Department of Labor, 1975, 1985, 1995, 2005a.

In general, labor force participation rates of older workers are declining in most developed countries. Exhibit 7.4 shows labor force participation rates in a variety of countries, contrasting males and females in developed and developing nations. For both sexes, rates of participation in the labor force above age 65 are generally lower in developed than in developing countries, probably because more of the developed nations have some type of pension available (Kinsella & Gist, 1995). The nature of a country's economy (whether it relies mostly on agriculture, manufacturing, modern technology

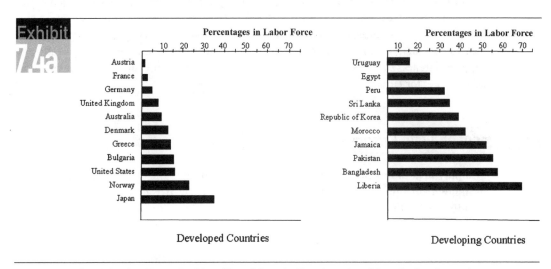

Labor Force Participation Rates for Men 65 and Over in Developed and Developing Countries
Source: Kinsella and Gist, 1995.

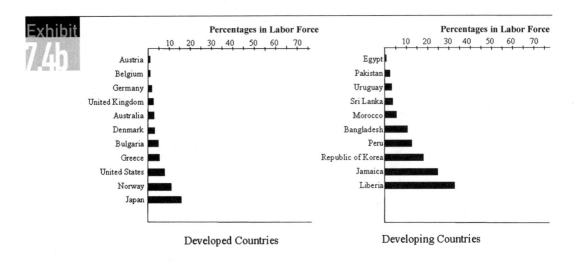

Labor Force Participation Rates for Women 65 and Over in Developed and Developing Countries
Source: Kinsella and Gist, 1995.

and information, or some combination of these) also shapes whether a society can make retirement available as an option. Differences in health also influence the likelihood that people over 65 will be employed. Cultural values and the roles of older adults in their families may further shape the likelihood that opportunities for employment will exist.

The second major pattern apparent in Exhibit 7.4 is that rates of labor force participation for older women are lower than those for men internationally. We must be cautious, however, because these statistics probably overlook many economic contributions of women to their families and societies through work in the **underground economy** (jobs such as home child care services or domestic work, paid in cash with no records kept) or family businesses. Whether this pattern of lower female involvement in the labor force will continue as women in developing countries have more education and more continuous employment remains to be seen. Women's labor force participation varies considerably among countries, probably reflecting cultural norms regarding the appropriateness of work at older ages for women and men and variations in demand in the market for labor.

Employment and Life Chances

Employment opportunities play a pivotal role in the life chances of individuals. Employment opportunities develop in part from early **life chances**—resources including education, social class, good health care, and a strong family—and unfold over the life course with consequences such as differing incomes, health status, and levels of social prestige. The opportunities to which individuals are (or are not) exposed, and the resulting differences in the types of occupations they hold, are a key to understanding inequality throughout life. Critical choices and opportunities early in life—specifically, education at the college level and beyond—have been shown to shape long-range outcomes for both women and men. "Winners" are those who, through

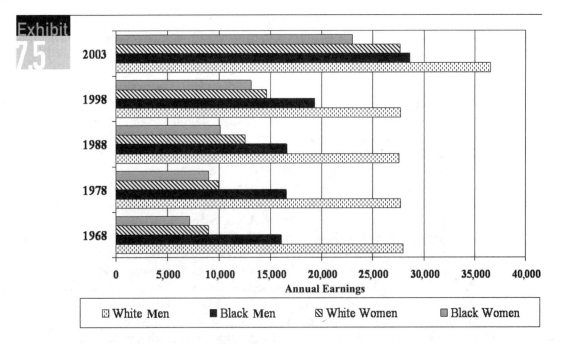

Earnings Inequality by Race and Sex, 1968–2003
Source: Infoplease, 2003; U.S. Bureau of the Census, 1998.

good fortune or hard work, achieve advanced education relatively early in life. Those who leave education systems at high school or before and do not return to build their educational credentials suffer lifelong disadvantage in competing for jobs and wages (Elman & O'Rand, 2004). An intermediate outcome belongs to those who return later for education; workers benefit from this, but by advancing their education later, they have fewer years to build the career and wage benefits available to those who had an earlier start (Elman & O'Rand, 2004).

Exhibit 7.5 presents information on gender and race inequality in earnings. From 1968 to 2003, inequality of income decreased somewhat, but differences remain. Moreover, the gap in earnings has been reduced not because women and Black workers are doing better, but rather because White men are doing relatively worse. Black women still fare the worst in terms of income, with White women and Black men doing slightly better. White men continue to hold the highest incomes, although of course this group (as all of the groups) shows considerable variation in earnings, job prestige, and other benefits that derive from employment.

Employment differences by sex and race/ethnicity continue to shape the working experience of adults, although differences in some areas are shrinking. Differences in the experience of employment and the access to jobs for women and men have shrunk in more recent cohorts. Blacks and the growing Hispanic and Asian populations also have had less access to jobs with higher incomes, employee benefits, and pensions. Gaps by race are also shrinking, but among older cohorts today, the employment experience across groups varies dramatically. Although we are progressing toward more equal opportunity in the labor force, differences in the occupations held by women and men, and by White and Black workers, persist (Wells, 1998).

Turning first to sex segregation in employment, there has been progress toward equality, but inequities persist. Why does **sex segregation of occupations** matter? Taking a broad view, Reskin and Padavic (1994) argue that "society as a whole pays a price when employers use workers' sex (or other irrelevant characteristics such as age and race) to segregate them into jobs that fail to make the best use of their abilities" (p. 46). In addition to these concerns, occupational segregation systematically restricts individuals' opportunities (life chances) within the labor market (Baron & Bielby, 1985). In a study of women in engineering, when women break this segregation by entering a nontraditional field, significant gaps remained in earnings between women and men. These gaps are diminishing among more recent cohorts entering the field, reducing the earnings inequality once women enter this male–dominated field (Morgan, 1998). While this trend is optimistic, women remain significantly under-represented in well-paid fields such as engineering and top administration (Morgan, 1998; Reskin & Padavic, 1994). The continued occupational segregation leads to lower lifetime earnings and reduction of other opportunities (skill development, professional networking, development of meaningful leisure activities, access to pension coverage), which are directly related to life chances in older adulthood.

The persistent effects of employment segregation on life chances are seen in the later-life employment and retirement options available to members of racial/ethnic minority groups. Jackson and Gibson (1985) show how limited life chances, because of both lower educational attainment and discrimination, result in disadvantage for Blacks throughout adulthood. Current improvements in opportunities have already taken decades and will take more time to reach fruition among future older cohorts of retired Blacks. In recent cohorts, many Black workers retired because of poor health, unemployment, or inability to find jobs (Jackson & Gibson, 1985). Many other older Blacks, even those in poor health, had to continue employment to maintain income in later life. In the past, a career as a day laborer or domestic, for example, often did not even carry the guarantee of Social Security and certainly lacked a pension, making continuing to work—as long as your health permitted—the only viable option. Jackson and Gibson also contend that a discontinuous employment history might make retirement less meaningful as a concept to Blacks in the United States.

Income differences during the working years are important, because they are correlated with later-life economic well-being. Lower earnings, discontinuous employment histories, and occupational segregation combine to significantly diminish the life chances of socially disadvantaged groups as they move through adulthood and into retirement. Chapters 8 and 9 show how these occupational opportunities (or their absence) play out in terms of differences in retirement decisions and income.

Productive Aging: Expanding Our Definitions of Work

For people who make it to age 65, life expectancy is 83 years and rising. Since many of those years are expected to be healthy, active years, there is a growing concern about what people can, should, and will do after they retire from paid employment. Attitudes regarding employment and retirement may be critical to deciding how individuals allocate this time. As discussed later in the chapter, the values of maintaining activity in retirement dominate U.S. cultural views of what constitutes a good and productive later life. One way of addressing the dilemma that not-working is devalued is to rethink our definition of work.

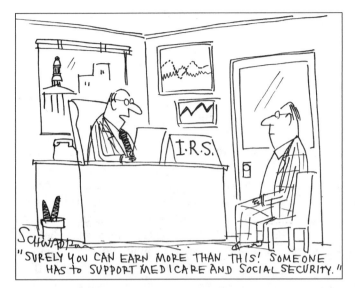

"SURELY YOU CAN EARN MORE THAN THIS! SOMEONE HAS TO SUPPORT MEDICARE AND SOCIAL SECURITY."

On a macro level, one of the great dilemmas facing developed and aging societies is the large amount of unstructured time provided by retirement. Is it useful to society to enable individuals to have this time without norms for utilizing at least some of it for social good? The growth of leisure industries, intended to provide enjoyable activities for those able to retire in good financial and physical health, does not confer the social status, build the social integration, and support the self-esteem that are associated with employment. Nor does it address the pressing social problems of most societies.

Researchers and policymakers are now considering how to tap the productive potential of an increasing population of healthy and educated individuals past the usual age of retirement, whose alternatives include both continuing paid employment (an alternative with growing momentum, given uncertainties regarding pension systems) and numerous voluntary activity options. According to a study by the Commonwealth Fund (1993), 10% of the nonemployed population over the age of 55 is willing and able to hold a job but cannot locate suitable employment. Even those who don't desire paid employment may seek interesting voluntary activities using their expertise and career experience to deal with the problems of society, such as poverty, illiteracy, or neighborhood decay.

Productive aging focuses on the overall productivity (both paid and unpaid) of the older population and the potential to tap unused productivity through broadening opportunities for paid, volunteer, and familial work. The productive aging approach also identifies existing structural barriers to full use of the productive capacity of the older population. Factors such as institutional ageism and age-based eligibility rules may promote inactivity for individuals who otherwise could be more productive (Caro, Bass, & Chen, 1993). It is important to point out, however, that older persons already contribute vast numbers of hours in volunteer work for their families and communities, work that currently gains little recognition in society (Commonwealth Fund, 1993).

The Occupational Life Cycle

The Occupational Life Cycle Model

The patterning of employment into the lives of individuals is a taken-for-granted aspect of the life course to most of us. But like many age-related phenomena, it is one that is socially constructed and subject to change. Most of us have a socially constructed model of an **occupational life cycle.** As an organizing concept, the occupational life cycle captures the interrelationship of individual lives over time with the social structure of employment and opportunity for advancement, prestige, and rewards. The dominant model in U.S. culture reflects the typical employment pattern of middle-class males in the mid- to late-20th century.

In this model of the occupational life cycle, a worker, upon completion of education or training, lands an entry-level position with a corporation. The worker, with the passage of time, advances through the ranks of that occupation, perhaps seeking additional training or changing companies along the way. The worker's earnings increase as he advances in terms of skill, experience, and responsibility, reaching a plateau in middle- or late-middle age. At that point, advancement may slow or cease in anticipation of retirement, which comes with health benefits and a solid pension (Doeringer, 1990). Research has demonstrated consensus among male workers regarding the ages at which promotions are most likely, with promotions less expected for workers beyond age 50 (Lashbrook, 1996). A random sample of Chicago-area adults confirmed that most people hold deadlines for completing school, entering full-time employment, settling on a career, and retirement; deadlines were less apparent among women than men, and there was little consensus on the ages by which some events (reaching a career peak, retirement) should occur (Settersten & Hagestad, 1996b). For example, retirement for women was suggested at ages from 40 to 75, a considerable range.

Although quite informal, this socially accepted model regarding the occupational life cycle is so ingrained into our way of thinking that we all take it for granted in personal planning and doing business. This model also translates into a macro-level expectation of how birth cohorts will transform into cohorts of workers for the labor market. What would happen, for example, if older workers in large numbers chose not to retire from their senior positions in their organizations? It could squeeze opportunities for advancement of younger workers, violating one of the core elements of the career model—advancement. What if large numbers of young adults were to take time off after training before initiating a career? This violation of expectations could create a labor shortage for employers, perhaps prompting recruitment of nontraditional workers or improvement of wages, benefits, and working conditions to attract the labor needed.

Although this model of occupational careers represented the experience of many middle-class men in retired cohorts today, questions have been raised as to whether it has ever characterized the labor force experience of other workers. Further, many wonder whether this model is still viable even for middle-class men in our changing economy. Layoffs from downsizing or corporate mergers, job automation via technology, and worker health problems may interrupt an orderly progression among middle-class men expecting to follow the traditional steps of this model (Doeringer, 1990).

On the generalizability of the model, there is ample evidence that the idealized occupational life cycle has never fit the experiences of employed women, workers with limited education, or groups who have experienced segregation or discrimination in employment. First, women continue to carry the bulk of responsibility for household work and child care, even while undertaking employment (Reskin & Padavic, 1994). Employed women often find themselves attempting to reconcile conflicting demands of family and job (Moen, 1994). The years of heaviest career building in the traditional model are also years of intense family responsibility (childbearing and care of small children). Second, jobs in the labor market that are occupied primarily by women have shorter career ladders, meaning that female workers have fewer opportunities to advance and attain higher wages, status, and benefits over time (Reskin & Padavic, 1994). In short, women hit their career ceilings sooner than men do on average. Third, the working lives of women have been and continue to be more subject to interruption by family-related needs, such as caring for a parent or child with health problems or changing jobs to follow a husband's higher-earning career path. Such interruptions typically diminish job and wage advancement significantly over time.

Similarly, the occupational life cycle model of the middle-class man does not fit other types of workers. How would it apply to migrant farm workers, for instance, who have no career ladder or guarantee of employment, minimal benefits, and no pension? How would the occupational life cycle model fit someone working as an exotic dancer in a nightclub, as a technician repairing office machines, as a waitress in a diner, as a carpenter, or as a telephone sales representative for a mail-order company? Clearly many jobs and companies, especially small businesses, do not offer the type of career trajectory that is generally associated with the occupational life cycle model, indicating that its usefulness is limited.

Contemporary Changes

The changing nature of the labor market also limits the usefulness of the occupational life cycle model. In prior cohorts, career workers were predominantly full-time and had incentives from pay and pension to remain with their employer, so that investments in training and knowledge specific to the company were maintained over time (Henretta, 1994). Increasingly, workers will face a career in which employer and occupation change may be the norm rather than the exception. Recent changes in the U.S. labor market include an increase in the number of smaller firms; less manufacturing, fewer labor unions, and more jobs in the service sector of the economy; outsourcing work to other countries; corporate mergers, takeovers, and downsizing; and the growth of what is called the **contingent labor force.** Contingent employees work as only day laborers once did, for the highest bidder for short spans of time (weeks or months to years). The difference is that contingent labor runs all the way from manual labor to the executive level. The world of contingent work guarantees little continuity, career building, or long-term company benefits, such as health insurance or a pension (Rupert, 1991). The movement toward contingent labor is part of a larger trend of companies limiting their long-term ties (and responsibility) toward their workers in the interest of remaining flexible and competitive in a rapidly changing global economy. Hiring someone on a contract to complete a particular project may be more efficient for the company than making an open-ended employment commitment, including pension benefits, and having to lay off workers if conditions change. Estimates of contingent labor are difficult to determine and have ranged from more than 20% to about 5% of workers in the late 1990s (U.S. Department of Labor, 2001; Rupert, 1991). Not surprisingly, a majority of those categorized as contingent say they would prefer more traditional employment (U.S. Department of Labor, 2001). Eventually this expanding variability in the patterns of employment through the life course may change the age-structured notions of when it is appropriate to have a job and to be retired, leading to the final demise of the occupational life cycle model (Henretta, 1994).

It seems clear that current changes in the labor market will mean that the occupational careers of individuals will be much less predictable and orderly in the future. For example, tenure in the current job among employed adults 65 and over in 2002 was 8.7 years, far from the duration that we think of in a "career job," and nearly 11% of workers 55 to 64 years old had been in their current jobs less than 12 months (U.S. Bureau of the Census, 2005a). We will see the end of the traditional occupational life cycle model as we have known it? Perhaps Riley's projection of adulthood as an intermittently shifting blend of education, leisure, and employment will become more realistic, with careers punctuated by breaks and returns to school for additional training or skill development (Riley & Riley, 1994). One challenging issue will be how individuals coordinate their occupations with roles in the family, especially parenting. The current situation is not optimal, especially for women, as completion of education, high demands from entry-level employment, and the care of children all overlap substantially in early adulthood. If life scheduling could arrange lower labor force demand during periods of intensive childcare responsibility (and if gender roles encouraged a more equal division of familial/household responsibilities), managing occupational and family roles might become less stressful for women.

One alternative in this new world of employment is for workers to anticipate **multiple careers,** in which an individual undergoes training and employment two or more times during adulthood, potentially in very different fields. Multiple careers theoretically reduce the risk of boredom for employees, accommodate changing labor market needs, and provide options to deal with skill obsolescence and a longer healthy life expectancy. Training might begin as it does now in late adolescence, followed by a 25-year career in a field. An individual could then experience a period of leisure before retraining for a second career. Multiple careers would require reeducation at mid-life, which has not been a normative pattern so far. It is also unclear whether there would be sufficient individual choice to make the multiple careers idea work in the manner described. Workers might be discouraged from selecting jobs requiring lengthy training and apprenticeship, such as medicine, under a multiple-career system. Downward mobility in earnings and prestige is likely to remain a risk in second-careers jobs (Ruhm, 1990).

The idea of multiple careers also seems to be premised on an undersupply of labor, so that workers have choices about jobs and ample salary and benefits to prepare for periods of leisure and training between them. If, instead, the supply of labor is abundant—either due to birth or immigration providing more workers or technology increasing each worker's productivity—contingent workers may be competing for scarce jobs while employers pay low wages and benefits and continue to ignore the needs and preferences of older workers. In contrast, if employers need to keep older workers on the job to meet their labor force needs when labor is in short supply, options such as multiple careers, part-time, or flexible schedules with better pay may become more prevalent than they are today.

With increasing healthy life expectancy, more people should expect a future with multiple careers, interspersed with periods of education or retraining (Myles & Quadagno, 1995). Rapid-fire changes in technology, jobs, and the economy suggest that flexibility may be a more highly prized quality in workers of the future. In this future, will retirement even be meaningful? That question can only be answered in the decades to come.

The Future for Older Workers

It could be argued that the individual, corporate, and societal decisions regarding the future of employment carry the potential for dramatically reshaping the way we organize the timing and sequencing of events in our lives. How the life course might change and what the place of employment will be within it decades from now are very difficult to predict, given the large flux in both the market for labor and its supply, and the accompanying changes in our notions of employment and its role in our lives. When science fiction writers speculate about possible futures, they often portray societies in which leisure abounds thanks to the labor of robots and other technological advances. Others describe a future where workers might be scarce and highly valued.

While the particular nature of employment and its connection to the aging of future cohorts is far from clear, we do expect the significant pace of change in recent decades to continue to re-form the occupational life cycle to something new and different, perhaps an individually specific pathway through family, employment, and educational roles that break all of today's norms for timing life events. Options such as flexible job scheduling, work from home in a 24/7 world, and regularly retooling skills to remain competitive may also prompt us to think differently about how work fits with family needs, education, and employer needs. As technologies evolve, continued or recurrent education may be required to remain competitive as skills become obsolete, and doubtless new career paths will open as others move offshore or end.

Older Workers and the Dynamics of the Labor Force

Researchers and policymakers discuss a group referred to as **older workers**. Often this term is not defined or is assigned varying ages of onset, because there is little agreement on a chronological age at which a worker is deemed "older." In fact, career trajectories vary, as do the demands of a job. Workers may be considered "older" at a much earlier chronological age if they are bricklayers or professional athletes than if they are public school teachers or Wall Street portfolio managers. The demands of the job, physical and mental, and the ages at which workers in the occupation reach their peak on the career ladder in terms of promotion and performance may be keys to defining when "older worker" status begins.

Also essential to understanding the older worker concept are the views of employers. We might argue that workers come to be defined as "older" when their employers start to treat them differently based on age—perhaps not considering them for promotions, training, or raises. When an employer stops investing in an employee because of age, the label of older worker has implicitly been attached, even if the judgment was made on seemingly individual criteria ("Walker isn't the 'go-getter' she once was"). The fate of older workers in the labor force depends on both the level of demand for labor in the marketplace and the views held by employers regarding the skills and productivity of older workers.

Workers over the age of 65, our socially constructed retirement age, are distributed differently in the labor market than their younger counterparts. Concentrations of older workers are found among the self-employed (e.g., self-employed dentists, accountants, or acupuncturists), in fields where substantial experience is valued (e.g., engineering or construction supervisors, heads of government agencies), and in declining occupations, where the age profile differs because few or no younger people are being hired (Cooperman & Keast, 1983). In both developed and developing countries, older workers are more concentrated in agriculture (a declining occupation) and less often found in jobs in the service sector (where growth is typical) than are younger workers (Kinsella & Taeuber, 1993). Is this pattern explained by individuals' moving out of clerical and service jobs and into agriculture as they age? For the most part, the answer is no. Again, the key lies in the dynamics of the labor market and the changing distribution of job opportunities presented to various cohorts. Shrinking occupational fields, such as agriculture and manufacturing, attract relatively few entrants from younger cohorts, because there are few opportunities. Entering cohorts turn instead to the growth sectors, such as service and high tech occupations. Such shifts in the labor market have marooned older workers in some fields that are in decline, further reducing their employment alternatives.

Skills and Employability of Older Workers

The employment options available to older workers depend in large measure on the overall supply of labor and the mix of skills relative to the demand. Specifically, the number of younger, "prime age" workers (perhaps ages 25–45) influences whether older workers are in high or low demand. Can we simply project the future demand for older workers based on the size of younger cohorts entering the labor force in the next 10–30 years? This younger worker/older worker algorithm would be fairly straightforward if the nature of employment and the number and kinds of jobs did not change over time. If job openings were stable, declining numbers of younger workers would simply signal an increasing demand for older workers. But social life is rarely so simple since both the numbers and the skills required shift constantly. So any given worker, young or old, faces a constantly changing array of opportunities in the marketplace for employment.

In addition, there remains the macro-level question of how many workers overall the economy needs to meet its goals. The answer to this challenging question depends on multiple factors, including the growth (or decline) of the overall economy and factors such as automation. Whether the market for labor will grow, remain stable, or shrink in the future is a subject of widespread disagreement, making it difficult to project the demand for older workers. Thus, the demand for older workers is related to, but not simply determined by, the number of younger workers available to fill jobs.

Another major influence on the demand for older workers is the perception of older people's competence and desirability as employees. Some of the most common **stereotypes of older workers** are that they miss more time than younger workers because of sickness, are less productive than younger workers, are more likely to suffer injury on the job, are not easily retrained, and are set in their ways. In fact, all of these stereotypes are untrue. Extensive data refute each of these claims against hiring or retaining older workers. Although it is true that a wide range of physical and mental capacities (speed, strength, visual acuity, reaction time) decline slightly with age, these changes are small until advanced ages and may be compensated for by greater experience, skill, or attention to the task (Welford, 1993).

In manufacturing, for example, employee productivity appears to increase with age up to 35–45 years, but this apparent increase may also be a result of less efficient employees leaving their jobs over time (Welford, 1993). Older workers have fewer work-related accidents, perhaps because of their greater experience. Results of studies on absenteeism

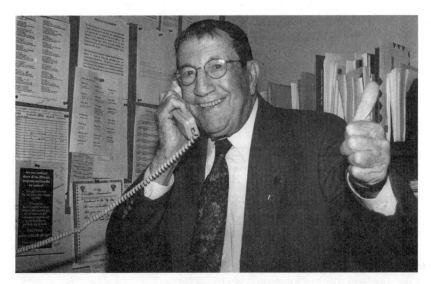

Older workers, like Richard Hoffman of the Ohio Department of Aging (ODA), often negate stereotypes by being among the most energetic, enthusiastic, and dependable employees in the workplace. Hoffman, pictured above, worked full-time at ODA until age 94. He started work there at age 66, after retiring from a full career in the aeronautics industry. (Credit: Mike Payne, courtesy of the Ohio Department of Aging)

are mixed, but managers perceive older workers as less often absent than younger workers (American Association of Retired Persons, 1995). As Robert Atchley (1994) argued more than a decade ago, "A majority of older people continue to function physically and psychologically at a level well above the minimum needed for most adult performance" (p. 280).

Less research has focused on the skills of office and managerial workers, because their tasks are more complex and difficult to measure than the speed and productivity of workers in manufacturing. A study of 12 diverse companies found that managers thought that age had an influence on skill and performance only for strenuous tasks. As Exhibit 7.6 shows, managers rated older workers (here defined as those over age 50) as better in terms of experience, judgment, commitment to quality, low job turnover, and attendance/punctuality while rating them poorer on flexibility, acceptance of new technology, ability to learn new skills, and physical performance in strenuous jobs (AARP, 1995). They rated older and younger workers about the same on another six traits, quite a mixed evaluation (AARP, 1995). In short, managers are no less subject to ageism than anyone else.

Some of the managers' negative views, however, remain an important influence on the hiring of older workers. In another questionnaire study, 1,600 middle- and top-level managers were asked to decide about hiring, promotion, discipline, and training one of two otherwise equivalent applicants—one young and the other older. These managers systematically favored the younger applicant over the older one. All voiced nondiscriminatory views on age, but older managers (over age 50) were more favorable toward the hypothetical older worker in hiring than the managers who were younger than age 50 (Rosen & Jerdee, 1985).

In addition, the perceived and real costs of providing benefits are sometimes a barrier to hiring, retaining, or retraining older employees. Experienced senior workers have often achieved substantial salaries, raising questions for the employer as to whether the work could be performed at less cost by a younger employee. Federally mandated

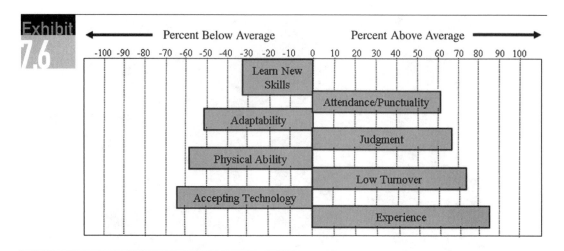

Manager Assessments of Older Workers' Performance by Attribute
Source: American Association of Retired Persons, 1995.

health benefits coverage has also added to the costs of employing older workers (U.S. Senate Special Committee on Aging, 1991). Employers sometimes weigh these added costs and decide against selecting an older applicant for a job or against keeping their older employees, as is discussed further below.

Special Programs for Older Workers

The literature on employment of older workers and retirees is replete with success stories of companies that have systematically hired older workers or rehired their own retirees to flexibly meet their labor force needs. Some companies have created options in which workers can continue some form of employment beyond the usual age of retirement, meeting the needs of both the worker and the employer (McNaught, 1994). Typically mentioned are the Days Inn Corporation, which substantially improved productivity and retention after hiring mostly older adults as reservation clerks (Miller, 1991). A second example is the Travelers Insurance Company, whose policy of hiring its own retirees to meet short-term personnel needs instead of using temporary help agencies, was in successful operation for many years. Other groups and organizations offer job banks or referral programs for older persons seeking employment (Fuentes, 1991). Many of these programs have been highly successful.

The problem that this short list denotes is that very few employers have considered options for using older workers—they have not had motivation to do so. In recent decades, the greater concern of employers has been how to reduce their labor force, often through early retirement incentives, rather than how to induce older workers to come back to or stay in jobs (Rix, 1991). The continuing negative attitudes of employers regarding the productivity of older workers have a lot to do with their reluctance to employ these experienced workers. Only recently, as the aging of the baby boomers reaches the doorstep, have employers begun to discuss the labor force challenges that will be faced following the retirement of these large cohorts in high-skilled positions. The question remains whether employers will be forced by a shrinking pool of available and skilled labor to reconsider how they can make use of older workers.

Rocking Chairs or Rock Climbing: Disengagement and Activity Theories

Theories often mirror the values of their creators and the norms of their social/historical times, reflecting and reinforcing culturally dominant views of what *should be* the appropriate way to do things. The two theories contrasted here follow this pattern of reflecting and reinforcing social norms. Both disengagement and activity theories postulate not only how individuals' behaviors and orientations change with advancing age, but also imply how they *should* change (specifying normative patterns of aging).

Disengagement theory, which was put forward by Cumming and Henry (1961), proposed that the process of **disengagement**—an inevitable, rewarding, and universal process of mutual withdrawal of the individual and society from each other with advancing age—was normal and to be expected. This functionalist theory argued that it was beneficial or functional for both the aging individual and the society that such a disengagement take place in order to minimize the social disruption caused by the older person's eventual death.

Cessation of work roles at retirement was a good illustration of this disengagement process, enabling the aging person to be freed of the daily responsibilities of a job, permitting the pursuit of other, more voluntary and flexible activities. Through disengagement, Cumming and Henry argued, society anticipated the eventual death of older people by removing them from roles such as those in the labor force and bringing new cohorts into full participation to replace them. Thus, the change was mutually beneficial.

Although focused primarily at the individual level of analysis, disengagement theory also had significant implications for the overall society. Developed during the period when mandatory retirement was common, the theory provided a positive spin on retirement, recasting it as a "functional" adaptation for the person and the society. To employers, the predictable withdrawal of older workers from various jobs meant that employers would be less likely to lose a critical employee unexpectedly, and senior jobs would become open to younger workers seeking promotions and better pay. In the family, disengagement from central roles such as child care meant that families would be less likely to lose a member with major responsibilities to kin upon their death.

Reaction to disengagement theory was swift and negative. To many of the activists and advocates involved in studying aging at that time, disengagement theory represented a threat to their goal of promoting more positive roles and a truly engaged life-style for older persons (Kastenbaum, 1993). Although the original theory was not stated in these terms, it was quickly interpreted as a normative statement ("people should disengage") rather than as a description of reality ("as they age, people do disengage").

Disengagement theory has had mixed success as a theory. Some argue that it was successful because it stimulated discussion and research (Hochschild, 1975), a major function of any theory. Yet it has been widely criticized as being unfalsifiable, a major failing contrast of any theory (Achenbaum & Bengtson, 1994; Hochschild, 1975). The theory states that disengagement is universal and inevitable, but that its form and timing vary among individuals (Hochschild, 1975). Thus, if a person is not disengaged at age 85 or 95, it may be only a matter of time until disengagement occurs, making it impossible to disprove its inevitability or universality. Cumming and Henry also labeled some individuals who continued to be actively involved as "unsuccessful disengagers," suggesting that being active and engaged was a dysfunctional response to a universal pattern of withdrawal (Cumming & Henry, 1961; Hochschild, 1975). The theory also allows for voluntary reengagement following withdrawal, further muddying the ideas of disengagement as universal and inevitable (Hochschild, 1975).

There are also problems of measurement: How do you determine whether someone is disengaged? What standard is used—the person's own earlier life or peer behavior? Does awareness of approaching death, advancing age, or both drive disengagement if it occurs? None of these questions has been adequately addressed (Hochschild, 1975). So although we may be able to identify the loss of social roles as common among individuals moving into advanced age, this loss does not necessarily signify an inevitable or beneficial process of disengagement.

Activity theory emerged, in part, in response to disengagement theory (Lemon, Bengtson, & Peterson, 1972). Activity theory also represents a normative view of aging—in this case arguing that individuals, in order to age well, must maintain social roles and interaction rather than disengage from social life.

(continued)

(continued)

"The essence of this theory is that there is a positive relationship between activity and life satisfaction and that the greater the role loss, the lower the life satisfaction" (Lemon et al., 1972). The activity theory mandate for a retiree was, therefore, to locate some other engaging activity to substitute for lost employment or family demands, maintaining levels of social involvement. In the case of employment, this activity must substitute for the goals (other than financial) that the job fulfilled for the individual (Atchley, 1976).

This theory has received considerable research attention. One early example is a study by Lemon, Bengtson, and Peterson (1972) that examined key elements of activity theory in a cross-sectional sample of future residents of a retirement community. That study found little connection between activity levels and satisfaction. The study may have been limited by the homogeneous nature of the sample (mostly White, middle-class, married, and interested in moving into a retirement community offering an "active lifestyle"). Beyond these issues, a problem with activity theory is establishing causation, especially using a cross-sectional research design. If we find that more active people are more satisfied, does that mean that activity causes satisfaction, that satisfaction promotes activity, or that some other factors (such as good health or high education) enhance both activity and satisfaction? From cross-sectional data, it is impossible to disentangle the causal puzzle.

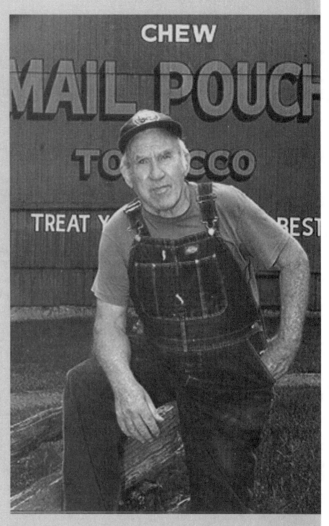

The late Harley Warrick, one of the last of the original Mail Pouch painters, defied disengagement theory by staying busier than ever painting and selling Mail Pouch birdhouses long after he climbed down the ladder from painting barns. (Credit: Mike Payne, courtesy of the Ohio Department of Aging)

Both activity and disengagement theories have fallen largely into disuse as theories, but they remain important guideposts regarding normative views on aging and examples of problems to avoid in theory development. Activity theory remains a dominant ideology of successful or productive aging and undergirds the behaviors of individuals and organizations that continue to believe that active aging is successful aging.

Think about these two theories and how they might reflect your expectations about your future aging. Disengagement suggests that you should and will retire from employment, lose friends to death without replacing them, take a less central role in your family, and perhaps withdraw from community activities as you age. You should, in other words, move toward the rocking chair as you move toward your likely date of death. Under the activity theory scenario, in contrast, you should maintain your active

(continued)

(continued)
involvement in your family and community and replace lost activities or friends with new ones to maintain full involvement as you age. Rock climbing would replace the rocking chair, as long as good health persisted.

What are the implications for the larger society if disengagement is an accurate description of social aging? How will life in our aging society, with more than 20% of the population over age 65, differ if older adults maintain active involvement? It is clearly an issue with implications for all cohorts.

Age Discrimination in Employment: Problems and Policies

In 1995 a federal jury awarded three pharmacists more than $2 million in back pay and damages in an age discrimination lawsuit against K-Mart. The jury found that the three pharmacists, who were between 62 and 65 years of age when they were fired, had been discriminated against by the company, which wanted to bring younger managers, pharmacists, and staff into its stores (K-Mart Pharmacists, 1995). From cases such as this one, we know that age discrimination in employment is far from a problem of the past.

Age discrimination occurs when an employer makes decisions on the basis of age that disadvantage its older workers in terms of hiring, promotion, training, wages, or other opportunities. Because age discrimination, stereotypical attitudes, and the "bottom line" of costs for labor certainly influence the demand for older workers, there are policies and laws prohibiting age discrimination in employment practices. The **Age Discrimination in Employment Act (ADEA),** originally passed in 1967 and amended significantly since then, prohibits the use of age in hiring, firing, and personnel policies for workers between 40 and 70 years of age (McConnell, 1983). By 1986, the ADEA prohibited mandatory retirement in all but a few occupations. It became illegal to force people to retire when they reached a certain age, and the percentages of workers facing mandatory retirement has declined rapidly (Fields & Mitchell, 1984). The continued need for lawsuits in recent years suggests the need for a closer look at the spirit, effectiveness, and enforcement of ADEA. Job losses among mid-career white-collar workers in recent economic downturns highlighted the remaining challenges of placing young older workers. In cohorts in the labor force unaccustomed to disruption, many of these workers faced difficulty finding new jobs in a constricting economy and were deemed overqualified for other jobs that might have provided some income.

Age discrimination is often subtle and difficult to prove in court. If a supervisor selects a younger employee over an older one for a training program, is this action age discrimination? Not necessarily, because the two employees undoubtedly differ on a variety of other work-related characteristics. But if the supervisor systematically selects younger over older workers for various opportunities, even when the qualifications of the older employees are equal or better, it is discrimination. Discrimination may be conscious or unconscious but is often predicated on negative assumptions by the employer concerning the attitudes and abilities of workers as they age. Proving age discrimination in court is often difficult, because employers claim legitimate reasons for failing to hire, promote, train, or increase wages to an older employee. The burden of proving age-related reasons for the treatment falls to those bringing suit, a burden that can be lighter if multiple employees shared an experience of discrimination (McConnell, 1983).

Even though mandatory retirement is now prohibited by the ADEA, the law allows for exceptions. Those exceptions are specific occupations in which age is considered a **bona fide occupational qualification (BFOQ)**. Examples include airline pilots, air traffic controllers, and some law enforcement positions. Why is it still legal to force people to leave these jobs at a certain age? Employers have convinced the courts that age has a predictable effect on one's ability to perform these jobs, and the consequences of inability to perform one of these jobs are potentially devastating. On the face of it, there is some logic to the BFOQ exceptions. However, recall the case presented at the beginning of this book of airline Captain Al Haynes, credited with saving hundreds of lives during a plane crash in 1989. All reports cited his experience as the basis for his ability to handle the crisis. Ironically, he was required to retire about 6 months after the incident because he had reached age 60, the mandatory age of retirement for airline pilots. Pilots have recently again moved to challenge the BFOQ standard for mandatory retirement from their jobs.

This example, and the very existence of BFOQ exceptions, raises two important questions: (1) Does age make a predictable, negative difference for performance in any occupations? (2) Has the ADEA been effective in reducing age discrimination? Although the first question cannot be answered definitively for all jobs, growing data on how differently each individual is affected by advancing age and on the importance of experience and effectiveness for many jobs suggest that age may not be a reasonable criterion for removing people from any kind of job. Those who argue in favor of retaining BFOQ exceptions point out that the alternative, testing the performance of each individual after a certain age, is costly and complicated. The fundamental question is which kind of mistake are we more willing to make—forcing potentially productive people out of jobs or retaining people on the job whose abilities may be declining? Thus far, BFOQ employers have chosen and successfully defended the former choice.

Turning to the second question, has the ADEA been effective in reducing age discrimination? Certainly it has had a legal impact in terms of ending mandatory retirement. Since most workers who had been employed under mandatory retirement left prior to the mandatory age even before the ADEA's passage (Fields & Mitchell, 1984), this change is largely symbolic. Many who have analyzed the policy have concluded that it provides more symbolic than real protection against other forms of discrimination as well. Atchley (1994) notes that the number of complaints of age discrimination reported to the Equal Employment Opportunity Commission have increased, but that the number of ADEA cases prosecuted by the government has dropped.

Age discrimination reflects our society's ambivalent feelings about older workers. These ambivalent views are reflected in the ideologies and underlying assumptions of two early theories attempting to describe retirement on the individual (micro) level.

SUMMARY

By the year 2012, the U.S. labor force is anticipated to include 162 million individuals, an increase of 12% over its 2002 size (U.S. Department of Labor, 2004a). At the same time, the composition of the labor force will become more diverse, as Hispanic, Asian, and Black population groups make up a growing proportion of workers. Women are expected to make up nearly half of the labor force (U.S. Department of Labor, 2004a). The growth in the overall labor force is slower now than it has been in some prior decades, forcing society to examine how labor market needs will be met. Will new technologies enable the economy to continue to grow with fewer workers, or will there be increasing pressure to keep older workers in the labor force? Either way, the future will bring changes in how we view work and retirement as part of social life and the individual life course.

Because employment helps to organize the sequencing of events in the lives of individuals on a micro level and the flow of cohorts into and out of the labor force at the macro level, any changes we devise in how work fits into the life cycle—either extending it, reducing it, or breaking it into different pieces—will have serious social and economic consequences. Although we cannot accurately predict what the demand for labor will be, the life chances that workers of diverse backgrounds have in the labor market will, in turn, shape their options as older workers and eventual retirees, a topic to which we turn in the next chapter. The current concept of the occupational life cycle is moving rapidly toward obsolescence, but a new model of employment in the life course is not yet clear.

For the present, older workers continue to face discrimination—a corporate mentality more interested in creating incentives to retire older workers than in developing them as a resource for the company. As contingent labor grows, will older workers be systematically removed from career employment into lower-paying jobs on the periphery? Will more workers entering the labor force encounter lives as transient employees, moving regularly between jobs and risking a pensionless future? With the population of older persons growing, society likely will address their needs, both economic and social, to avert some of the worst problems. It remains unclear, however, whether the coming labor market will be an ally or the nemesis of older workers.

WEB WISE

U.S. Department of Labor
http://www.dol.gov

The U.S. Department of Labor (DOL), created by Congress in 1913, is responsible for securing the adequacy of workplaces in America. This comprehensive Web site offers information about the DOL and its programs and an opportunity to explore department agencies. The "labor related data" option links to the Bureau of Labor Statistics Web site described below. Media releases, the history of minimum wage, and the budget for fiscal year 1998 are also topics to explore. A DOL search function is also available.

Bureau of Labor Statistics
Employment and Training Administration

http://stats.bls.gov
The Bureau of Labor Statistics (BLS) is a national agency within the U.S. Department of Labor. The BLS gathers, assesses, and disseminates data in the field of labor economics.

The agency's Web site offers overviews of surveys on employment trends, productivity data, and projections surrounding the labor force, industries, and occupations. The 1997 economy is presented in terms of labor force statistics, productivity, and price indexes; the option to view the data graphically is also available. This site provides opportunities to explore other federal statistical agencies, as well as publications and research papers, and listings of recent archived news releases.

KEY TERMS

activity theory
age discrimination
Age Discrimination
  in Employment Act
  (ADEA)
bona fide occupational
  qualification (BFOQ)
compression of
  employment

contingent labor
  force
disengagement
employment
labor force
labor force participation
  rates
life chances
market for labor

multiple careers
occupational life cycle
older workers
sex segregation of
  occupations
stereotypes of older
  workers
underground
  economy

QUESTIONS FOR THOUGHT AND DISCUSSION

1. Defining work as paid employment has implications for how society views other activity and rewards it (or fails to reward it). What consequences would arise and which groups would experience the most change if we broadened our definition of and recognition for work beyond the labor market to other productive activity?

2. Nobody in 19th-century companies manufacturing buggy whips thought they would ever be without a job, but clearly this is not a high employment area today. What kinds of jobs can you think of that are (a) likely to shrink or disappear, (b) likely to grow and develop, or (c) likely to expand in response to an aging population in a technology-driven world?

3. Identify three social problems where the energies of retired adults might be put to good use to help society. Outline the kinds of programs that might attract these individuals to give back to their community, state, or country. What might these programs do and what challenges would they face?

4. The employment careers of women are starting to resemble those of men by being more continuous. How might older worker issues be similar or different for women and men in the next few decades?

Retirement

8

If retirement from the labor force marks the passage into old age, then the old among us have grown considerably younger in recent years. (Quinn & Burkahauser, 1990, p. 307)

Defining Retirement

Col. K retired from the military after 30 years of service. She receives a military pension and has recently begun a full-time consulting business based on her military expertise.

Basketball superstar Michael Jordan retired from that sport in 1993 at age 30. He subsequently undertook a career in professional baseball, but later "unretired" and returned to basketball in 1995 at age 32, retiring again a few years later.

Mr. L, 70, receives a pension from the large accounting firm where he worked for 30 years. For 3 months of every year, Mr. L is a self-employed, full-time tax preparer for long-time clients and his family. The remaining 9 months, he enjoys an active leisure lifestyle.

Ms. J, age 58, has had a spotty record of employment throughout her adult life, working temporary and part-time jobs when she could find them. Having more trouble than usual in the past few years in finding work, she has given up looking for jobs and begun to call herself "retired" when people ask. She'd work again if she could find a job, because money is scarce.

Mr. S, age 76, has operated a community pharmacy in his stable community for decades. He started receiving Social Security benefits at age 65 and now takes required payments from his IRA plan, but continues to work 40 hours per week, with no intention of quitting.

Would you categorize any or all of the above persons as "retired"? How do we decide? It is useful to establish some common ground about the boundaries that define retirement in order to develop both policies and research on retirement. As the preceding examples show, the definition is not as simple as it first appears.

Before we can discuss criteria for when retirement occurs or whether an individual is retired, it is necessary to think about what retirement means. Atchley (1976) described several ways in which we use the word **retirement**. It may refer to the event or ceremony marking departure from a career or employment in a particular job, a phase of the occupational life cycle preparatory to such a departure, a process of separation from employment, or a social role (the "retiree" role). We use the term retirement interchangeably to refer to all of these diverse meanings, making it imprecise.

The central focus in this chapter is on retirement as a life stage and as a process of separation from employment. Recognizing some ambiguity in how the concept is used, we can now turn to the questions of when retirement begins and when an individual is considered retired. We can answer these questions in one of two ways: using self-definitions (answers to straightforward questions, such as "Are you retired?") or using objective, standardized indicators. Ekerdt and DeViney (1990) have outlined several such indicators that have been used by researchers to establish whether someone is retired—among them, (1) receiving a pension, (2) total cessation of employment, (3) departure from the major job or career of adulthood, or (4) a significant reduction in hours of employment. As illustrated in the cases described at the start of this chapter, many workers today do not make a clean break from employment by moving from full-time jobs one day to no employment the next, our traditional view of how retirement occurred (Atchley, 1976). Instead of a clear-cut event, retirement has become somewhat more blurred than crisp as a life transition, and we may need several criteria to constitute a working definition of retirement (Mutchler, Burr, Pienta, & Massagli, 1997).

Although there is no agreement about exactly how to measure retirement status, two objective criteria are part of most definitions: receipt of a pension (public or private) and diminished activity in the labor force at some advanced age for reasons other than death (Gendell & Siegel, 1992). Within these general guidelines, researchers and policymakers then set more precise limits, depending on their purposes and the data available. Because not everyone uses the same definition, it is important to pay attention to which boundaries of retirement are being used in any given discussion, since not all definitions are equivalent.

The Social Construction of Retirement

Where did retirement come from? Did it always exist? The fact that retirement is a social construct is easily seen by looking at employment and leisure throughout history. Retirement did not always exist in Western societies and is still not common in many developing nations around the world (Kinsella & Phillips, 2005). Researchers date the start of large-scale retirement to the close of the 19th century (Quadagno, 1982), arising from a mix of social and economic changes.

Throughout most of history people from all social classes were required to work in order to ensure the survival of themselves and their kin (Quadagno, 1982; Reskin &

Padavic, 1994). Labor started early in life, because childhood was not recognized as a separate stage of life to be protected from labor, and continued until death or disability prevented it (Plakans, 1994). Even the nobility of Europe had duties to perform in connection with their station in life and could not do whatever they wished with their time. In fact, elders in many cultures around the world have held responsibility for leadership or other pivotal roles to very advanced ages (see Amoss & Harrell, 1981, for some examples).

Retirement was not entirely unknown prior to industrialization in Western cultures. Occasionally, landowning farmers would have contracts with their inheriting sons to provide care for them (and their widows) once they retired and turned over operation and ownership of the farm. Wealthy British men could retire to their country estates, undertaking a slower, but not entirely leisurely, life-style. "Retirement in 'modern' society is unique only to the degree that it is associated with massive intergenerational income redistribution through a state bureaucracy. Retirement, itself, is not new" (Quadagno, 1982, p. 199). Historically speaking, however, the option of most people having a block of unstructured time at the end of the life cycle is new.

Four social conditions set the stage for the emergence of retirement as a social institution (Atchley, 1976; Cooperman & Keast, 1983; Plakans, 1994; Quadagno, 1982). First, the society must produce an economic surplus (usually via industrial production) sufficient to support its nonemployed population. Second, there must be some mechanism in place (such as pensions) to divert that surplus to the needs of these nonemployed members of the society. Third, the culture must hold positive attitudes toward not working for pay, legitimating other pursuits as acceptable or desirable. Fourth, people must live long enough to accumulate an acceptable minimum of years of productive employment to warrant support during retirement (Atchley, 1976). The development of retirement was enabled by the creation of public and employer pension systems. Employer pensions first appeared in the late 1800s. Pension benefits to workers were considered a reward for merit and a gift from a magnanimous employer (Quadagno, 1988); there was no sense that employers owed their retirees any support. Initially, few employers offered private pension options. In the post–World War II era, however, pension programs grew rapidly in a strong economy, expanding in the 1940s and 1950s to cover a wider range of occupations. Retirement incentives, such as pension programs, grew up during periods when labor was in ample supply, as larger youthful cohorts were continually entering the labor force (Cooperman & Keast, 1983). The availability of pensions continued to grow until the 1980s; since then it has leveled off or declined in many fields (Employee Benefit Research Institute, 2004).

The first retirement programs in developed countries were regulated and highly structured. Pensions were not available until reaching the age of eligibility or years of service standard in their employer's plan (Kinsella & Phillips, 2005). There was no Social Security, and relatively few people had access to company pensions. When companies did develop pensions, they typically paired them with mandatory retirement policies in order to have greater control over moving senior workers into retirement and replacing them with younger workers. Based on legislation described later in the chapter, the United States and many other countries have moved away from this clearly structured system by ending mandatory retirement, except in certain occupations where capacities, such as good vision or speedy reaction time, are still used to justify mandatory ages of retirement. In less developed countries, however, where family-based businesses or agricultural economies

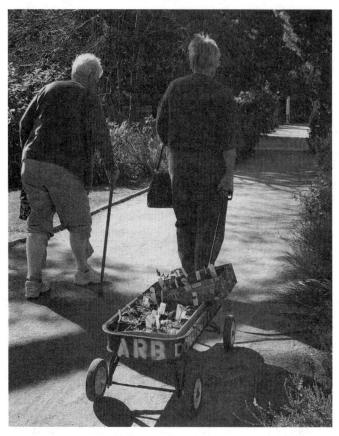

A range of activities in retirement are looked upon favorably—and enviably—by society. (Credit: E. J. Hanna)

predominate, retirement as a status remains less structured and less common (Kinsella & Phillips, 2005).

Worker attitudes toward retirement were slower to change than were pension policies; Atchley (1976) contends that sequential cohorts of workers have become more positive in their attitudes toward retirement. The idea of retirement had to contend with a strong work ethic that suggested that the worth of an individual was tied to her or his productivity, most specifically in the labor force. Retirement is now generally accepted as an appropriate stage of the adult life cycle and as a legitimate, earned privilege (O'Rand, 1990). The legitimization of leisure has accompanied and reinforced positive attitudes toward retirement, as long as one maintains a high level of personal activity and social involvement (Ekerdt, 1986). Normative support for a leisure life-style has reduced the appeal of continued employment, and numerous studies suggest that retirement has been accepted as a new phase of life in most Western societies (Atchley, 1994). Even as its meaning continues to change, however, questions have been raised regarding whether the concept of retirement has ever been truly meaningful for minority, economically disadvantaged, and female workers, who often have experienced discontinuous labor force histories and more often continue employment into old age because of financial need (Calasanti, 1996b; Gibson, 1996).

As some of the expected security from employer pensions falls subject to corporate bankruptcies and Social Security funding is again the subject of political debate, studies of baby boomer cohorts suggest that the relatively young social construct of retirement is under reconsideration. A recent study of 10 nations suggests that views of later life, including the place of retirement within it, are being rethought as economic conditions and life expectancy shift over time (HSBC/AgeWave, 2005).

Theoretical Perspectives on Contemporary Retirement

In the past, mandatory retirement—by providing a formal, universal, and manageable exit from the labor force for all people reaching a certain age—solved a number of problems for industrializing nations. In a macro-level view, retirement operates for corporations and societies as "a mechanism for adjusting the supply of labor to the demand" (Atchley, 1976, p. 123). According to the functionalist perspective, the functions retirement fulfills for society include controlling the flow of labor into and out of the labor market, making room for younger workers to be hired at lower wages with the promise of future advancement, smoothing the flow of labor over time, and facilitating the removal of older, more highly compensated workers (Atchley, 1976; Johnson & Williamson, 1987).

From a conflict perspective, however, retirement looks very different. A conflict perspective begins with different assumptions and asks different questions. Who benefits most from the existence of retirement as a social institution? Who controls the process and timing of retirement? Matras (1990) describes the contraction of employment through retirement as engendering a "struggle for employment" between workers and employers. In this struggle the power is largely in the hands of employers, who control what groups work and receive what wages and benefits. According to John Myles (1984), politics, not demographics, determine the conditions of life for older people. The exclusion of older workers from employment is not a necessary result of changing demographic realities in an aging society, but instead an act of discrimination. According to the conflict perspective, the social construction of retirement as a time of life without employment builds an army of unemployed but able workers, who serve as a mechanism to control the current labor force participants by posing the threat of replacing them if they are difficult or demanding (Matras, 1990). This argument is supported by research showing that many retirees would consider working again under acceptable conditions.

It is clear that the policies at the societal level (such as the age of eligibility for full Social Security benefits) and at the corporate level (pension eligibility and special early-retirement options) are intended to manipulate the retirement decisions of individuals to serve the needs of the corporation or the society as a whole. Conflict theorists point out that employers can and do utilize such policies to manipulate the labor supply to achieve their own goals. Through the lens of conflict theory, retirement pits relatively powerless workers against the interests of a powerful organization that may no longer require or desire their services.

Hardy and her colleagues (Hardy, Hazelrigg, & Quadagno, 1996; Hardy & Quadagno, 1995) studied auto workers who had taken either regular early retirement or special **early retirement incentive programs (ERIPs),** created to downsize the work force. Auto workers are a good case study because their unions have a long history of strong and flexible pensions. Many of the autoworkers in Hardy's sample feared for their jobs because they knew that their employers planned to close some plants and decrease the labor pool. Taking an available "voluntary" early retirement option (if eligible by age and years of service to the company) avoided the risks of layoff if a worker's plant was among those closed and seemed to guarantee a degree of economic security. The workers' decisions, made under threat of layoffs, appear to be far from truly voluntary retirements. By creating such conditions, employers continue to control the retirement decisions of their employees, even though mandatory retirement is no longer legal and the decisions to retire appear to be purely voluntary.

The process of retirement has been described as having both **push and pull factors:** pushes (e.g., poor worker health, family caregiving demands), which in a negative fashion increase the odds of retirement, sometimes involuntarily, and pulls, such as leisure plans, which are more positive factors in movement toward retirement. The relative mix of pushes and pulls in any retirement may ultimately relate to worker satisfaction with the transition and life after retirement (Schultz, Morton, & Weckerle, 1998).

The Role of Social Security

The creation of the U.S. Social Security Administration in 1935 enabled retirement to become a reality for the majority of American workers (see chapter 9 for further discussion of this program). Social Security has been important in helping to institutionalize and promote retirement in three related ways. First, the existence of Social Security makes retirement socially legitimate as a transition and stage of the life cycle. Second, Social Security benefits enable individuals to retire by providing a reliable source of income to the vast majority of U.S. workers. The percentages of people insured (for retirement and survivor benefits) by Social Security increased between 1980 and 2003: for men from 76% to 98.8% and, even more dramatically, from 63.8% to 93.7% among women (U.S. Bureau of the Census, 2005a). As a consequence of this growth, increasing percentages of older adults receive benefits upon eligibility, rising from 69% of age-eligible persons in 1962 to 90% in 2002 (Social Security Administration, 2004a).

Third, Social Security for many decades encouraged retirement by creating financial disincentives to continued employment, especially full-time employment. One such disincentive is called the **earnings test**. In 1995, Social Security reduced retirement benefits to any individuals aged 65–69 with earnings above $11,280 by $1 for every $3 of additional earnings; thus, the earnings test was essentially a penalty for work after retirement (Social Security Administration, 1995). Rules of the earnings test have been relaxed, so that it

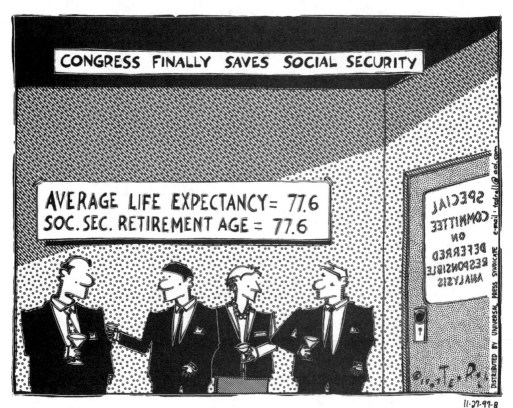

RALL © 1997 Ted Rall. Reprinted with permission of UNIVERSAL PRESS SYNDICATE. All rights reserved.

now applies only to earnings by workers taking early retirement (currently below about age 66). In 2005, an "early retiree" (i.e., someone taking benefits before age 66) can earn up to $12,000 (the lower limit) before the earnings test begins to withhold $1 from the Social Security benefit for every $2 earned over this lower limit. There is also an upper limit, such that when this early retiree earns more than $31,800, Social Security then reduces the benefit beyond this amount by $1 for every $3 earned, reflecting a diminishing penalty for employment by higher earners. These limits have risen significantly in each year since 2000, reducing the effect of the Social Security earnings test as a disincentive to retirement substantially (Social Security Administration, 2004b).

Although Social Security was created to enable workers to retire, not all of its provisions clearly work in that direction. Policy changes in Social Security have started to encourage workers to stay in the labor force longer by raising the age of eligibility for full benefits. Ironically, this change is occurring in an era when private industry, through pension programs, has been encouraging early retirements. As Exhibit 8.1 shows, Social Security eligibility ages are important. Currently workers can take early (reduced) benefits at age 62 and full benefits at age 66. These are, not coincidentally, the peak ages at which workers start their Social Security benefits, with the trend having moved more toward 62 in recent decades. This trend has, however, flattened recently (age 62 retirements were down slightly in 2003), as uncertainties about retirement income sources prompt greater caution among workers. By the year 2022, a worker will have to be 67 (rather than 66) in order to retire with full Social Security benefits. The purpose of increasing the age was to control the costs of the system by shortening the number of years that individuals receive benefits. This change also increases the financial penalty for early retirement at age 62, since Social Security spreads out the same expected dollar amount of benefits over a longer span of years. For example, benefits for taking retirement at age 62 will be reduced from 80% (when the full benefit age was at 65) to 70% (for full benefit eligibility at 67) of the full benefit amount, because of the small reduction assessed for every month that retirement is taken early.

This age increase is not widely understood by the public. Results from the 2004 Retirement Confidence Survey show that only 18% of survey respondents answered correctly regarding the age at which they would be eligible for full benefits under Social Security. Most people thought they would be eligible at an age younger than that designated under the current policy, and 21% didn't know when they would be eligible. The most common incorrect answer, age 65, indicates that many people still do not know about the 1983 policy changes (Center for Retirement Research, 2004).

Although intended to move the "normal" retirement age upward, analyses done to date suggest that the increased age for full Social Security benefits may have little effect on the timing of retirement (Quinn & Burkhauser, 1990). Incentives to keep working have already been implemented, such that Social Security benefits are higher if taken at age 70 than if taken at age 66 or 67. Congress and advocates have brought the age of receipt of full Social Security benefits to the table again as various approaches are made to reform the system to control the costs of supporting the large cohorts of the baby boom (Espo, 2005).

The Role of Employer Pensions

For workers expecting pensions from their employers, the provisions of those programs and the size of benefits are central to retirement decisions (Bender & Jivan, 2005; Schultz

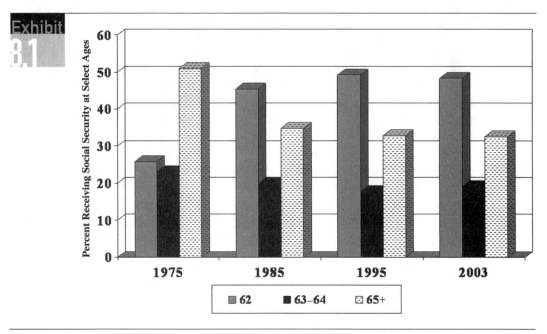

Age at Initial Receipt of Social Security
Source: Social Security Administration, 2004c.

et al., 1998). Increasingly in recent years, the stability of the company's promise to pay benefits through future decades have come into question, as corporate mergers, bankruptcies, and other issues have resulted in dramatic changes in benefits received versus those expected. Advocacy groups, such as the Pension Rights Center, point out the high level of risk involved from underfunded employer pensions, with defaults accumulating at the Pension Benefit Guarantee Corporation (PBGC), the government agency that works to protect pensions as the FDIC does for bank accounts. The PBGC does not guarantee 100% coverage of an individual's expected pension benefits if the employer's program goes into default (Pension Rights Center, 2005).

From the perspective of a worker, **employer pensions** have been thought of as compensation deferred from their working years or a reward for past productivity. Although we often think of pensions as providing an incentive to retire (or to retire early), policies that provide larger benefits if the worker delays retirement another year (or more) can also create an incentive to continue employment (Fields & Mitchell, 1984). Pension provisions have a stronger effect on decisions about retirement timing than does Social Security (Hogarth, 1991), with workers often evaluating various scenarios to calculate their best balance between free time and income.

From the viewpoint of an employer, pensions look quite different (Burkhauser & Quinn, 1994). Pension programs are designed as policy tools to be used by the employer to modify its labor pool as needed over time. Many pension programs both enhance employee loyalty during certain earlier spans of the career and later facilitate departures from employment, both goals frequently sought by employers (Hardy et al., 1996). Employers can build provisions into their pensions that create incentives to exit at a certain age by shrinking the value of a pension if it is deferred. In special circumstances (such as a need to reduce a work force suddenly because of economic stress or merger), employers may add incentives, making the pension more attractive and encouraging mature employees to depart early (Hardy et al., 1996). Pensions may also contain antiwork policies, such as financial penalties to workers for transferring to part-time jobs with the same employer after retiring or denying older workers training or opportunities for advancement (Burkhauser & Quinn, 1994).

The use of pension programs as a policy tool is clearly demonstrated by the recent trend to accomplish corporate downsizing and layoffs through early retirement incentive programs (ERIPs). It is no coincidence that these programs flourish during difficult economic times with an oversupply of labor, when it is less costly for an employer to pay pensions than workers' salaries. Early retirement incentive programs are one solution to having too many employees if demand for goods or services drops. Incentives in some programs are high, including a dramatic increase in both the monthly and lifetime value of a pension and coverage under the employer's health insurance until the age of eligibility for Medicare (Hardy et al., 1996). Although the cost of ERIPs is often high and employers cannot legally choose which employees to retain (such as those with rare or specialized skills), ERIPs are viewed as more humane, better for the corporate image than layoffs, and as causing fewer legal problems for the company.

How the availability and size of a pension influences the decisions of individual workers and the overall trends toward early retirement are complexities beyond the scope of this chapter. Suffice it to say that pension programs are incredibly detailed and diverse. How pensions will change in the future is unpredictable, but changes will certainly be carefully crafted to benefit employers at least as much as retirees (Quinn & Burkhauser, 1990). Changes to pension programs often reflect the changing balance of power between workers and employers in a fashion similar to salary fluctuations. As the supply of labor (including global labor) grows, workers are in a less advantageous position to negotiate for generous pension programs. If employers need to hire and retain highly skilled workers in short supply, however, they may need to offer more extensive benefits, including more generous pensions. To limit their costs and their long-term commitment to funding pensions, many employers are switching to employee-funded and -directed pensions (e.g., 401(k) programs) (Quinn & Burkhauser, 1990). In these programs, employees choose from several investment options and contribute, along with their employers, to a pension "nest egg," which is really an investment in stocks and bonds outside the company's control. Advocates suggest that this change fits well with the American ethic of individual responsibility. Individual workers "own" the fund, but they also undertake whatever risk arises from a downturn in the stock market or poor management by the pensioner (Quinn & Burkhauser, 1990). In addition, this change means that employers have less leverage over when their employees retire, because they are less able to manipulate provisions of this type of pension program to get people to retire when the company wishes (Quinn & Burkhauser, 1990).

Trends in Retirement

Women's Retirement

Projections to 2012 from the Bureau of Labor Statistics suggest that women will constitute 47.5% of the total labor force, a slower growth than that seen in the past several decades, but approaching half of all workers (U.S. Department of Labor, 2004b). Perhaps more significantly, however, an increasing proportion of women will be labor force participants during most of their adult lives (Guy & Erdner, 1993). Despite the significant participation of women, the legacy of presumed disinterest in employment has slowed the study of retirement among women until fairly recently. Historical evidence from the 1800s (Quadagno, 1982) suggests that women living and working then often continued employment into old age because of financial need, even if the jobs available to them were difficult or demeaning. Has the retirement situation improved for women since the early industrial era?

As discussed early in this chapter, women have not followed men into early retirement—at least not the cohorts retiring so far. One reason may be that many of the women in those cohorts entered the labor force later or had more interrupted participation than their male peers, making them both less anxious to withdraw from employment and less likely to be eligible (due to years of service) for employer pensions. As described in chapter 9, there is a gender gap in pension coverage, even without considering women's lesser time in the labor force, so that unmarried women face a different economic landscape if they consider retirement. Early retirement by unmarried women, given fewer economic resources and a longer life expectancy than unmarried men, may be much less economically appealing.

As more of each female cohort participates in the labor force, more women will face eventual retirement. As a result, retirement may encompass different social concerns and meanings in 2050 than it did in 1950, when nearly all retirees were men. The world has indeed changed since Cumming and Henry declared, "Retirement is not an important problem for women, because … working seems to make little difference to them. Retirement is a man's problem" (1961, pp. 144–145).

Early Retirement

Retirement as a stage of life has been increasing at both ends, through increased longevity and earlier retirement. In 1950, before Social Security had its early retirement option, retirement was mandatory and less socially accepted; the average age for receipt of Social Security retirement benefits was 68.7 for men. By the 1980s, the mean age of receipt of Social Security benefits for both men and women had dropped about five years (Gendell & Siegel, 1992). Interpreting the results for women should be done cautiously, since the women who were entitled to retirement benefits from Social Security in the 1950s and 1960s were a select subset of all women. Using other data, Gendell and Siegel (1996) demonstrated a similar pattern for Black workers. Examining the data in Exhibit 8.2 shows that the decline in average age for both women and men has persisted but has not slipped to lower ages. There is much speculation that retirement ages may climb again among baby boom cohorts, ending the slide toward ever-earlier retirement ages among the most economically secure.

Early retirement has become an international phenomenon. Some experts argue that early retirement seems illogical, given increases in both longevity and health well into the seventh and eighth decades of life (Kohli, 1994). Throughout the world, increasing numbers of people are retiring for ever-lengthier periods of time during which they encounter few demands on their time and limited opportunities to contribute to societal productivity. Many countries have passed legislation to raise the age of eligibility for benefits to counteract or minimize the early retirement trend, including some countries where retirement was permitted at even earlier ages (e.g., 60). In the United States we can no longer say that 65 should be identified as the normative age

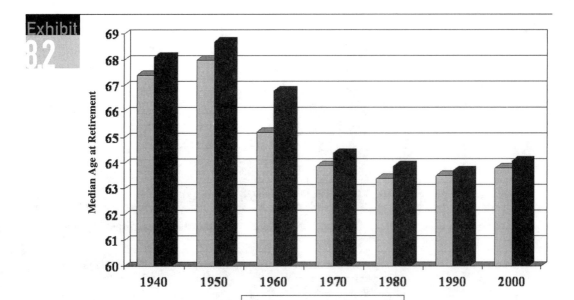

Median Age at Retirement by Sex
Source: Social Security Administration, 2004c.

for retirement, because more workers retire at age 62 than at 65 or 66 (Burkhauser & Quinn, 1994). Yet 65 retains its significance and use as a boundary to later life.

Recent data show that retirement at early ages is declining in the United States and slowing in European countries (Organisation for Economic Co-Operation and Development, 2000). If uncertainty in the labor market increases, if fewer workers have (or trust) employer pensions, or if Social Security benefits decrease, then average retirement ages may increase to 65 or beyond. Alternatively, improvement in the economy may encourage workers or reduce employer disincentives to continuing employment. Any increased age for full Social Security benefits will probably fall most harshly on workers who have had poorer life chances—women, minorities, and the less educated—while early retirement may prevail for those more advantaged. Data on early retirees, for example, show that 20% of them have significant health problems limiting their capacity to work and significantly more held blue collar jobs (Leonesio, Vaughn, & Wixon, 2000). Raising the age of retirement would doubtless expand this percentage of "at risk" workers. If, on the other hand, economic cycles and technological change reduce the demand for labor, older workers may continue to be encouraged to take regular or early retirement. In sum, the future of early retirement rests with social and economic forces beyond prediction today.

Variations in Retirement Trends

As discussed in chapter 7, the life chances of persons in different social groups vary in the labor force. It is not surprising that those who are most advantaged during their years in the labor force also have the greatest number of options regarding ending their employment via retirement. Those who most freely choose to retire are those who can

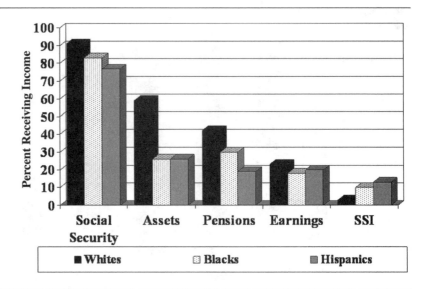

Percentages Receiving Income From Sources by Race/Ethnicity, 2002
Source: Social Security Administration, 2004a.

afford to retire, but who may also have the option of continuing employment. These opportunities are not equally distributed in U.S. society. How do life chances ultimately influence the choices workers face regarding retirement?

Social class and race/ethnicity are other important sources of variation in the conditions facing individuals who are approaching retirement. Those with sporadic employment histories or who became a part of the underground economy are seldom covered by Social Security or employer pensions. These individuals are often unaware as they approach later life that they have worked for years without Social Security contributions being made on their behalf. Exhibit 8.3 shows the percentages receiving any income from major sources, but does not indicate the amount of income. Fewer Black and Hispanic retirees receive income from Social Security, employer pensions, or money generated by assets. Too poor to contemplate early retirement, many of these individuals continue employment as long as their health permits and opportunities are available, often at menial and physically difficult jobs. Retirement, if it comes at all, arrives with the need to cease employment because of poor health or lack of a job and the acceptance of Supplemental Security Income (SSI) or similar welfare-type assistance. Exhibit 8.3 shows that only 3% of older White Americans receive SSI, compared to 10% and 13% for older Blacks and Hispanics. As this graph shows, it is important to not generalize about "the elderly" from the experience of middle-class individuals with pensions and other resources, since not all adults have had equivalent opportunities through the employment structure upon which retirement income is based.

A study of over 11,000 people in 10 countries revealed cultural variations in orientations toward old age and retirement. Despite very different views, the study showed that people in all countries rejected age-based restrictions on employment, with many indicating they planned to work beyond their country's traditional age of retirement (HSBC/AgeWave, 2005).

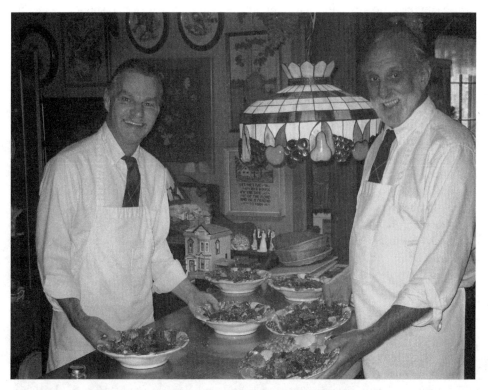

Retirement at early ages is declining in the United States. (Credit: E. J. Hanna)

Individual Retirement

In addition to its importance to the economy, for corporations, and for the larger society on the macro level, retirement is also a key micro-level life cycle transition for individuals and couples. Since mandatory retirement is illegal (with a few exceptions), one might expect increasing variation in when and how workers withdraw from full-time career employment. For most workers, however, this decision is not freely made. Most workers, for instance, cannot decide at age 45 that they wish to retire and be able to do so with economic support from the society or their employer. Despite the acceptance of the social construct of retirement as a life stage and as a legitimate part of the occupational life cycle, a surprising number of workers at ages approaching retirement (51–61) have no plans for the transition or its timing (Ekerdt, DeViney, & Kosloski, 1996). A variety of factors shape the decisions about whether and when to retire.

Further, the orientation toward retirement is based in general attitudes regarding key goals, challenges, and gratifications to be found in retirement. Data from the 10-country study mentioned earlier found that, while Americans focused on later life for spiritual fulfillment, positive attitudes, and private pensions, respondents in other countries differed significantly in their focus (HSBC/AgeWave, 2005). Adults in Brazil focused on relaxation, religion, and support from children; Mexican respondents identified work, financial stability, and personal responsibility as priorities; and Japanese respondents identified work, positive attitudes, and responsibility. Decisions about when and why to retire seem to be based partly in culture.

Determinants of the Retirement Decision

Often we think of retirement as determined by age, and in fact an individual's age does play a role by determining eligibility for retirement programs and pensions. The earliest research on retirement behavior in the 1940s focused on mandatory retirement policies and poor health as causes for male workers to leave their jobs via retirement (Quinn & Burkhauser, 1990), typically viewing retirement as a negative event in a worker's life. A few decades later, attention turned to the critical role played by retirement income as an enabling factor in retirement. While economists continue to focus on pensions and Social Security benefits, many other factors—health status, job satisfaction, family responsibilities, and the retirement of a spouse—are considered central to retirement decisions today (Quinn & Burkhauser, 1990; Ruhm, 1996).

In thinking of the **retirement decision**, we assume that every worker reaching an age at which retirement is common periodically considers this array of factors to decide whether to retire this year, next year, 10 years in the future, or never. In fact, the process of reaching this retirement decision is probably not as orderly as researchers once presumed and may involve a variety of individual factors (how much they like their coworkers, the difficulty of their commute, changes in the cost of living or health care, what activities they anticipate during retirement) that remain largely unmeasured (Hardy et al., 1996). Research has focused on more standard items—such as health, availability of pension and other retirement income, marital status, and employment history—which are available for secondary analysis in large national surveys (Quinn & Burkhauser, 1990).

Among the most highly researched topics are financial factors, which are often quite complex in their effects on retirement decision making (Fields & Mitchell, 1984). The size of a monthly pension benefit and its rules (e.g., based on age or years of service for eligibility), the monthly dollar value of Social Security benefits, and workers' expectations about the adequacy of these main sources of income over the future years of retirement help to shape individuals' decisions regarding the timing of retirement. A worker might, for example, balance the value of current earnings and any added benefits to a pension or Social Security from another year of work against the cost of a lost year's worth of pension and other benefits and leisure time sacrificed if she continues employment (Quinn & Burkhauser, 1990). It is unclear how well typical workers understand the economic intricacies involved, such as figuring the growth in cost of living over a 20–30 year retirement or its potential for erosion of buying power if their employer pension is a fixed dollar amount. Recently this uncertainty has been augmented by growing numbers of employers closing retiree health benefit programs or failing to fund their pension funds adequately.

It was not until the 1970s that researchers began to investigate retirement among women (Slevin & Wingrove, 1995). Given lifelong differences in employment patterns for women, concerns were raised that utilizing a male model of the retirement decision would inadequately represent the factors that influence women. Retirement decisions among women are influenced by a variety of factors that are often ignored in studies of men, including family caregiving responsibilities and (for those who are married) their spouse's health (Weaver, 1994). For example, Ruhm (1996) found that married women with heavy caregiving responsibilities more often withdrew from employment and were much more likely to give family reasons for their decisions. In some studies of women's retirement, financial issues were much less important than health and family factors in determining when retirement occurred (Weaver, 1994). For married couples, a subset of women continue to work after their husbands retire, but some research suggests that wives time their retirements to that of their husbands, but that the opposite is not true (Slevin & Wingrove, 1995). Continuing to work after a husband retires may be due to women being younger and thus not yet eligible for retirement benefits, or continuing to work may be a financial necessity. Interruptions in married women's labor force participation, such as breaks for child rearing, may also mean that they are less ready to retire at the same ages as their husbands (Feuerbach & Erdwins, 1994). Women's attention to couple and family issues, and men's relative inattention to these issues in retirement, suggests that cohorts recently retiring have not moved very far from our stereotypes of women as primarily rooted in the family and men in their careers. It will be interesting to see whether the dynamics of retirement among women will become more like those of men as more women in coming cohorts of retirees have experienced career trajectories involving fewer and shorter interruptions for family work and as wages for women have risen. It will also be interesting to see whether family-related issues become more central to studies of male retirement.

Decisions on whether to retire and when to retire are also related to the availability of continued employment. As mentioned earlier, significant subsets of older adults continue employment beyond age 65 (Social Security Administration, 2004a). There is a resurgent interest in both health and labor-market barriers to continued employment (Quinn & Burkhauser, 1990). Many older workers say they would prefer to work part-time. What they actually mean is that they would like to reduce their hours but remain at the same wages—preferably in the same job. Employers seldom offer the same wages to part-time workers, so few workers can gradually retire through movement to part-time employment in their same jobs (Quinn & Burkhauser, 1990), sometimes called "phased retirement (see Exhibit 8.4). Instead, the retirement decision is most often an either/or decision of continued full-time employment or complete withdrawal—at least from a primary employer. Such a retirement may not be final, however, because many people become reemployed after retiring from a long-term job, as we discuss later in the chapter.

A significant number of men and women participate in the labor force while receiving either Social Security retirement benefits or income from an employer pension (Herz, 1995). Some describe this combination as "work after retirement," but it may be more complicated than that. Employment with a pension is highest for the youngest group of men (ages 50–54) and drops substantially for those 62 and over, the age of eligibility for early Social Security benefits. Employment among the younger pensioned individuals (under age 62) has been increasing since the mid-1980s, perhaps reflecting the continued employment of men leaving their career jobs through early retirement incentives but not yet ready to withdraw completely from employment.

Our thinking about retirement may eventually evolve into a series of decisions on whether to seek a new job once the current job ends (Doeringer, 1990). Fields and Mitchell (1984) have proposed a variety of possible models to substitute for the either/or retirement process, including intermittent work, gradual reduction of hours, and varying levels of part-time employment after leaving a primary career (see Exhibit 8.4).

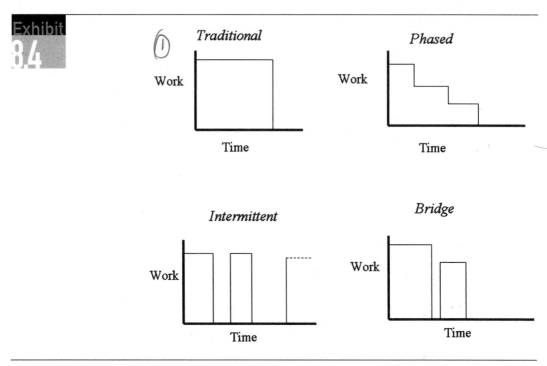

Exhibit 8.4

Alternative Retirement Patterns

Employment After Retirement—Bridge Jobs

We think about retirement as an abrupt transition, moving from full-time career employment one day to no employment the next, as in the traditional pattern in Exhibit 8.4. In fact, it is not so simple. A growing percentage of older workers find their career jobs disappearing before they are ready to retire, requiring them to seek what are called **bridge jobs**—jobs to carry them over between a career job and full retirement, often with lower pay and fewer benefits (Burkhauser & Quinn, 1994; Doeringer, 1990; Quinn & Kozy, 1996). Ruhm (1990) reports that half of all workers leave their career jobs and take other employment before fully retiring, with the highest percentages in this pattern found for minority and women workers. Employers continue to offer relatively few options for flexible retirement, clinging to the occupational life cycle that strictly separates the working phase of life from that of retirement. Among innovators, Mc-Donalds created a McMasters program, intended to attract retirees to employment on a part-time basis for fast-food restaurants at low wages. This typically represents substantial downward mobility for a former manager or professional, but may provide needed income for someone not yet eligible for retirement income; such programs benefit employers by the greater reliability of older (versus teenage) workers. Chapter 7 also described companies using their own retirees to meet labor force needs in specialized programs.

Many older workers find new jobs, construct self-employment options, or locate bridge jobs that move them more gradually from full-time employment to complete retirement (Quinn & Burkhauser, 1990). One study found that more than 25% of retirees from a career job continued in the labor force, most for at least two years and many in substantially different types of employment (Quinn & Burkhauser, 1990). This pattern helps explain the growing numbers of people with both pensions and jobs. Ruhm (1990) describes job-stopping as increasingly similar to the period of labor force entry, wherein a worker holds several jobs on the way to a career job of longer duration.

Mutchler and her colleagues (1997) describe this newer pattern as blurred rather than the crisp transition of traditional retirement. Departure from employment may involve stepping through a number of jobs as individuals wind down their involvement with the labor force. The contradictory messages coming from private employers through incentives and downsizing ("retire early") and from the government via increased Social Security eligibility ages, reduced penalties for work in retirement, and removal of mandatory retirement ("retire later") may mean that bridge jobs are an increasingly prevalent form of gradual exit from the labor force (Quinn & Kozy, 1996).

Retirement Consequences for Individuals and Couples

Early researchers (in the 1940s and 1950s) studied the consequences of retirement with clear expectations. They anticipated, based on their orientations as middle-class men steeped in the work ethic, that retirees would experience stress upon separation from employment and lose their core identities as male breadwinners. Since mandatory retirement was much more prevalent at the time, it was feared that workers were being unwillingly "put out to pasture" before they were socially or economically prepared. It was with a great deal of surprise, therefore, that they found that most retired men were not unhappy or maladjusted (Atchley, 1976). Most early studies of retirement satisfaction showed that retirees were largely happy with their situations, not the stressed and "roleless" outcasts that had been expected (Atchley, 1976).

A longitudinal study of 800 workers found no change in self-esteem and a decline in depression among those who retired, suggesting stability or positive outcomes from retirement (Reitzes, Mutran, & Fernandez, 1996). Not all retirees enjoy retirement equally. Those who retire in good health, who have adequate income, and whose decision to retire was truly voluntary fare better, as do those with strong social networks and activities planned during retirement. The work ethic, as we will see in upcoming discussion of continuity theory, is transformed into the "busy ethic" of an active leisure in retirement for many of these advantaged individuals.

While negative outcomes have not been shown for the majority of male workers, the evidence for women is more mixed. Although most of the research has focused on men, an analysis of both men and women showed that women are less satisfied in retirement, partly due to other major life events (illness of self or spouse, relocation, divorce, or widowhood) happening near the time of retirement (Szinovacz & Washo, 1992). Recent analyses by Szinovacz and Davey (2004) show that the women who retired abruptly due to spouse disability experienced greater depression than men with similar experiences as caregivers, a result that seems to contradict gender-based expectations.

These mixed findings may also be related to the poorer economic security of retiring women, especially if they are widowed (Guy & Erdner, 1993). Calasanti (1996a) points out that women's satisfaction in retirement is shaped by their experiences in the labor force, which systematically differ from those of men. For women in traditionally female jobs, Calasanti (1996a) found that only health influenced their satisfaction in retirement. Using only the experiences of male workers (often middle-class White male workers) gives an unrealistic picture of how the experience of retirement influences workers in other groups.

Research using the 2000 wave of the Health and Retirement Study (HRS) examined satisfaction of retirees with retirement itself and in comparison to their pre-retirement circumstances. Few individuals (7.5%) said retirement was not at all satisfying; about 60% said it was "very satisfying." Half reported that retired life was better than life before retirement (Bender & Jivan, 2005). Not surprisingly, individuals who experienced push factors, such as poor health or being forced in some way to retire, reported less satisfaction.

Another study examined retirees' perceptions of whether their exits were voluntary or involuntary. Analyzing three waves of the longitudinal HRS sample, researchers asked self-identified retirees whether their retirement was "forced." Nearly a third of older workers perceived their retirements as forced, with several of the typical push factors (i.e., poor health, family caregiving, or job loss) bringing about retirement when it was not expected or desired.

Examination of those who said their retirements were not voluntary showed that they were in a more tenuous economic situation, perhaps lacking the time to accumulate the resources to allow them to feel secure in retiring (Bender & Jivan, 2005; Szinovacz & Davey, 2005). Workers who chose to retire and were able to choose the timing of this transition have fared better than those whose health, employment circumstances, family pressures, or other personal factors forced their retirement at a time not of their choosing. In the study of auto workers mentioned earlier (Hardy & Quadagno, 1995), those who had anticipated retirement and perceived it as a true choice were more satisfied afterward than those who felt pushed to retire by their employment situation or health problems.

In addition, it is important to examine the context of retirement within the life course perspective. Kim and Moen (2002) examined psychological well-being over a 2-year period of older adults who continued to work, were newly retired, or had been retired for some time. They found that the context in which these employment-related changes occurred (i.e., marital status, income adequacy, subjective health, sense of personal control) made a difference for both women and men. Temporal issues (recentness of retirement) made a difference in depression and morale only for men. Recently retired men, described as being in a "honeymoon phase," fared better in psychological well-being than longer-retired men, but there was also significant influence by the contextual factors. Women did not experience a similar change in psychological well-being in conjunction with their transitions to retirement. The authors conclude, "Our findings indicate that retirement is not simply a state but a complex process, embedded in prior psychological resources as well as gendered experiences" (Kim & Moen, 2002, p. 219).

Rethinking Retirement for the Future

Changes in Policies and Political Attitudes

The U.S. government has already taken policy steps, including abolishing mandatory retirement and raising the age of full entitlement to Social Security benefits, intended to increase the likelihood of employment into later years of life. The business community has so far not followed suit by modifying pension programs and employment policies to encourage older workers to remain, even in a modified capacity. Business' short-term interests still point to removal, rather than retention, of workers past their early 60s (Rix, 1991). Although the alarm has sounded about the aging of the baby boomers and smaller cohorts to follow, a variety of political forces and attitudes shape retirement for future cohorts and, indirectly, employment prospects for younger cohorts.

As mentioned earlier, proposals have been put forward to raise the age of entitlement to Social Security beyond the target age of 67. One such proposal argues for "equivalent retirement ages," whereby the age of entitlement would be shifted to keep the ratio between years in retirement and working life constant (Chen, 1994). Such a policy would shift the age of entitlement for Social Security benefits upward as life expectancy increases and, presumably, as healthy life expectancy expands. This would keep the retirement stage more fixed in length, rather than permitting its continued expansion as longevity increases. Other proposals simply suggest mandating 70 as the age of eligibility for full Social Security benefits, further penalizing early retirement financially.

Despite policy changes encouraging later retirement (Quinn & Burkhauser, 1990), the interest in early retirement remains strong in most developed countries (Guillemard, 1996). The synergy between income maintenance programs and the institutionalization of retirement should not be underestimated. Workers lacking financial support do not see retirement as a viable option if it would mean poverty! And dismantling or significantly altering what has now come to be an expected part of the life course will be far from simple.

Applying Theory

Continuity Theory and the "Busy Ethic"

A central tenet of Western cultures for centuries has been the importance of employment—the **work ethic.**

> The work ethic, like any ethic, is a set of beliefs and values that identifies what is good and affirms ideals of conduct. The work ethic historically has identified work with virtue and has held up for esteem a conflation of such traits and habits as diligence, initiative, temperance, industriousness, competitiveness, self-reliance, and the capacity for deferred gratification. (Ekerdt, 1986, p. 239)

Although sometimes attributed to the Puritans, the work ethic has a long cultural heritage from a time when labor by all was necessary to survival, and pride in successful employment was central to identity (Plakans, 1994). The work ethic has long been viewed as a pivotal force, driving men (and, more recently, women) to seek employment and job-related achievement as one basis of self-worth.

But how do individuals adjust when retirement removes the status and achievement engendered by employment?

Perhaps a partial answer to this question can be found in continuity theory, an individual-level theory spawned (along with activity theory) from the reaction to disengagement theory. Central to continuity theory is the idea that adults, in adapting as they age, attempt to preserve and maintain existing self-concepts, relationships, and ways of doing things (Atchley, 1989). Activity theory argued for equilibrium—replacing a lost activity or relationship with an equivalent. "Continuity theory assumes evolution, not homeostasis, and this assumption allows change to be integrated into one's prior history without necessarily causing upheaval and disequilibrium" (Atchley, 1989, p. 183). Faced with change, aging adults select alternatives consistent with who they have been and what they have done in the past. Internal continuity enables individuals to connect current changes with their past, sustaining the sense

(continued)

(continued)

of self. External continuity is maintained by "being and doing in familiar environments, practicing familiar skills and interacting with familiar people" (Atchley, 1989, p. 185).

Consistent with the tenets of continuity theory, David Ekerdt (1986) posited a moral imperative for involvement during retirement, which he calls the **busy ethic.**

> Just as there is a work ethic that holds industriousness and self-reliance as virtues, so, too, there is a "busy ethic" for retirement that honors an active life. It represents people's attempts to justify retirement in terms of their long-standing beliefs and values. (p. 239)

He argues that people legitimate retirement and leisure by being highly occupied—keeping busy—much as they did during their years of employment. Rather than unlearning the work ethic, people transform it into the busy ethic, giving content to the retiree role once considered void of normative expectations. The result is a moral continuity between employed and retired statuses that answers many questions about the appropriateness of retirement as a life stage. As a stepchild of the work ethic, Ekerdt argues, the busy ethic lets retirees approach leisure in the same organized and purposeful manner in which they previously approached employment. Retirees don't actually have to pursue constant busyness but should at least talk about their activities and plans to be busy in the future. This busyness represents a high degree of continuity in the lives of individuals, who substitute community work, socializing, and leisure pursuits for a schedule made busy by employment. It structures time in a much more socially acceptable and work-consistent manner than would an ethic of nonconformity and self-indulgence, therefore providing a sense of continuity to individuals and to society. The busy ethic, then, gives middle-class retirees a type of continuity at retirement, minimizing (according to the theory) the risks of disruption and distress.

Those planning activities for future cohorts of the elderly may want to keep the notion of continuity in the forefront. If continuity is important, then older adults who have retired will probably seek activities in which they can gain both the sense of

(continued)

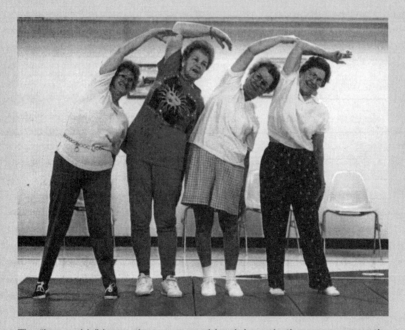

The "busy ethic" has retirees approaching leisure in the same energetic, organized, and purposeful manner as they approached employment. (Credit: Mike Payne, courtesy of the Ohio Department of Aging)

(continued)
busyness and the feelings of accomplishment for-merly provided by employment. These needs may help explain why some adults eschew participation in today's senior centers, where gossip, arts and crafts, lunch, and bingo often represent the core of the day. If such activities do not provide a sense of continuity for individuals who have retired, perhaps rethinking the activities available at senior centers to include meaningful volunteerism and opportunities for part-time employment will make them more rel-evant to future cohorts of retired Americans.

Changes in the Economy and the Nature of Work

The productivity of the labor force depends on a number of factors, including the use of advanced technologies such as computers and robotics, as well as the degree of fit be-tween a job's demands and the skills and abilities of a worker filling it. And one thing is for certain—the labor market is changing. Many types of jobs require high levels of skill and continuous upgrading of education or training so that workers remain current with new developments. Other jobs are becoming deskilled, as machines take over the tasks of workers, who simply service and maintain the equipment. For example, engineers and architects are now significantly assisted by computer software that replaces some tasks formerly done by humans. The resulting deskilling of jobs often results in lower wages and makes workers more easily replaceable, because their particular training and knowledge of the business so rapidly become obsolete (Auster, 1996). These changes are so fundamental that it remains unclear how they will ultimately shape the needs and the size of the labor force. Given all of the uncertainties, it is difficult to predict the degree to which older workers may be encouraged to continue in current jobs, be retrained into new employment, retire, or move to part-time work.

Employers are changing their policies to move away from lifetime employment of workers. The odds of receiving a pension from a single lifetime employer are limited by trends such as contingent employment. By using contingent labor, employers limit their current costs and also their investment in particular workers over the long term. Employees may pay a price, as retirement may become impractical for contingent work-ers, who lack pensions and may have been less able to save except to fund gaps between contracts (Quinn & Burkhauser, 1990).

These changes also reflect the goals of large-scale business and industry as they com-pete in a global marketplace for both goods and labor. Locking a business into long-term obligations with hundreds or thousands of workers in one country limits its capacity to respond to lower wage rates or abundant skilled labor elsewhere in the world. In addition, employers are starting to think more flexibly about the site of employment, as more in-formation-based jobs can be performed at home or in less-expensive office space halfway around the world. The ramifications of these changes for how individuals move through and exit from their working lives have not been fully explored. Although we tend to focus on the big employers and how they are changing, most U.S. workers are employed in smaller businesses, not the corporate giants. Only 36% of workers are employed in firms of 2,500 workers or more (U.S. Bureau of the Census, 2001), and smaller firms have al-ways had more difficulty offering benefits such as pensions to their workers.

Attitudes about work and retirement seem to be moving in a direction supportive of a flexible view of moving into and out of the labor force in a less structured fash-ion. Exhibit 8.5 shows the percentages of working-age adults (18–39 and 40–59) in 10

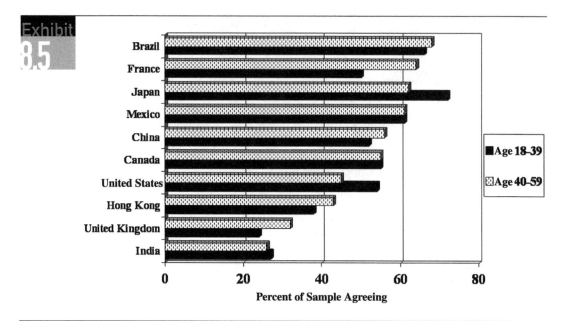

Exhibit 8.5

Percentage Agreeing That Alternating Periods of Work and Leisure Is the Ideal, by Age and Country
Source: HSBC/AgeWave, 2005.

countries supportive of going back and forth between periods of work and periods of education and leisure as the "ideal plan" (HSBC/AgeWave, 2005). Support for this idea ranged from a low in India to a high in Brazil, with the United States among countries whose populations are less favorable to this possibility. There are age differences, but they aren't systematic—sometimes the younger adults are more favorable, sometimes those closer to retirement. The study's authors suggest that this is part of a new vision for later life that includes significantly more flexibility of roles and their timing, including when—and whether—retirement is chosen by individuals.

Robert Kahn (1994) has suggested a rethinking of how we define and organize work. He concurs that the concept of **productive aging** should be expanded to include activities such as family and household duties and volunteerism undertaken by older and younger persons. Given the preferences many workers have for part-time jobs, Kahn also suggests that we re-engineer work time into four-hour work modules that can be flexibly combined into full- or part-time options. This more flexible approach would avoid a false dichotomy between the 35- to 40-hour full-time status and any other type of schedule (i.e., part-time, retired) that now seems to be built into the thinking of employers. This type of innovative thinking may give us clues to how retirement may evolve into an entirely new, socially constructed pattern in the future, where work, training, and leisure are variably combined through time, much like Riley's rethinking of an age-integrated life course (see chapter 4).

SUMMARY

We are already seeing the policy underpinnings of a changed conception of retirement, as Social Security raises entitlement ages and reduces penalties for working while receiving benefits. As policy discussions continue regarding the fate of Social Security (see chapters 9 and 12), we face continuing questions regarding the future of retirement. As the break between employment and retirement becomes less clear, we may one day cease to celebrate this passage in the way we now do—with gold watches and parties—and simply bid farewell to workers of all ages as they move on to their next employment opportunity. With a dynamic labor market, dynamism in individual lives, and changing meanings of work and retirement, the best prediction we can make is one of change—either modest or major—in the future of these social institutions.

Individual retirement, influenced by a broad array of personal dimensions as well as financial issues, continues to be a welcomed stage by most retired people. Suggestions that early retirement is fading and that cohorts of the baby boom are voicing hesitation to retire reflect the power of financial insecurity in the overall equation of whether it's safe to retire. As the first of these individuals reach early retirement age under Social Security in 2008, the changes will begin to be revealed.

WEB WISE

Center for Retirement Research

http://www.bc.edu/centers/crr

The Center for Retirement Research promotes research on current retirement issues from some of the leading scholars and regularly provides publications that represent cutting-edge information that may be of interest. A recent visit to the site found featured topics including Social Security reform, success of 401(k) retirement programs, health care costs, and "what makes retirees happy."

National Academy of Social Insurance

http://www.nasi.org

The National Academy of Social Insurance is an organization to promote understanding and informed policymaking on social insurance, including Social Security, Medicare, workers' compensation, unemployment insurance, and private employee benefits. The NASI conducts research and writes reports, and the Web site is searchable for detailed information on the topics within its area of interest.

KEY TERMS

bridge jobs	earnings test	retirement decision
busy ethic	employer pensions	work ethic
continuity theory	productive aging	
Early Retirement Incentive Programs (ERIPs)	push and pull factors	
	retirement	

QUESTIONS FOR THOUGHT AND DISCUSSION

1. Given the dynamics of lives and the labor market, does the concept of retirement make sense? Think about the diverse circumstances (i.e., familial,

economic, health) individuals face as they approach retirement ages as you consider alternatives.

2. Employer pensions have been a cornerstone of enabling large numbers of people to fully withdraw from employment at retirement. As pensions become less reliable and baby boomers show some hesitancy to retire, consider whether they'll be able to find good quality employment, either bridge jobs or post-retirement employment. What are the barriers and benefits for an employer?

3. David Ekerdt points to what he views as a mainstream adaptation to retirement in his concept of the "busy ethic." What constitutes a "good retirement," and does society currently enable all people opportunities to achieve a good retirement?

4. Chapter 6 explored some significant changes in family structure and relationships that are likely to reshape the future. How might changes in families influence decisions regarding retirement or activities of retirees?

E-Elders

The computer revolution and the exponential growth of the Internet are among the most recent in a long line of technological innovations that have touched the lives of current older adults. The oldest old have seen the development of home electrification, air travel, interstate highways, "smart houses," portable recorded music, cell phones, and microwave ovens, to name only a few. How are older adults responding to these major transformations of the social and electronic worlds? Do older adults embrace or reject the electronic revolution? Do the reactions of older adults to the emergent cyber-world support or refute stereotypes of older adults being resistant to learning innovations, including new technologies? Although we don't yet have all of the answers to these questions, some studies of older adults and the use of electronic technologies, most specifically personal computers, give us some clues.

Exposure and Expansion

Examples of older adults using the Internet are increasingly visible. A quick search of "Books in Print" database shows that publishers are starting to market books on computers for Seniors, with two new ones appearing in early 2006. Web designers and advocacy groups have begun campaigns to make online resources more accessible to older adults (Benbow, 2004). National studies show that older adults increasingly have computers available in their homes, and use them (Rogers, Mayhorn, & Fisk, 2004). But many questions remain, including whether this growth reflects older adults adopting these new technologies or whether new cohorts of computer-users are "aging into" the population and raising the figures. It appears that the trajectory of increase in computer use has to include significant adoption of the technology by those who have been retired for many years. The most persistent myth, despite lots of cartoons and jokes in the media about getting children or grandchildren to operate electronic gizmos, is that older adults can and do use these technologies (Rogers et al., 2004).

How do older people use computers? There are an increasing number of ways that computers are useful, including supporting people with services, connecting them to friends and family via e-mail, and increasingly addressing health care. Managing life with limitations, an older woman with failing eyesight and mobility limitations was able to remain in her home with the support system available via her computer. She used online food orders sent to her grandson some distance away to continue her independence (Setton, 2000). Communication with friends and family is a key use of computers. After a retirement community training class, one trainee said, "I have friends all over the country." Another stated that the course "improved my outlook on life. I really can learn something new and it makes me feel more up-to-date." Contrary to some stereotypes, other students in the course expressed concerns about becoming "computer junkies" (White, McConnell, Clipp, Bynum, Teague, et al., 1999). Studies that have monitored users found a decrease in loneliness and a sense of mastery after learning something new and innovative (White, et al., 1999). Despite positive reactions among older adults, there remain persistent negative attitudes toward older people taking—and succeeding in—computer training (Morrell, Mayhorn, & Echt, 2004).

Only recently have programmers and Web site developers directed creative attention to the needs of older people. While product development for older adults has caught up with that for younger markets, there is a growing thrust in designing online services and products that are appealing and accessible for older people. As the age of the population shifts and a growing portion of the market for electronic goods will be over 65, businesses focusing on the new technologies will need to be careful not to cut off one-fifth of their potential market.

Utilization and Benefits

There are varying estimates of the utilization of personal computers and the Internet by adults over age 65. National estimates from 2001 showed that about one-fourth of households (23.4%) headed by people over 65 included a personal computer, compared to over half (51.6%) of all households. Even fewer (17.7%) of the 65 and older households had Internet service, so older adults lag behind in home access to computers and use of the internet (Administration on Aging, 2001).

In recent years developers are continuing to create Web sites specifically oriented to older adults, including sites such as "Goldngal: the Cyberspace Granny," "SeniorNet," "Thirdage.com" and a range of others, including some you'll find at the end of the chapters in this book (see Furlong, 1997; Setton, 2000).

Advocates for the new technologies cheer the vast potential for practical and innovative uses of computer technology for the older population. Internet access can reduce the social isolation of individuals with mobility limitations that keep them at home much of the time. Older people with health problems can also use the Internet to access sources of information about health and treatments (Vastag, 2001), and increasingly "telemedicine" allows health conditions to be monitored at home via measurement equipment (e.g., a blood pressure monitor) that can be attached to a desktop computer to feed regular readings to the physician. The Internet can enhance autonomy among older adults in the community or in long-term care by linking people to information about services and organizations and by encouraging the creation or maintenance of social networks (Deatrick, 1997; Hunt, 1997; McConatha, McConatha, & Dermigny, 1994; Redford & Whitten, 1997; Setton, 2000).

Limitations

Access to the world provided by the personal computers and the Internet may be hampered for older adults in two ways. First, physical or cognitive limitations may make technology harder to access. Limited vision or hand dexterity because of arthritis or stroke, for example, make use of standard computers difficult without additional modification, such as voice recognition software. Handheld devices, with even smaller keys and screens, are even more challenging to use (Scialfa, Ho, & Laberge, 2004). These additions may be costly or add to the challenge of using the computer (White et al., 1999). Many of today's older adults have little or no experience using a keyboard, which makes typing itself a challenge and discourages some people from trying to learn more. Research on the willingness and capacity of older adults to learn computer skills is ambiguous (Kelley & Charness 1995). Although older adults take more time to learn software and make more errors during training courses (White et al., 1999), most older adults are quite capable of learning the skills (Morrell et al., 2004).

Second, the issues of the so-called digital divide remain influential in the use of computers by low-income elders. A fundamental cause of this divide is economic. High initial costs of computer equipment for the home, plus the costs of Internet connections, make the expense of getting connected too high for some low-income people, including older adults on low fixed incomes. To help address the digital divide, many senior centers or community program sites now have desktop computers available to use at no cost, enabling wider use of favored programs, such as e-mail contact with friends and family living far away. However, the best way for older adults to have access is not to hope for an open desktop at the senior center but to have a personal computer at home with Internet access. We are still far from equal access to computers for old or young in American society.

Economics and the Aging of Society

The future of old age is uniquely tied to the future history of our welfare state. ... Politics, not demography, now determines the size of the elderly population and the material conditions of its existence. (Myles, 1989)

The Role of Economics in Aging

The economic structure of a society has a profound influence on the lives of its citizens. The economy affects, and is affected by, politics, social policy, and work and retirement patterns. These interrelationships make it difficult to discuss one social institution without the other. As we explore the economics of aging, it is important to understand how our social policies relating to work, retirement, and income maintenance in later life at the macro level shape, reflect, and sustain the economic circumstances of older people. This link between social policy and the economic situation of older people is not unique to the United States. "Despite enormous national differences in social structure and political ideology, state-administered Social Security schemes are now the major source of income for the majority of elderly in all capitalist democracies" (Myles, 1989, p. 322). While an in-depth analysis of the intersections among ideologies, market economies, and the welfare state are beyond the scope of this book, we must acknowledge that political processes, power, and agendas play a pivotal role in shaping the economic situation of older people.

Economic factors influence our lives as they unfold through time in many ways. This chapter examines both the economic status of the older population, primarily in the United States, and how older persons as a social group in turn influence the economy. We start by exploring the complex world of policies to provide income support to the older population and their implications for economic well-being.

Policy and the Economic Status of Older Adults

Income Maintenance Policies

In many countries, older persons are protected by **income maintenance systems**—public, private, or combined systems for supporting the poor, ill, and elderly using public monies or funds generated through employment. The idea of providing income to maintain older persons in their later lives, after they are no longer involved in the labor force, grew from many roots. Central among these roots was the British system of Poor Laws from the 17th century. Poor Laws defined older persons as among the **deserving poor**—citizens lacking the means to support themselves through no fault of their own. Poor older adults and other paupers who were considered deserving of society's support (those who had worked hard, saved, not drunk or gambled away their money) received either a modest pension or food and lodging in a workhouse or poorhouse run by the community (Quadagno, 1982). From this beginning has evolved a set of public and private programs in many countries that are intended to maintain at least a minimal flow of income to older persons who have retired or become economically dependent (Kinsella & Phillips, 2005; Schulz & Myles, 1990).

Since its creation, the U.S. system to support the deserving poor has kept changing between pensions and poorhouse support because of concern that providing a cash income from public coffers (called a pension) would discourage personal saving, undermine the duty of family to provide support, and ultimately increase the financial burden to the community. The poorhouse, a truly unattractive alternative, was believed to encourage personal and family responsibility compared to pensions (Schulz & Myles, 1990). This familiar debate about maintaining individual and family responsibility for the care of dependent elders and other deserving poor persons has a continuing legacy today. Western societies still struggle with the tension between individual and collective values regarding provision for dependent populations. Concerns persist today that remotely comfortable levels of government benefits will undermine the responsibility of families and individuals for their own financial support.

The interest of governments in establishing income maintenance policies is not purely altruistic. As Schulz and Myles (1990) point out, countries that develop industrialized economies need ways to deal with those who are unable to participate as workers for reasons of advanced age, disability, and so forth. Having some income maintenance system, whether it involves benefits based on need (e.g., disability programs or Supplemental Security Income [SSI], discussed below) or public/private pensions based in employment, enables governments to avoid upheavals from masses of disenfranchised persons. "Very simply, market economies need ways of providing for those who cannot participate in markets; labor markets need welfare states or people will die or revolt (or both!)" (Schulz & Myles, 1990, p. 401). Thus, as many countries industrialized and urbanized, it was clear that issues of income maintenance would have to be addressed.

Instead of general policies including all ages, many societies established separate programs of income maintenance for older persons and for children, disabled adults,

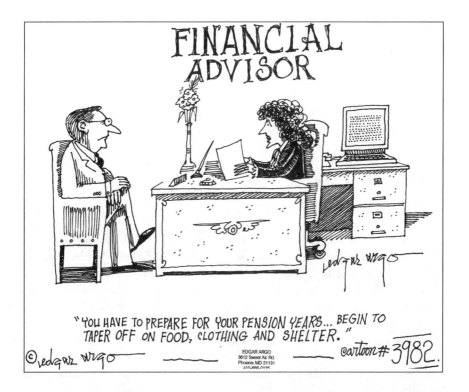

"YOU HAVE TO PREPARE FOR YOUR PENSION YEARS... BEGIN TO TAPER OFF ON FOOD, CLOTHING AND SHELTER."

and other deserving groups. Until fairly recently, programs to assist the elderly have drawn high levels of support from both the public and politicians (Hudson, 1978). Support from the older population and their family members swells the constituency with an interest in seeing that income maintenance is continued. In recent years, however, income maintenance for older persons has become a controversial issue internationally, largely because the aging of populations raises the price tag for these programs.

Income Maintenance in the United States

Two distinct premises underlie the income maintenance system in the United States. The bulk of income maintenance is predicated on the idea that benefits are earned through prior productivity. Leading examples are Social Security retirement benefits and employer pensions, which are based directly on having made a significant contribution in the paid labor force (or being a dependent of such a contributor). By reaching a specified age (or number of years of employment), one becomes eligible for benefits—a system known as **age eligibility**. Additional programs, such as the SSI program for poor and disabled older adults, are based on need. When individuals establish that their resources fall below a certain level, they receive benefits based on criteria of **need eligibility**.

SSI, a major need eligibility program for income maintenance in the United States, supported about 6.9 million beneficiaries in 2005 (nearly 2 million of them 65 or older) with the average recipient's monthly benefit being $579 (Social Security

Administration, 2004d). Although SSI is administered by the Social Security Administration, it uses need eligibility criteria—in contrast to the age eligibility basis for retirement benefits—to determine who receives support. Because such need entitlement programs carry the stigma of welfare, they are embraced by neither taxpayers nor benefit recipients. In either age or need eligibility, the fundamental ideology behind income maintenance is that older people are economically dependent through age and (possibly) poor health and are deserving of public support, rather than being left to rely entirely on their families or their own resources.

International Views on Income Maintenance

Although Americans tend to be most familiar with domestic programs such as Social Security, income maintenance for the elderly is a feature of social policy in most countries of the world (Hoskins, 1992). In 1940 only 33 countries had retirement systems in place, but the number had grown to more than 165 by 2000 (Kinsella & Phillips, 2005). Most countries began with a minimal benefit, enabling workers to survive when the health problems common with aging made them unable to earn a living. Percentages receiving coverage in these programs range from 90% or more in some developed countries to some developing countries that only cover government workers (Kinsella & Phillips, 2005). The generosity of benefits also varies widely across countries and for women and men within these countries, with the U.S. programs doing worse than some other countries in keeping older adults out of poverty (Holtz-Eakin & Smeeding, 1994).

Programs of the social insurance type (similar to U.S. Social Security) predominate among the industrialized nations (Schulz & Myles, 1990). Most **social insurance** programs share the traits of national coverage with compulsory participation, benefits related to earnings or length of employment, contributions from workers and employers, a benefit intended to meet minimum needs, and mechanisms to adapt this benefit to inflation (Schulz & Myles, 1990). Programs in less developed nations may take very different forms, such as mutual benefit societies among occupational groups or compulsory savings programs, called provident funds, to meet a variety of needs including, but not limited to, retirement and disability (Schulz & Myles, 1990).

Income maintenance in the United States rests on a number of different programs and sources (Social Security, employer pensions, personal savings and IRAs, SSI, other benefits such as food stamps and housing subsidies) rather than on an integrated system of benefits used in some European countries. Many European countries have universal social insurance retirement pensions with relatively high minimum benefit levels (Holtz-Eakin & Smeeding, 1994).

Sources of Income

The image used by the Social Security Administration in describing income maintenance for retired Americans is a **three-legged stool**. If any of the three legs is missing, it is impossible for the stool to provide support—it falls over. The three legs (or sources of income) are retirement benefits from Social Security, payments from employer pensions, and income from assets and personal savings. The device of the three-legged stool

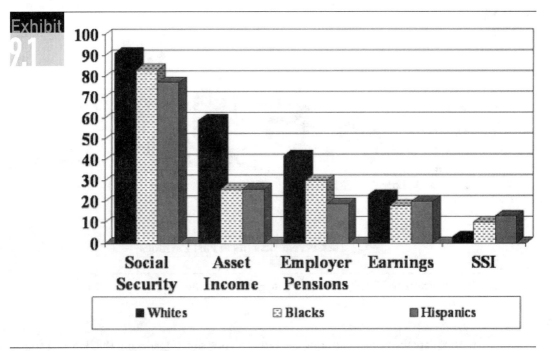

Percentage of Older Adults Receiving Income From Various Sources by Race/Ethnicity, 2002
Source: Social Security Administration, 2004a.

represents the view of its creators that Social Security was not designed to provide an adequate standard of living by itself, but rather to serve as one component of a system of support. Exhibit 9.1 shows the percentage of older adults receiving income from various sources in 2002 by race/ethnicity. This chart does not reflect the *amount of money* coming from any source, which could be minimal or quite large, but just whether any income came from the source. Clearly, the most common income source is Social Security, and some of the remaining sources (e.g., assets, SSI) vary significantly across the groups.

Critics point out that this stool is rather precarious for many older persons, because most people have stools with only one or two legs (Borzi, 1993); that is, they lack an employer pension, personal savings/assets, or both. In the aggregate these three components, plus earnings, constitute the bulk of the income to households headed by an older person or couple (Social Security Administration, 1994). As Exhibit 9.1 shows, the income maintenance system actually has four legs, since earnings continue to be important for about one in five older adults (Social Security Administration, 2004d). This aggregate view of income can be quite misleading, however, because there are striking differences in who gets income from what sources in later life. Before examining these inequalities, let us take a closer look at the three basic components of income maintenance.

Social Security: Background and Contemporary Issues

Social Security, initiated in 1935, developed in the context of the Great Depression and the **Townsend Movement**—a 1930s social movement that advocated granting $200 monthly pensions to older people and requiring the funds to be spent within 30 days

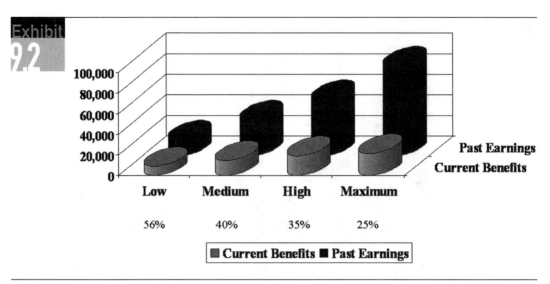

Exhibit
9.2

Social Security's Redistributive Effects Based on Past Earnings for Age-65 Retirees, 2004
Source: Reno, 2005.

to stimulate the economy during the Great Depression (Quadagno, 1982). Many young people supported both the Townsend Movement and Social Security at its outset, since most older adults at that time relied on their kin for financial support. For families, the start of a public pension program reduced their financial burden at a historically critical time, the depths of the Great Depression.

The fundamental premise of the Social Security program is that of a social insurance program, in which society shares, rather than individuals undertaking, the risks of growing economically dependent through old age or disability. As with any insurance system, some participants benefit more than others from Social Security, by virtue of higher benefits (from higher earnings while working) or by living longer (receiving benefits for more months). Alternatively, some individuals pay into Social Security through withholding and recoup few benefits, because they die before or shortly after becoming eligible for benefits.

A second critical aspect of Social Security is that it serves an **income redistribution** function, returning a higher percentage of prior income (called the replacement rate) to poorer individuals and a lower percentage to high-earning retirees (Jones, 1996). This redistribution, shown as a comparison of prior earnings to current benefits in Exhibit 9.2, is important to reducing poverty, because fewer individuals with low or inconsistent earnings histories have private pensions or savings to augment Social Security (Reno, 1993, 2005). This redistribution function is also politically controversial, because it is somewhat in conflict with the "contributory" basis of the program—the idea that benefits are linked to prior contributions to the system. One of the proposed changes to Social Security would reduce this redistribution function, which would be harmful to low-income workers who rely more heavily on Social Security in later life.

Social Security is now a massive program, equal to 4.5% of the gross domestic product in 1999 (Lee & Haaga, 2002). The dollar amounts paid by the program, which include the influence of inflation over many decades, have grown dramatically since the 1940s, as shown in Exhibit 9.3. Because of the huge number of recipients and the dollar amounts, any

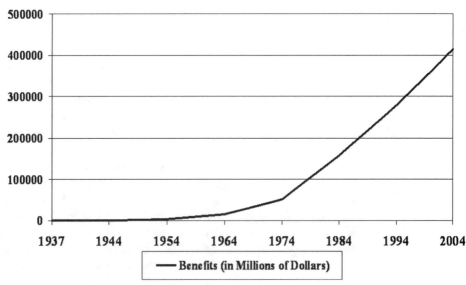

Growth in Social Security Payments, 1937–2004
Source: Social Security Administration, 2005.

changes in the program's provisions or funding have a significant effect, not only on individual retirees and other recipients, but on the overall economy and the federal budget.

As shown in Exhibit 9.4, retirees are not the only recipients of benefits from Social Security. At various points after its initial approval, dependents of workers (spouses, children), survivors of beneficiaries, and the younger disabled (pre-retirement age) were

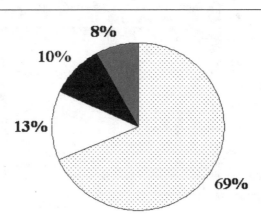

Types of Social Security Beneficiaries
Source: Cauthen, 2005.

added to Social Security, so that now funds are distributed not only to retirees or the older population, but also to younger persons (Social Security Administration, 2004d). The largest component of dollars paid out by the program and the largest number of recipients, however, are still retired workers.

Many experts agree that Social Security has been highly effective in reducing poverty among the elderly both in the United States and in other countries. Data drawn from the Luxembourg Income Study of U.S. and Western European countries, displayed in Exhibit 9.5, show that Social Security–type benefits dramatically reduce the percentage of older adults below 50% of median national income, a standard employed here since there is no standardized "poverty level" across nations. The black bar shows the percentage of each country's older adult population below the country's median national income, and the gray extension to the bar shows what this percentage *would be* without the benefits from the country's Social Security benefit program (Wu, 2005). For example, while the percentage of older adults below median income would multiply several times over in Sweden without its Social Security system, it would double in the United States. Many of these European countries have lower percentages of older adults falling into low-income ranges than the United States, and for many of these countries the benefits received are substantially re-sponsible for this success. This success has its limits, however, because there remain many older persons with incomes just above the poverty threshold (Quinn & Smeeding, 1993). In addition, certain groups continue to face higher risks of near-poverty or poverty-level incomes than others, as we examine later in this chapter (Quinn, 1993).

One area of ongoing concern centers on the **adequacy of benefits** to support those relying on them and the equity of benefits across various groups. Under current provisions, monthly benefits to divorced and widowed women are often their sole source of income and are often well below the poverty level, raising the issue of adequacy

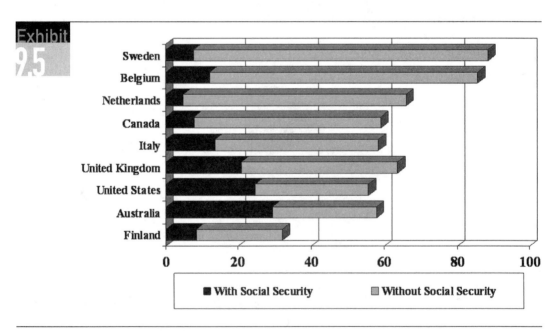

Population Below 50% Median Income From Social Security Benefits
Source: Wu, 2005.

(Burkhauser & Smeeding, 1994; Weaver, 1997). Many of these poor are part of the one-third of recipients for whom Social Security is 90–100% of their overall income (Munnell, 2004). Currently married couples, especially those with one high-earning worker, fare better in terms of Social Security benefit returns relative to contributions compared to unmarried people (Weaver, 1997). Proposals have been put forward to adjust the benefit amount for married couples downward to permit a more adequate benefit to widowed or divorced women without raising the total costs of Social Security (Burkhauser & Smeeding, 1994; Sandell & Iams, 1997).

Concerns regarding **equity of benefits**—the degree to which fairness exists across groups—are also voiced for married women who have contributed as workers to Social Security, about half of whom receive benefits (as spouses) that are no larger than had the women never held jobs at all (Quinn, 1993). Under current policies, single-earner couples benefit more than dual-earner couples and single persons because of the way benefits are calculated for retirees and their dependents (Harrington Meyer, 1996). These inequities in the returns to beneficiaries compared to what they contributed reflect the outdated notion of the male breadwinner and economically dependent wife as the typical family pattern. Although reforms have been discussed and researched for decades, the policies have not been modified substantially to address adequacy and equity of benefits under Social Security (Herd, 2005).

Debates about the foundations of Social Security have escalated in the face of the so-called pig in the python of the baby boom. As these large cohorts move inexorably toward the age of entitlement for Social Security benefits, fears have escalated regarding the ability of smaller cohorts of workers to provide the financial support needed to maintain them (Lee & Haaga, 2002; Munnell, 2004). What will the effects of societal aging be on the future of Social Security? The contemporary debate regarding Social Security is more fundamental than those in prior years, when modest

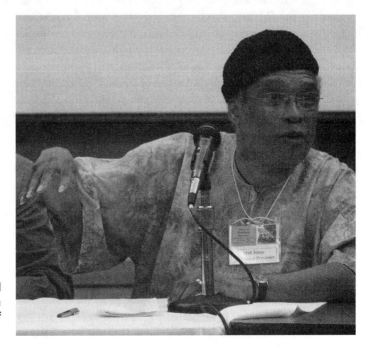

Political processes, power, and agendas play a pivotal role in shaping the economic situation of older people. (Credit: E. J. Hanna)

adjustments, reflecting politically expedient compromises, adapted the program to changing societal needs. Today's debate has included several fundamental issues: the social insurance premise, using age as a basis for entitlement, redistribution of income, and the funding mechanism for the Social Security program (Munnell, 2004; Myles & Quadagno, 1995).

Data from the Social Security Administration's projections show that the ratio of workers to beneficiaries will decrease from 3.4 in 1990 to 2.0 in 2030 and will drop even lower by 2050 (Jones, 1996). Although the system has primarily been pay-as-you-go, with funds contributed by today's workers mostly going to support today's retirees, excess funds have always been kept in the **Social Security Trust Fund**. Changes enacted in 1983, the last major alteration of the Social Security system, built in growth in the trust fund in anticipation of the needs of the baby boom cohorts (Jones, 1996). As contributions are collected from paychecks and employers, extra monies are funneled into this trust fund, which will build up until about 2013. After that time, the retirement of baby boomers will begin to deplete the surplus, and the trust fund, barring additional changes, is projected to run out of money around 2040, although this latter date is a constantly moving target (Munnell, 2005). Depletion of the trust fund does not mean that Social Security will be without funding, because it will continue to receive payments from current workers.

This spending of the trust fund and reduction in the worker-to-retiree ratio will require lowering benefits (i.e., raising retirement age, changing formulas for benefit calculation) or increasing revenues (i.e., increasing economic productivity, increasing FICA deductions, or raising taxes on benefits received) or some combination of these approaches. Although the alarm has long been raised in Washington about these issues, political efforts to change the system at the beginning of George W. Bush's second term have yet to result in any changes being enacted. This campaign has succeeded in raising national awareness of the Social Security issue and the challenges involved in restructuring. The most hotly debated suggestion focused on changing Social Security to permit some portion of contributions to be invested in stocks and bonds, which may yield higher returns than the government bonds used for the trust fund. These proposals are referred to as **privatization of Social Security** or personal accounts, depending on your political leanings. Advocates prefer the risks of the stock market to the returns of the current system, especially given the steady and prolonged rise in the stock market until the early 21st century. Moving toward privatizing Social Security would also reduce both the social insurance and redistribution aspects of the program (Rix & Williamson, 1998) and could have unknown effects on the stock market.

Critics of privatization point out two major concerns with current proposal. First, privatized accounts would provide no protection for individuals who, in seeking high returns, invest their money poorly or are swindled by con artists. Social Security and the SSI program currently protect people against such risks. Second, the transition to a more privatized system could incur additional costs, as one generation pays twice: once to finance their own retirement and again to pay for the benefits of those older adults already in the existing Social Security system (Starr, 1988).

Alternative scenarios for addressing the funding crisis include adjusting ages for benefit eligibility upward, increasing contributions through payroll taxes, converting Social Security from an age entitlement to a need entitlement program, or recovering benefits from high-income retirees through taxation (Goss, 1997). Other proposed

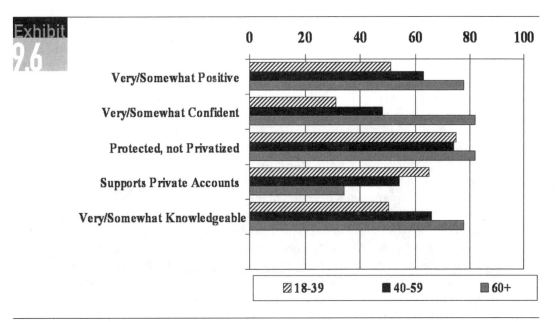

Attitudes Toward Social Security by Age
Source: AARP, 2005b.

changes not receiving such public attention would change the rules about how benefits are adjusted for inflation, which amounts to an invisible reduction in benefits (Munnell, 2004). Most of these proposals face practical or political problems that keep them from being ideal solutions (Myles & Quadagno, 1995). For example, an increase in the retirement age could increase the risk to disadvantaged workers, who both face higher rates of health problems limiting their employment and rely most heavily on Social Security as part of their later-life income. In fact, Congress has moved by raising the age of entitlement for full Social Security benefits to 67 (by 2027), and raising taxes on higher-income elders to recoup some of their Social Security benefits. Whatever final plan emerges will reflect a lengthy and very political debate.

Attitudes about the Social Security system have become a political battleground. Although many younger people doubt that Social Security retirement benefits will be there for them when they retire (Borden, 1995), the program continues to enjoy considerable social support, because most of us have at least one relative, neighbor, or friend receiving Social Security benefits (Day, 1993b). As Exhibit 9.6 shows, about half of younger adults are generally positive about Social Security, with approval increasing in higher age groups. Only about one-third of younger adults are confident of receiving benefits, compared to half of baby boomers and over 80% of those 60 and over. Ironically, while younger adults were supportive of the idea of private/personal accounts, they also responded very positively to a question asking whether the Social Security system should be "protected, not privatized." Finally, younger adults admitted to being less informed regarding Social Security than their older counterparts, with the 60 and over age group claiming to be most informed (AARP, 2005b). What would families do if Social Security suddenly disappeared? Most people do not wish to contemplate the answer, and thus they support some version of the program.

Employer Pensions

Employer pensions—retirement income systems sponsored or organized (and often financed) by employers—represent a complex legal, fiscal, and policy area. The details of pension design and financing are beyond the scope of this chapter, and the magnitude of their importance in the overall economy is staggering. In 2003 employers spent $569.1 billion on pension programs (Employee Benefit Research Institute, 2004). Paired with the vast accumulations from individual 401(k) and other personal savings, these funds constitute a major component of financial capital in stock and bond markets. Since access to a private pension is often the difference between an economically secure old age and a more marginal existence, both individuals and the larger society must be concerned about how pensions operate and their soundness.

Jobs usually come with or without a pension attached to them, so the type of occupation an individual undertakes influences the prospects for an eventual pension. For some types of programs an individual must work a minimum number of years to become eligible, or **vested,** for eventual pension benefits. Thus, not everyone employed in a job covered by a pension will receive a pension from that employer. The likelihood of being covered by a pension thus depends on a variety of factors, including occupation, education, union membership, frequency of job change, and gender. Exhibit 9.7 shows the percentages of people in various groups who lack pension coverage using a very broad definition (from current primary or secondary job, from a previous job, or from an IRA account). Drawing all of these sources together, women are more likely than men to lack pension coverage, but the gender gap is decreasing. In addition, low-income workers are more likely to lack any pension coverage than their counterparts earning $30,000 or more. The gap between White and non-White workers is fairly small and there are some interesting age differences, indicating that baby boomers are more likely to lack pension coverage (in most cases) than cohorts preceding or following them.

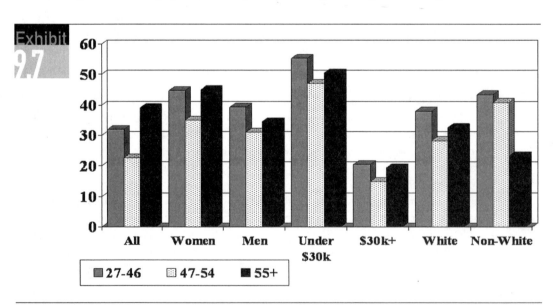

Exhibit 9.7

Percent of Labor Force Lacking Any Employer Pension Coverage, 1993
Source: Lichtenstein and Wu, 2000.

Since employers generally seek to minimize pension costs, sometimes at the expense of the pensioners, the federal government has passed legislation (the Employee Retirement Income Security Act of 1974, or **ERISA**) that controls how pensions are offered and funded. This law and its subsequent amendments mandate how funds must be collected and credited to employees, how employees become vested, and how pension funds are managed. The legislation was prompted by the failure of a number of pension funds, leaving the retirees without promised resources (Salisbury, 1993). Now pension funds have some protection through the Pension Benefit Guarantee Corporation (much as the FDIC insures funds in banks), which, as discussed in chapter 8, is under financial pressure due to a large number of corporate pension defaults.

One basis of economic insecurity among older widows has to do with the rules for employer pensions. Because pensions are earned by individual workers, a pension often ended when the worker died. Since most pensioners in past cohorts were male and few wives were eligible for their own pensions, this major source of income would end abruptly for many widows, throwing them into poverty. In 1985 legislation was passed requiring all pensions to offer survivor options and mandating that both spouses approve in writing a choice of single or survivor options (Miller, 1985). If the survivor option is chosen, the monthly pension amount is decreased, but the pension continues to support the survivor after the pensioner dies. In fact, pensions are becoming such an important part of family wealth that they are increasingly viewed as jointly earned property, to be allocated like other property in divorce settlements (Women's Initiative, 1993). A recent analysis of data from the Health and Retirement Study regarding survivor benefits (Johnson, Uccello, & Goldwyn, 2005) found, however, that 28% of men and 66% of women decline survivor protection. Many of those making this choice seem to have weighed the costs and benefits of their choices. As those authors point out, annuities such as those received from 401(k)-type programs are not covered by the legislation on survivor benefits and may also disappear upon the death of the holder.

One major trend in pensions is away from **defined benefit** systems. In a defined benefit pension system the employer controls a worker's pension. The employer invests and controls a common fund under rules defined by ERISA. Benefit amounts are guaranteed on a formula based on the number of years an individual has worked and his or her salary, or related factors (Smeeding, Estes, & Glasse, 1999). Under such systems workers can know exactly what their pension amount will be and whether it will grow with the cost of living. Issues may arise when the worker changes jobs, since these programs are held and managed by employers—pensions may be frozen and often benefits are forgotten and go unclaimed.

 Growing more common are **defined contribution** pensions, familiar to some as a 401(k) plan. Defined contribution is a system in which the worker, the employer, or both contribute to a fund held by an independent financial entity, so that the money belongs to the worker and is subject to the stock and bond markets to determine benefit amounts. Benefits at retirement are not guaranteed, but may depend on the trends in the stock and bond markets near the time of retirement (Smeeding et al., 1999). Payment may come as a lump sum to be invested or as an annuity, paid over the life of the retiree and/or the spouse. Under this system the worker often has control over investment choices (and thus can take risks with it if she or he so chooses), and may either succeed or suffer depending on the vigor of the stock market and individual investment choices (Gale, Iwry, Munnell, & Thaler, 2004). Employers have less responsibility to oversee the fund, but also have lower control over the timing of retirement, since they don't control the funds or provisions for their receipt. Over the past 25 years, however, defined contribution plans have grown from supplemental programs to the primary pension to the only pension available to most workers (Gale et al., 2004).

Personal Savings/Assets

Savings and other **assets** accumulated during one's life are the third leg of income maintenance in retirement. As we saw in Exhibit 9.1, asset income is less available to Blacks and Hispanics than to Whites over 65 (26% versus 59%) (Social Security Administration, 2004d). Assets are all the resources people own that can be converted into money, including home equity, cash savings, IRAs, stocks, and bonds. Assets "provide housing, serve as a financial reserve for special or emergency needs, contribute directly to income through interest, dividends, or rents, and help to enhance the freedom with which individuals spend their income" (Schulz, 1992, p. 37). Most older persons have savings or assets of some type, although a large percentage of assets do not generate income. Exhibit 9.8 shows the difference by age in overall assets held (known as net worth). Net worth increases dramatically for mid-life and older adults, with lower amounts appearing for those 75 or older. However, the great majority of this net worth is tied up in home equity rather than savings, stocks and bonds, or other more liquid resources. In short, the great majority of net worth does not generate income to older adults.

Like other resources, savings and assets are unequally distributed among the older population, and this inequality has grown in recent years (Quinn, 1993). Accumulation of assets is only made possible by having surplus resources to save or invest, limiting the likelihood that lower-income persons will develop independent assets to utilize in later life. In a few cases, assets are inherited from kin, but most people who develop assets do so through their own productivity in the labor force. Thus, inequality in asset accumulation is a reflection of income inequality during the working years.

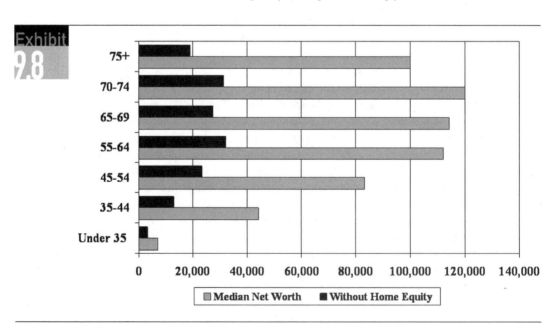

Median Net Worth by Age
Source: U.S. Bureau of the Census, 2003b.

In summary, the three-legged stool of income maintenance for older people is a very shaky structure for a majority of older adults today, and it is significantly more wobbly for some groups than for others. Social Security is undergoing major changes, private pensions are only available to some members of the older population, and few older adults have substantial savings or assets beyond home equity.

Economic Well-Being of Older Americans

So, how are older Americans doing economically? Armed with an understanding of the three legs of the income maintenance stool, let us next consider the effectiveness and long-term impact of this structure on the economic status of older people. The adequacy of these strategies and policies in maintaining some level of economic well-being for older people is an important, complex, and multifaceted question. Future policies are being shaped by today's debates, which in turn shape all of our economic futures.

As we have seen, groups in the older population vary widely in their sources of income. This heterogeneity plays an extremely important role in answering the question about the economic status of older people, and we will review major sources of, and explanations for, the variations in a later section. Another basic influence on our answers regarding the economic status of older Americans is which definitions or measures we use to examine the data.

Alternatives for Measuring Economic Well-Being

Two measurement issues are involved in answering our question about how well or poorly older people are doing financially. First, there are many definitions of economic status, including income, assets, and in-kind income. Poverty level offers another kind of measure of economic well-being. In any measure, the number and nature of financial resources we include in our analysis influence our results. We will review each of these measures and the sometimes conflicting conclusions they allow experts to draw about the economic status of older people. Second, the statistics we use to describe the economic well-being of older adults—such as means, medians, and measures of variability—will similarly shape the conclusions.

Measures of Economic Status

Some economists have suggested that economic well-being encompasses not just income, but also economic responsibilities (such as family support and tax liabilities) and economic resources (such as home ownership and medical insurance). Usually, however, it is measured more simply. One obvious way to assess people's financial situation is to find out about how much income they receive. Salaries and wages, interest and dividends, and income from public or private transfers (such as Social Security and unemployment compensation or child support payments) are traditionally included in definitions of income. Comparisons across age groups reveal that older people have lower incomes than younger adults, and that people over 75 are more disadvantaged than the 65–74 age group. In 2003 the median household income for persons 65 and older was about $23,787; for all adults median income was significantly higher (about $43,318); for people 75 and older, median income was only $19,470 (U.S. Bureau of the Census, 2004b).

Individual or household income is only one measure of financial resources available, and the picture of the economic status of older people is more complete, and more complex, when we consider these other indicators. Two other measures commonly used in discussing the financial situation of older people are assets and in-kind income.

When assets are included in the calculation, a much more positive picture emerges than if we look only at income. As demonstrated earlier, this is primarily because so many older people own their homes and can count the equity among their assets. With all appropriate cautions about variability in the older population, Smeeding (1990) reports an "impressive level of wealth among the older population" (p. 366). Home ownership by older persons is higher in the United States than in many equally developed European countries (Holtz-Eakin & Smeeding, 1994). Interest-earning assets (savings accounts, savings bonds, and certificates of deposit) constitute another 29% of total wealth, followed by rental property, stocks, bonds, and mutual funds (another 17%) (Holtz-Eakin & Smeeding, 1994).

Assets are important not just as a reserve; they also can provide income through interest and dividends. For example, asset income constitutes almost 20% of total income for those in the highest fifth of the income range, but under 3% income for those at the bottom of the income scale (Federal Interagency Forum on Aging Related Statistics, 2004). Consistent with lower lifetime incomes and fewer sources of retirement income, about one in four adults over 65 have no equity in a home, but the figure rises to one out of three widows living alone (Radner, 1993). Not surprisingly, those with the highest incomes also had the greatest store of wealth in assets.

Another way to examine economic well-being is to examine in-kind income. **In-kind income** includes non-cash benefits that contribute to income by reducing expenditures. Publicly funded medical insurance (Medicare) is an example of in-kind income. Subsidized housing and food stamps are other familiar examples of such non-cash benefits. The inclusion of in-kind income in calculations of economic well-being has an enormous impact on the outcome of those analyses. In one study that used an "expanded income" measure (income plus some other cash and non-cash benefits, including health insurance, realized capital gains, public housing value, and net equity), older people as a group were found to be as well-off as the non-elderly (Smeeding, 1990). This is quite a different conclusion from the one we would draw from the data on median personal income or assets exclusive of home equity. One dilemma of such inclusive measures has to do with the role of health benefits. When people are seriously ill, gaining a lot of in-kind benefits from Medicare and/or Medicaid, these large amounts are sometimes added to calculations of their "incomes" to figure economic well-being. Even though no money comes to them, such seriously ill people appear wealthy because they receive such high levels of in-kind health care benefits. Such variations in how income is measured reinforce the need for caution in drawing conclusions about income unless you understand the definitions and measurements used to generate the results.

Rates of Poverty

While measures of financial resources answer one kind of question about economic well-being (how well-off are older people?), poverty rates answer another kind of question about economic health: How large or small is the proportion of older people who are in extreme financial jeopardy? Poverty rates tell us the proportion of the population living below a minimum level of income defined as necessary for survival. The poverty threshold is the income level below which people are categorically defined as "poor"; this threshold is linked to eligibility for many safety-net (need eligibility) programs in the United States. For example, food stamps are available to people whose income is less than 130% of the poverty threshold. The poverty rate (the proportion living below the poverty threshold) is thus not a measure of how many resources individual people have, but of how many of them live in an untenable financial situation.

Researchers and policymakers often use poverty rates and trends to chart how effectively programs and policies address social ills, redistribute resources in ways society desires, and improve the financial situation of various groups. The poverty rate among elderly Americans was 28.5% in 1966, compared to 10.2% in 2004, reflecting substantial improvement. Because of the many ways people use poverty statistics, and because of the many competing agendas that can underlie those uses, it is important to understand the way the U.S. government calculates poverty.

The original poverty level was based on the cost of food needed to meet minimal nutritional requirements. The cost of food was calculated based on 1962 prices when the index was initiated, and that amount was multiplied by three (based on data from a 1955 survey which showed that food represented one-third of the average family's budget) to arrive at the official poverty threshold. These levels now are calculated for individuals and households of various sizes and reflect increases due to inflation. Individuals or households whose incomes fall below that level qualify as poor. In 2003 the poverty threshold for a family of four was $18,810; by 2005 the equivalent figure had grown to $20,144—a slow growth related to inflation rates (U.S. Bureau of the Census, 2005c).

The poverty threshold formula is open to serious criticisms. First, food costs are based on minimum consumption and were originally developed for emergency periods; no one was expected to survive on these menu plans for a long time. Second, different food plans were developed for different kinds of households. The plan for a household in which the head of household is under 65 allows for higher food costs than if the household is headed by someone over age 65. The result of this different food plan for older people is a lower poverty threshold, meaning that older people have to have lower incomes than younger people to be considered poor and to quality for need entitlement programs. For example, a single individual under age 65 had a poverty threshold of $10,160 in 2005, compared to a mere $9,367 for a single individual aged 65 or older. (U.S. Bureau of the Census, 2005c).

A final focus of criticism is the multiplier of three. The idea that food represents about a third of a family's budget, which was apparently the case in 1955, is quite unrealistic today. Most families require much more than three times their food budget to meet all of their other needs, including housing, utilities, and transportation (U.S. Bureau of the Census, 1993). Housing takes a much higher proportion of the budget and food a lower proportion than in 1955 (even though food costs are higher today). Moreover, families at different levels of living will have different expenditure patterns; for poor families, necessities such as housing and food will consume a higher proportion of the total budget than in middle-class families of the same size.

The impact of the approach to calculating the poverty threshold is to keep that threshold artificially low, meaning that people have to be extremely poor in order to be categorized as living in poverty. Questions about how poverty is and should be calculated are receiving significant attention from researchers, policy analysts, advocates for older people, and the government agencies that produce poverty statistics (Citro & Michaels, 1995).

Reflecting these concerns about the adequacy of the poverty threshold formula, poverty rates are now reported for 100%, 125%, and up to 200% of the poverty line. Those falling within 100–150% of the poverty threshold are often referred to as "near poor." In 2004,

10.2% of all older people lived below the poverty line; however, raising the poverty level to just 125% of the threshold increases this group to 16.9% of adults over 65. Thus, hundreds of thousands of older people who are not categorically poor according to the official poverty threshold are nonetheless economically vulnerable. Smeeding (1990) has termed the group between 100% and 200% of the official poverty level the "'tweeners," those not poor enough to qualify for safety net programs but too poor to be financially secure (p. 372).

Another study reinforces the need to be cautious about concluding that poverty is not a serious problem for older adults. Rank and Hirschi (1999) examined not just the annual rate of poverty (a cross-sectional, snapshot view), but the likelihood that someone would experience an episode of poverty at some time in later life. In a large, longitudinal study, they followed individuals from age 60 and found that 35% experienced an episode of poverty by the time they reached 85. Some of the individuals in the study were at greater risk of becoming poor, especially those with less than high school education, those who were unmarried, and those who were Black. A married White man with more than high school education had a 14% risk of ever experiencing poverty by age 85; risks for a married Black man who didn't graduate high school reached 60%, and soared to 88% for his female counterpart (Rank & Hirschi, 1999). The life course perspective shows a different picture of the problem of poverty among the elderly than cross-sectional views.

People concerned about how our government defines poverty also question the way income is and should be measured to determine poverty status. Traditionally, income was defined as direct money income, from sources such as wages and salaries, Social Security, public assistance, interest and dividends, and pensions. Current discussion and alternative calculations focus on the inclusion of in-kind income sources and net worth. Analyses based on these alternative definitions can illustrate the impact of in-kind benefits such as government transfer programs on the poverty status of the population. Such analyses can also fuel debate and pave the way for policy changes.

These kinds of analyses underscore the complexity of answering questions about economic status. The very different conclusions that can be drawn—all of them supported by facts and figures—suggest that answers and conclusions can be easily shaped by ideology, vested interests, and political agendas. If an 85-year-old widow subsisting on SSI in her modest house appears to be economically secure because the cost of a temporary nursing home visit is considered "income," we all need to develop a critical eye for the statistics we see on the economic well-being of the elderly. Statistics can be crafted to support almost any point of view. Data-based but ideologically motivated statements about the economic status of older people have stereotyped them as "greedy geezers," responsible for the federal deficit, and a drain on the welfare of children. You are now better prepared to be look more cautiously at the bases for such statements. Whatever definitions and measures we select, comparing subgroups within the older population will also reveal the importance of not generalizing about older adults as a category.

Economic Well-Being and Inequality Among Older People

Most researchers agree that there have been striking improvements in the economic well-being of the average older American in the past three decades (Quinn & Smeeding, 1993).

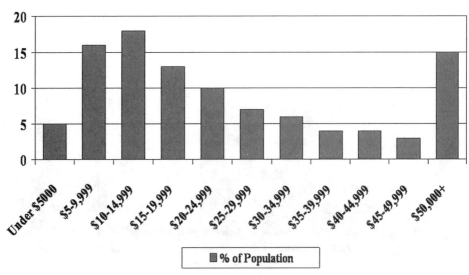

Income Distribution of the Population 65 Years and Over in 2002
Source: Social Security Administration, 2004d.

Poverty rates among older people have fallen sharply since the days prior to some of the age-based entitlement programs. In 1959, 35.2% of older people lived below the poverty level; in 2004 the figure had dropped to 10.2%. This success, in turn, provides support to political and social agendas seeking to reduce government entitlements to older people. However, despite the historical decline in poverty among older Americans, significant variation exists in the economic status of older adults, including pockets of severe economic distress in certain social groups (Quinn & Smeeding, 1993). Exhibit 9.9 shows a wide variation in levels of income and a concentration of older adults at the low end of the income distribution. Perhaps surprisingly, the modal (largest) income category is between $10,000 and $14,999, and that individuals over 65 with incomes over $50,000 constitute only about 15% of older adults. Over half have incomes under $20,000 per year.

These wide income variations are mirrored in the differing rates of poverty for different groups within the older population. Exhibit 9.10 shows that the overall poverty rate masks enormous differences. Being Black, being Hispanic, being female, and being unmarried are related to greater economic disadvantage. The poverty level for married people over 65 is under half of the average, with unmarried men and women both showing higher percentages who are poor or near poor. The poverty rate for older Blacks and Hispanics is above 20%, compared to 9% for older Whites. If we include the near poor individuals, poverty among Black and Hispanic elders is above 30%.

In addition, older age is associated with economic disadvantage. Exhibit 9.11 shows median income by age category, marital status, and sex. Moving from younger to older cohorts, you find lower median income amounts, with consistently higher incomes among married individuals (compared to unmarried age-peers) persisting into advanced old age. Even among the unmarried, there is a consistent difference between men and women. Also keep in mind that the percentage of each age group that is married grows

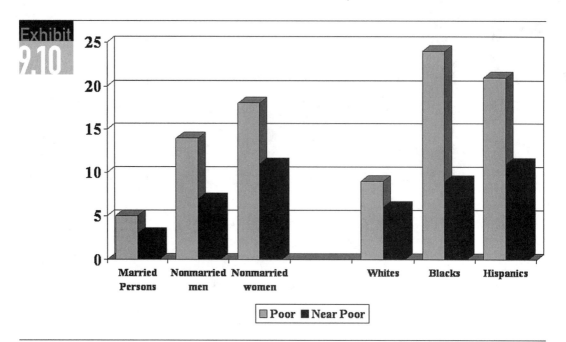

Percent of U.S. Older Persons in Poverty by Marital Status, Sex, and Race/Ethnicity, 2002
Source: Social Security Administration, 2004d.

smaller as you move from the 65–74 cohort to the 80 years and over cohort in the chart. Given the gender differential in widowhood, the concentration of persons in these age ranges shifts from predominantly married couples (65–74 years) to predominantly widowed women (80 and over).

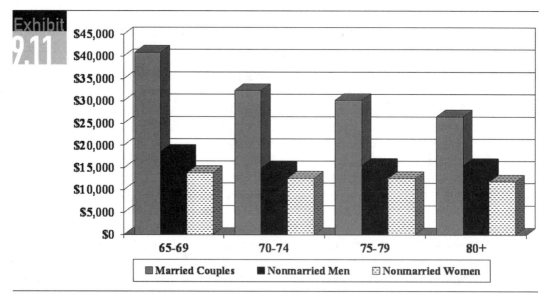

Differences in Median Income by Age, Sex, and Marital Status, 2002
Source: Social Security Administration, 2004a.

As mature cohorts reach age 65 or retirement, each one in recent years has included a higher percentage of people with Social Security benefits and income from pensions and assets. So when we state that the aggregate economic well-being of the older population has improved, it is mostly because poorer members of the oldest cohorts have died and have been replaced by more affluent individuals moving into the 65 and over range. It is usually not the case that the economic fortunes of specific persons have improved (Quinn & Smeeding, 1993). Nor is it the case that individuals or couples, as they advance in age, necessarily move to lower levels of income. An analysis by McGarry and Schoeni (2005) found that nearly half of the differences in economic well-being between the married and widowed is due to economic conditions that predated the death of the spouse; remaining differences are due to high health costs in the last years of a spouse's life, loss of her or his income, and continuing high health costs for the surviving spouse. Some additional erosion of buying power is possible if income sources don't adjust for inflation or if health or family problems require consumption of assets that had been providing income. So in interpreting cross-sectional data such as these, it is important to avoid the life course fallacy.

Effects of Population Aging on the Economy

So far we have considered the impact of aging (along with gender, race/ethnicity, and marital status) on the economic well-being of individuals. Questions at a more macro level of analysis examine the impact of societal aging on the economy of the nation as a whole. Population aging can have an effect on aggregate economic activity, the size and composition of the labor force, aggregate labor force participation rates, productivity, and the structure of demand and consumption (Matras, 1990). Here we will consider some of these effects of societal aging on the economy.

Spending and Saving Over the Life Course

How will societal aging affect savings behavior in the U.S. economy and the pool of assets in pension funds and privately owned assets? If future cohorts behave like current ones, the already low level of savings by individual Americans could drop even more. However, we can't necessarily predict the savings behavior of future cohorts from the activities of aging cohorts to date.

Economists posit an **economic life-cycle hypothesis** of saving and spending. According to this hypothesis, rational economic planners (all of us, presumably) accumulate assets of various types, including personal savings, home equity, and pension wealth, in anticipation of a change in behavior in later life as we become less economically productive at retirement. The hypothesis argues that we defer some of our consumption (in pensions and IRA accounts) to support ourselves in later life, spending down these assets as we move through later life (Holtz-Eakin & Smeeding, 1994). A person who adapted perfectly to the life-cycle hypothesis would end up with absolutely no resources left at the time of death, but this outcome seldom occurs. Economically secure people often die leaving an estate, whereas the less advantaged often outlive their money, requiring assistance to pay for basic needs and long-term health care before they die. Others start with significant resources, which can be consumed by costs for health or long-term care services.

Research shows that the oldest age groups have fewer accumulated resources than do slightly younger cohorts over age 65, suggesting either that they are spending down their accumulated resources or that there is a cohort difference (i.e., they started out with fewer resources at age 65 than do current cohorts). People doubtless do spend down their resources with age as they "consume" pensions and other resources, but not as quickly as the life-cycle hypothesis suggests (Holtz-Eakin & Smeeding, 1994). While most people do not add to their accumulated assets in later life, most work to hold onto the resources accumulated in earlier years to meet expected or unexpected needs (a new car, health care expenses). If the life-cycle hypothesis is accurate for most people, the aging of society should reduce private assets, the stock of money in pension funds, and thus the capital available to the economy for investments in new capital or research. While this sounds dire for the health of the economy, let us turn next to examining the somewhat limited research on consumption patterns of older adults.

Consumption Patterns

Researchers have analyzed how patterns of saving, spending, and consuming vary by age and other social variables. The amounts and types of spending by older adults may seem of little relevance to the rest of us. However, as the society ages and older consumers become more than one out of five Americans, the degree to which they can afford to consume desired goods and services (discretionary income) will have a major impact on the overall vigor and size of the economy, indirectly influencing everyone. Spending by individuals over age 65 now constitutes 14.6% of all consumer dollars (Paulin, 2000). Choices made by this large consumer pool will also help to determine the mix of products and services available in the economy.

Early studies on the older population showed that a significant percentage of income is spent on basics—food, health care, utilities, and housing—with discretionary spending on leisure and recreation varying substantially by income level (Goldstein, 1960). Poorer households could ill afford the travel or recreation consumed by the middle class; as with poor people of any age, nearly all of their incomes went for necessities (food, shelter, transportation). It has been argued that one of the reasons that Social Security passed in 1935 was the hope that consumption by benefit recipients would help spur the economy, which was mired in the Great Depression (Quadagno, 1988).

Other studies of consumption indicate that the consumption pattern remains largely unchanged for low- to moderate-income households. Fixed costs still constitute a major component of spending by older consumers. A 1992 study by the United States General Accounting Office, for example, estimated that half of older homeowners spent at least 45% of their incomes on property taxes, utilities, and home maintenance. Among married couples (with their larger incomes), only about 30% of expenditures are for housing-related costs (Nieswiadomy & Rubin, 1995). Other necessary expenditures, such as food and health care, also represent larger percentages of the more modest incomes of unmarried women compared to married couples. In all, Nieswiadomy and Rubin (1995) found that current cohorts of retired couples spent only 3%–5% of all consumer spending on entertainment.

A more recent analysis of the Consumer Expenditure Survey between 1984 and 1997 compares expenditures for big ticket items and recurring expenses for those 65–74 and 75 years and over to determine whether preferences and behaviors changed over time (Paulin, 2000). While older consumers spent fewer dollars than those under 65, the trends over time in spending for shelter, food, and other items did not change dramatically across the

The Stratified Life Course and Economic Diversity

As we have seen, groups within the elderly population differ substantially in rates of poverty and on more positive measures of economic status, with married couples faring better than unmarried adults and Whites faring better than Hispanics and Blacks. What brings about these systematic differences, which tend to appear regardless of the measure used to evaluate economic well-being? The answer has to do with choices and opportunities throughout the life cycle—prior life chances.

These differences must be considered from a life-cycle perspective, as the consequence of differences in life chances (including education, health, family, and labor force experiences), consequent access to various types of resources (income, family support, pensions, and assets), and provision of income maintenance programs (O'Rand, 1996). Thus, life chances associated with earnings potentials and access to pensions have long-term consequences for economic well-being in later life. Sociologists and economists have used the notions of **cumulative advantage** and **cumulative disadvantage** to describe this process whereby individuals who have early opportunities for success (better life chances) most often build on that success to perpetuate their advantages into later life, while those with disadvantages also carry those

disadvantages forward through sequential life stages, often resulting in later-life poverty (Crystal & Shea, 1990; O'Rand, 1996). Structural barriers to full employment in some groups within a society (women, minorities, those with less education) will inevitably result in their greater financial need in old age, barring income maintenance policies that correct for those distinctions through income redistribution.

> One interesting implication of a life cycle perspective is that, in the long run, the well-being of the elderly may be more efficiently served by concentrating on programs whose impact occurs long before old age-programs like education, training or health…. [Such programs] can have great impact on the income, assets, and health status of the elderly-to-be. (Quinn, 1993, p. 21)

As evidence of this argument, studies continue to confirm that women with children earn lower wages, even after differences of education, experience and job type are taken into account (Waldfogel, 1997). This and similar life-course events shape labor force choices, savings, and a range of other behaviors over time. The tendency, then, is for those who have been advantaged in early stages of adulthood to continue that advantage into later life, with economic disadvantage also following persons as they age. Common exceptions to these patterns of continued advantage or disadvantage in later life are individuals whose resources are depleted

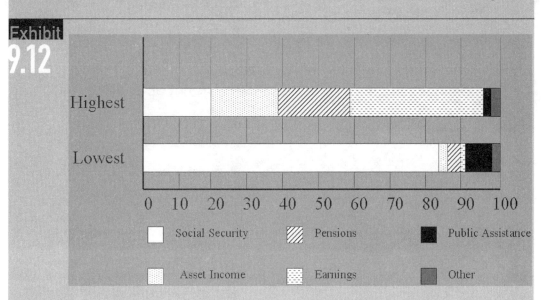

Exhibit 9.12

Shares of Aggregate Income in Lowest and Highest Income Quintiles
Source: Federal Interagency Forum on Aging and Related Statistics, 2004.   *(continued)*

(continued)

suddenly by health problems and women who experience increased risks of impoverishment following widowhood (Quinn & Smeeding, 1993).

Both race and health influence the accumulation of wealth by affecting life chances: Blacks and those with chronic health conditions generally have lower assets in later life than their more advantaged age peers (Shea, Miles, & Hayward, 1996). Older Blacks are less likely to own homes or have high home equity amounts as they approach later life, giving them fewer resources for the future (Myers & Chung, 1996). Life-course events, such as marriage, divorce, and childbearing, can also influence individuals' long-term economic status. For example, a study of pre–retirement-age women showed that those who had been divorced or widowed had significantly lower incomes and assets than those who remained in first marriages. Even if the divorced or widowed women had subsequently remarried, their economic well-being was lower (Holden & Kuo, 1996).

Life chances and life experience translate into various groups' being more or less likely to have income from the major sources discussed earlier. Exhibit 9.12 shows that individuals in the highest one-fifth of the income distribution are far more likely to have income from assets; clearly, those most economically secure in later life were earning incomes enabling them to save during their working years (Federal Interagency Forum on Aging Related Statistics, 2004). Older persons in the lowest quintile of income receive over 80% of their income from Social Security, whereas those in the highest quintile receive about 20% of their income from Social Security. Thus, the income sources, as well as the income amounts, of economically secure individuals differ substantially from those who are least economically secure.

Although life chances are associated with membership in particular social groups and categories, the system is not completely deterministic; individuals sometimes do beat the odds and do very well—getting excellent jobs, good incomes, and substantial pensions despite membership in a group that fares poorly on average. The notion of life chances simply points out that, to date, individuals in different groups have had different odds of moving successfully through the events of the life course in ways that result in economic security in old age. These different odds—patterned

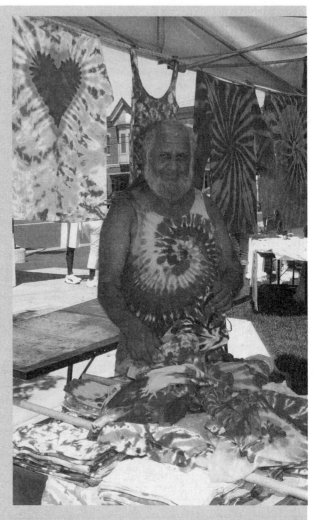

Differing opportunities for economic security in later life offer one kind of diversity among older persons. (Credit: E. J. Hanna)

by race, ethnicity, and gender—are the product of our history and social structure.

Differing life chances for economic security in later life is one kind of diversity among the older population. But diversity can have different meanings and implications. Is diversity a positive, negative, or neutral fact of life in our society? Should we promote diversity or seek to reduce it? Obviously the answer to that question depends on what kind of diversity and on the ideology of the people discussing it. In the case of economic status, a high degree of diversity may be a negative reflection on our society and may call for policies to reduce differences.

age groups, with most following parallel spending patterns through economic upturns and recessions. In general, trends and preferences in spending for these age groups did not change substantially over the 13-year period examined in this research.

One component of consumption that is not entirely predictable is health care. Health care costs, which have varied depending on Medicare's coverage and copayment levels since 1965, were about 12% of total expenditures by retirees in the late 1980s (Nieswiadomy & Rubin, 1995). (See chapter 11 for more detail on health care costs.) Those who can afford to do so seek to control this unpredictable cost by buying insurance that supplements any public or private programs to which they are entitled, including an increasing share of those 65 and over (Paulin, 2000). Concerns regarding the high cost of health care and the potential for costly catastrophic illnesses may prompt older adults to hold onto savings and suppress current spending, thereby influencing the consumption patterns of the older population in areas other than health care.

Experts disagree on whether consumption patterns will shift substantially in the next decades, as new cohorts enter later life. Johnson and Williamson (1987) claim that the improved health and financial status of current and future retirees, as well as their potentially increased leisure time, will result in new products and services targeted to this market. Their side of this debate suggests that specialized products and services, as well as senior-oriented leisure, will be an expanding market as societal aging continues. For example, people over age 60 make up 35% of the consumers of vacation cruises (Cruise Lines International Association, 1996). If that percentage remains constant as the population ages, shouldn't enterprising shipbuilders be preparing now for the growing number of customers?

On a less optimistic note, as more people survive to ages at which assistance is needed in household tasks and personal care, how much should home health care companies anticipate growing over the next several decades? This question is complicated further if each succeeding cohort has later onset of disability than its predecessors. It remains unclear how quickly or vigorously such markets will shift, in part depending on the level of financial security of the older cohorts of the future.

On the other side of this debate, some researchers voice concerns regarding restricted consumption by the older population. As society ages, this group wonders whether the economy will slow if older consumers keep cars and durable goods (such as refrigerators) longer than do younger adults (Kneese & Cooper, 1993). Will the aging of society have a negative effect on consumerism? Again, the answer will turn on whether aging or cohort effects are more potent in these behaviors. Spending and consumption patterns of future aging cohorts may be based more on per capita income and the choices available; we cannot assume that because a society ages, its rate of consumer spending automatically drops (Easterlin, 1996). Future cohorts may be more free-spending or more tight-fisted with their money, depending in part on their lifetime experiences with money and the economy, their expectations of their futures, their levels of disposable income, and social policies in force during their later lives (for example, will Social Security and Medicare benefits be more limited than today, requiring that more income be devoted to necessities?).

One thing that is clear is that businesses and marketers have discovered the "gray market" for products and services (Minkler, 1991b). This discovery has had the dual effects of recognizing and meeting the needs of this population, but has also resulted in a focus on the affluent among the older population, downplaying the continuing economic marginality of some subgroups within the older population (Minkler, 1991b). Both the senior lobby and private corporations have contributed to the notion of the older population as a vast, untapped resource for marketing goods and services. The fact that we now see older models in advertisements, even for products not oriented to older adults, is a signal that the gray market is no longer as marginalized by business (Minkler, 1991b). It remains important, however, for the marketplace to be responsive to the needs of a wide range of older consumers, not just the wealthiest. Many predict significant expansion of private sector products and services and public/private collaborations (see Cutler & Timmerman, 2004–2005).

Prospects for the Future Economic Status of the Elderly

Predicting the economic well-being of future cohorts of older persons involves many unknowns. Critical among these unknowns are the potential changes in public and private policies for income maintenance and the overall health of the economy. Under a worst-case scenario, the economy would face sustained growth in the elderly population, continued trajectory of early retirement, increases in the costs of care (both medical and personal assistance), a smaller working-age population, a less productive work force (dominated by older workers and less educated youth), and a stagnant level of economic growth (Szanton, 1993). In less negative scenarios, one or more of these factors shifts to moderate the impact of an aging population.

Although we do know that the aging of society will likely proceed, barring an unexpected increase in fertility, many of the other elements in that worst-case scenario are hotly debated by experts and may deviate dramatically from current trends (Szanton, 1993). For example, the size of the productive work force can vary considerably in a given country depending on immigration policies and shifts toward higher average ages of retirement, due to incentives to continue working or fears regarding economic insecurity. How close we come to the worst-case scenario is yet to be determined.

Although we have seen improvement in the economic fortunes of recent cohorts, there is no guarantee that this improvement will continue for future cohorts. The cohorts born in the 1920s have been dubbed the **"good times" generation,** because of the way in which historical events have shaped their lives and their retirement incomes (Moon & Smeeding, 1989). The good times generation are a privileged cohort, because they were in their prime working years during the economic boom following World War II, worked during the period in which private pension coverage was expanding, and benefited from the windfall of a dramatic increase in the value of real estate during their lives (Holtz-Eakin & Smeeding, 1994). The coincidence of so many favorable circumstances is unlikely to repeat for future cohorts.

What also seems likely, however, is that inequality will continue to be problematic among the elderly. In contrast to many other countries, the piecemeal system of income maintenance in the United States leaves some individuals much less protected than others in old age. By attempting to create incentives early in life to work hard and achieve, our income maintenance policies mostly reward high achievers and do less for the unfortunate or unmotivated. As a nation, we will probably be revisiting several pieces of our income maintenance policies in the next few decades, with the outcomes from those political processes shaping the economic well-being of all of us as we age in the future.

SUMMARY

Economic well-being is one area in which it is especially critical to avoid discussions of "the average" older adult. It is clear that economic well-being has improved on the average, but many sizable groups continue to experience high rates of poverty and economic marginality. Lifelong advantages and disadvantages embedded in the labor market and public and private policies of income maintenance result in individuals whose economic histories, for good or ill, follow them into later life to result in security or insecurity. In general, wealthy older people are not suddenly impoverished after retirement, nor are the poorest older persons likely to be in poverty for the first time as a result of retirement. As James Schulz (1992) eloquently put it,

> The issue is not whether ... we can have better pensions and services for the aged. The issue is whether we want a higher standard of living in our retirement years at the expense of a lower standard in our younger years. Whether we like it or not, the "economics of aging" begins for most of us quite early in life. (p. 201)

The choices of a graying consumer market regarding saving versus spending, and on what types of goods and services, will have a significant impact on the larger economy in years to come. The economy cannot afford to ignore such a large group of consumers and continue to gear merchandise for the youth market only. Whether consumption among older adults will be for necessities only or for leisure and optional goods will depend, to a great extent, on how much disposable income is provided by the public and private systems of income maintenance.

On the societal level, older persons constitute a growing percentage of the population. Income maintenance programs place large and growing demands on both the public and private sectors. We can undoubtedly anticipate some modifications of these policies that will affect future cohorts. The issues facing the United States and most other countries with aging populations are much the same. Can our economies support a growing number of economically dependent adults for increasingly lengthy periods of retirement and still survive in worldwide competition? These issues are likely to challenge political and economic leaders for years to come.

WEB WISE

United States Census Bureau

http://www.census.gov

The United States Census Bureau collects and disseminates data about demographics, the population, and economy of the United States. This site offers information about the Bureau, including its organizational structure and employment opportunities. The current U.S. population and world population data are also available as well as current economic indicators and information on businesses and income, and labor force statistics. A manual and subject search option is provided. A "just for fun" function is also offered, and is an interactive approach to learning about geography and statistics.

Social Security Administration

http://www.ssa.gov

The Social Security Administration provides a great deal of information on various topics, including Social Security (SS) benefit information and forms, how to apply for services, direct online services, SS budget and planning, and SS laws and regulations. Quick access to the Office of Research, Evaluation and Statistics, which offers continuing data and research examinations of old-age, survivors, and disability insurance (OASDI) and Supplemental Security Income (SSI) programs, is offered. In addition, current SS information, the most requested top 10 SS services, and frequently asked questions are presented. Lastly, separate educational pages for children ages 6–12, teens, teachers, and parents are offered.

Center for Policy Research, Maxwell School, Syracuse University
NIA-Sponsored Research Projects

http://www-cpr.maxwell.syr.edu

The Center for Policy Research (CPR) is part of the Maxwell School of Citizenship and Public Affairs, Syracuse University. CPR conducts research and related projects in areas including aging and income security policy. This Web site offers information about Syracuse University, the Maxwell School, and CPR. It provides links to quickly access the Center for Demography and Economics of Aging and the CPR Aging Studies Program. Users can also explore National Institute on Aging–sponsored research studies as well as other economic- and income-related projects.

Luxembourg Income Study

http://www.lisproject.org/publications/wpapersg.htm

This key international study has generated interesting, comparative data across several nations on income, pensions, assets, and living arrangements of older adults. This page provides titles and abstracts of the most recent publications from this database. Topics vary over time, and analyses are performed by leading economic researchers in many countries.

KEY TERMS

adequacy of benefits	economic life-cycle hypothesis	need eligibility
age eligibility	equity of benefits	privatization of Social Security
assets	ERISA	social insurance
cumulative advantage	"good times" generation	Social Security Trust
cumulative disadvantage	income maintenance systems	Fund
defined benefit	income redistribution	three-legged stool
defined contribution	in-kind income	Townsend Movement
deserving poor		vested

QUESTIONS FOR THOUGHT AND DISCUSSION

1. Considering life chances and the pattern of cumulative advantage and disadvantage, what steps are you taking and plans are you making in your current stage of life that will influence your economic security in later life? In taking the long view, what are the major unknowns about how this will turn out?

What choices have you already made and what opportunities granted or withheld from you will determine this outcome?

2. Social Security has for years battled to reach the goals of adequacy and equity. But they are sometimes inconsistent. Both reflect middle-class American values. Should one of these goals be more important than the other? Should they be weighted equally in policy changes? Explain why you think your choice is best.

3. Imagine yourself at a family gathering where your uncle asks about your classes this semester. When he hears that you are taking a course in aging, he lets you know in no uncertain terms that he thinks older people are selfish and a huge drain on the economy, living comfortably and demanding more than their fair share while giving back nothing. How would you respond to him?

4. Now that you know a little bit more about the social construction of poverty, do you think that the definition is adequate? Are the assumptions fair? What would be the advantages and disadvantages of not changing the standards for measuring poverty for older and younger people?

Aging and the Health of Individuals

We can have a dramatic impact on our own success or failure in aging. What we can do for ourselves, however, depends partly on the opportunities and constraints that are presented to us as we age—the attitudes and expectations of others toward older people, and on policies of the larger society of which we are a part. (Rowe & Kahn, 1998, p. 18)

The health status of an older person is the result of many factors, including lifelong health habits (including diet and exercise), heredity, and exposure to occupational and environmental hazards. The quality and availability of health care throughout life also plays a role in health in later life. Many of these influences on individual health are, in large measure, socially shaped or constructed. As the quote above suggests, health behaviors are affected by societal values and by the practices and habits of the people in one's immediate social world, such as families and peers. For example, a person's food preferences and eating habits are clearly shaped by one's family experiences regarding food. Our growing awareness of the importance of exercise is another example of how societal values can influence individual values and behaviors. Your attitudes about exercise are probably quite different from those of your grandparents. Your health in later life will be influenced by this broad range of individual and social factors. This chapter explores those influences and looks at some information about the health status of older people to get an idea of how aging is related to health. In chapter 11, our focus shifts to the policies and practices within the U.S. health care system that shape access to and quality of health care for older adults.

Physical Aging

Why do we grow old? What happens to health as we grow older? Is there an inevitable increase in illness and poor health that accompanies age? To answer these questions, we can compare the health status of older people overall to that of younger cohorts. However, we also need to look at variations within the older population. Indeed, the degree of diversity in health among older people suggests that age itself may not be a very strong predictor of health problems. Variations in health status across cultures provide further evidence for the idea that age is not the most powerful influence. For example, Americans experience a progressive age-related increase in blood pressure, but in Japan and China resting blood pressure changes very little well into old age (Alessio, 2001). We examine many of these variations in health status throughout this chapter.

To set the stage for discussing these cultural and social variations in health, it is useful to know that there is extensive research on the physiology of aging. This specialized topic is beyond the scope of this book, but interested students can look to the numerous sources that describe physical changes that accompany age and the array of biological theories that seek to explain how and why the human organism ages. An example of such a source is *Human Aging: Biological Perspectives* (DiGiovanna, 2000). A recent issue of *Generations* (Spring 2000) focused on genetics of aging, covering the genetic influence on disease, new research on telomeres and alleles (some of the mechanisms operating at the cellular level to influence the aging of an organism), cloning, and cell transplantation. The human genome project will have incredible implications for our understanding of the genetic basis for aging. Physician George Martin (2000) draws attention to the clinical, ethical, and social consequences of "'new genetics' ... the present explosion of information concerning the structure and function of the human genome" (p. 10).

X Keep in mind that there are normal physical changes that accompany aging, such as a reduction in collagen that results in wrinkling of the skin and decreased elasticity of veins and arteries, which can reduce the ease and efficiency with which blood flows through the circulatory system. The timing and extent of such changes are highly variable among individuals, and they do not inevitably produce disease or disability. There are, however, diseases that become more common as we grow older, such as arthritis, heart disease, and Alzheimer's disease. Age can be a marker for physiological declines and increased likelihood of some diseases, but its role as a *cause* is not at all clear. Physiological aging—normal changes that accompany the passage of time—is highly variable. As discussed in chapter 1, Rowe and Kahn (1997) brought this variability to light in their distinction among successful, usual, and pathological aging. This breakthrough changed our thinking about physiological aging, paved the way for "a new gerontology" (Blazer, 2006), and continues to generate considerable research. Recent refinements have focused on clarifying the multiple dimensions of **successful aging,** including the avoidance of disease and disability, engagement with life, and high cognitive and physical function (Rowe & Kahn, 1997). Other current research is examining the factors that predict successful aging (Depp & Jeste, 2006).

Obviously, we must be cautious not to assume that age-related patterns are solely or even primarily caused by age. Some older adults get certain of these diseases, others

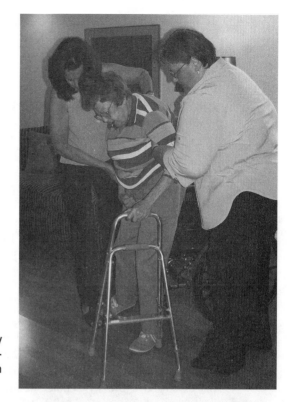

The timing of age-related decline and disability is highly variable, and some older persons demonstrate a great deal of strength and elasticity in their 70s, 80s, and beyond. (Credit: E. J. Hanna)

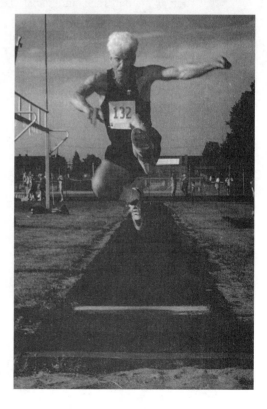

(Credit: Mike Payne, courtesy of the Ohio Department of Aging)

do not—so clearly age is not a cause or almost everyone would get these diseases as they aged. Beyond this, the patterns of illnesses we see for older adults in the United States do not necessarily hold true for other cultures, as mentioned above regarding high blood pressure. This illustrates that physical aging is only one of several factors that influence health and disease for older people. Compare, for example, the relative absence of breast cancer among Japanese women to its exponential increase with age among American women. In the United States in 2000, an average of 29.2 women per 100,000 died of breast cancer; the rates of this cancer mortality increase noticeably with age. Among women aged 55 to 64, the death rate was 59 per 100,000; that rate more than doubles (to 151 per 100,000) for the 75 and older group. Based on these numbers, we might conclude that something about the passage of time—simply living a certain number of years—increases the likelihood of breast cancer. However, in Japan in 2000, only 14 women (of all ages) per 100,000 died of breast cancer (World Health Organization, 2006), less than half the U.S. rate for all women. The fact that the breast cancer mortality rate is so much lower in Japan suggests that cultural factors—the context in which the passage of time is taking place—are at least as important as age.

Throughout this chapter we look at the health of the older population as a way to get a glimpse into what happens to the health of individuals as they age. The averages and patterns among the older population as a whole mask a great deal of individual variation. We can all think of examples of healthy, active 80-year-olds, and frail 65-year-olds in poor health. For any individual, health is a product of many factors—the genetics discussed above; life-style choices related to exercise and diet; and social characteristics such as gender, race, and social class. Because these latter characteristics reflect both individual and social forces, we use them as a way to disaggregate information about the entire older population. By presenting some information about groups within the older population, we can get some idea of the kind of variation seen among individuals. The diagram in Exhibit 10.1 is a simple representation of the multiple forces that influence an individual's health.

The Health Status of Older People

To develop a profile of the health of older people, we need to clarify how health is defined and measured. Even though health includes more than the absence of disease, much of the national data focuses on diagnosed illnesses and impairments, chronic conditions, hospitalizations, and doctor visits. We might argue that we have traditionally tracked indicators of the absence of health rather than health itself. Few national surveys include emotional, spiritual, and social well-being, mirroring our emphasis on the medical model of thinking about health. The major feature of the **medical model** (which is discussed in detail in chapter 11) is its focus on the diagnosis and treatment of disease, rather than a more holistic perspective on the physical, psychological, and social dimensions of health and wellness.

Recently, however, there has been increased interest in positive health behaviors such as prevention and health promotion, including nutrition, exercise, and

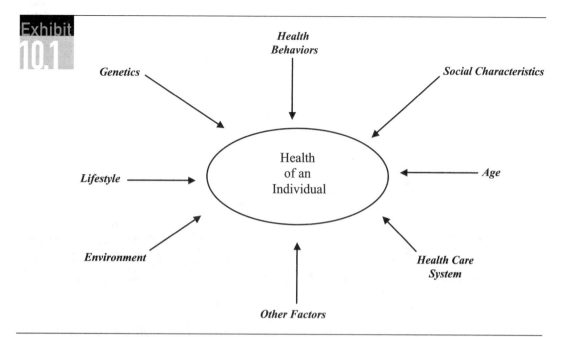

Exhibit 10.1

Factors Influencing an Individual's Health

smoking cessation. Health promotion and disease prevention is the explicit goal of a major U.S. initiative called Healthy People 2010. This public health effort seeks to improve quality of life and life expectancy for all Americans, emphasizing physical activity, healthy weight, mental health, and avoidance of tobacco (Healthy People 2010, 2006). One recent national report provides data on one of these health indicators: leisure-time physical activity among U.S. adults (U.S. Department of Health and Human Services, 2005). Exhibit 10.2 shows a steady increase with age in the proportion of people who are physically inactive. However, the increasing likelihood of inactivity is gradual until people reach the oldest age group (75 and over). Further, it is not known whether any cohort differences are reflected in these age-related data. People raised in earlier cohorts may have had different patterns of physical activity or inactivity even when they were younger. So whether this reflects inactivity that results from health limitations or simply a continuation of lifelong patterns is unclear.

Despite growing data that identify health positively, a strong focus remains on disease-based measures indicating absence of or limits on health. The following sections summarize some important trends in this area. We also provide information on the mental health of the older population, on their self-assessed health status, and on their ability to perform the major tasks of everyday life.

Prevalence Rates for Chronic Conditions

One of the most common measures of the health of the older population is the prevalence of chronic health conditions, such as diabetes and arthritis. **Chronic**

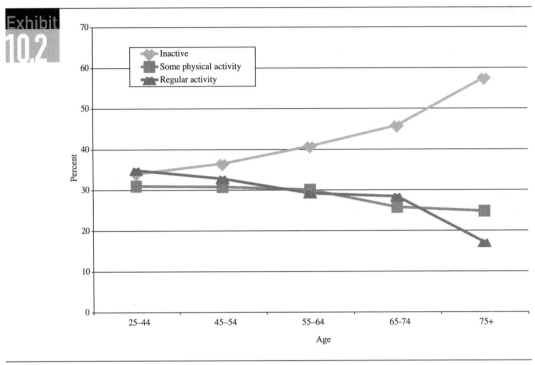

Leisure Time Physical Activity by Age in the United States, 2003
Source: U.S. Department of Health and Human Services, 2005.

conditions are health problems that last for an extended period of time and are not easily or quickly resolved. In contrast, an acute condition appears suddenly and changes quickly. Influenza is an example of an acute condition. Here we focus on chronic conditions, since they become more common as we age. Prevalence rates indicate what proportion of a given group has a certain condition or diagnosis. These rates, which say something about how common a condition is, can be reported as percentages, telling us how many people per 100 have the condition. For health problems that are less frequent, prevalence rates are often reported per 1,000—how many people per 1,000 in the group of interest have the specified condition. Exhibit 10.3 shows the prevalence (expressed as a percentage) of several common chronic conditions among men and women ages 55 and older. Comparing the darker bars with the lighter bars in this chart shows that all four of these conditions become more common with age. In general, hypertension and hearing impairments are more common than heart disease or diabetes among older men and women.

There are some interesting gender differences shown in Exhibit 10.3. Women have higher rates of hypertension and diabetes than men, but men have higher rates of heart disease—the number one cause of death in the United States among adults. This conclusion is consistent with the general observation that older men have higher rates of the most life-threatening conditions, but older women have higher rates of illness and disability overall. This pattern has been summarized (and probably oversimplified) in the statement, "Women get sick; men die," which reminds

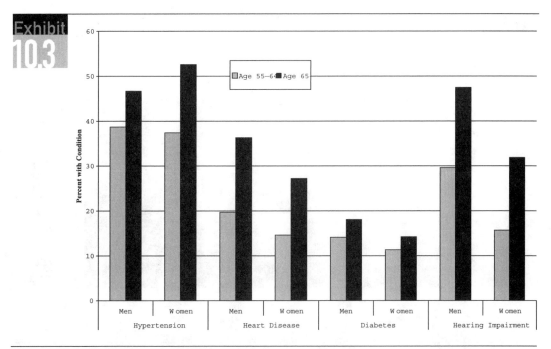

Exhibit 10.3

Percent of Older Population with Selected Conditions by Age and Sex: U.S. Average 2000–2003
Data Source: Schoenborn, Vickerie, and Powell-Griner, 2006.

us of the life expectancy differences described in chapter 3. Later in this chapter, we discuss a number of social forces, including differences in gender socialization regarding undertaking risky behaviors (e.g., drug use, high-speed driving), attention to bodily symptoms, and seeking help for health problems that contribute to this pattern.

Functional Ability

Another important indicator of the health status of the older population is the degree of limitation in people's ability to carry out their activities of daily living. Knowing about older people's health conditions is informative, but in order to plan meaning-ful and effective services, we need to know how these conditions affect people's lives. Measures of **functional ability** or **functional limitation** (these terms are used here interchangeably) serve that purpose. These measures evaluate older persons' ability to get through the day by asking about what activities of daily life they are able to perform, how difficult a given activity is for them, and whether the help of another person is needed to accomplish a given task. The most common measure of functional ability is the Activities of Daily Living and Instrumental Activities of Daily Living (ADL/IADL) scale, developed by Katz, Downs, Cash, and Grotz (1970) and refined by numerous researchers (Freedman, Martin, & Schoeni, 2002; Glass, 1998; Kovar & Lawton, 1994; Lynch, Brown, & Harmsen, 2003). This measure assesses the extent to which an indi-vidual needs help with basic personal tasks such as bathing, eating, and getting dressed

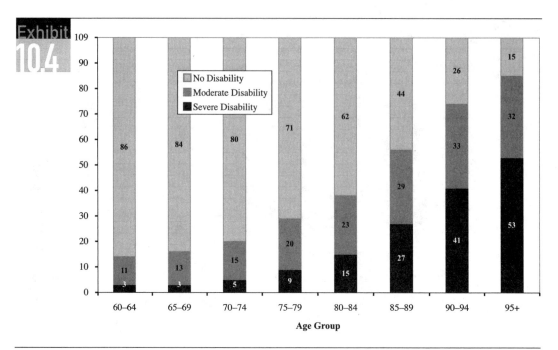

Percentage Distribution of U.S. Population by Disability Status and Age, 1995
Data Source: Mehdizadeh, Kunkel, and Ritchey, 2001.

and with household and independent living tasks such as preparing meals, shopping, and transportation. Some version of this measure of functional capacity is used for a wide range of purposes, including determining eligibility for services, evaluating the appropriateness of care plans for people receiving assistance, describing the health status of the older population, and projecting future challenges to the health are system.

Based on the ADL/IADL scale, Exhibit 10.4 shows the proportion of people at various ages who have different levels of limits in functional ability: no disability, moderate disability, and severe disability. People were placed in these categories based on the kinds of activities with which they need assistance. The severe limitation category includes people who need help with the most basic activities, such as bathing, getting in and out of bed, and dressing. The moderate category includes people who need help with activities such as shopping, meal preparation, and walking. Even though the proportion of people who have severe disability goes up noticeably with age, the majority of older people under age 85 have little or no limitation in their ability to perform the personal and home management activities of daily life. At age 85, most older people have at least a moderate level of disability, requiring some assistance.

Another way of measuring functional ability is to look at a person's self-reported capacity to perform specific physical tasks. Exhibit 10.5 gives information about what proportion of the older population in different racial and ethnic groups has difficulty with some of those tasks. In general, non-Hispanic Whites and Asians have the least amount of difficulty, non-Hispanic Blacks have the most difficulty, and Hispanics experience a comparatively moderate amount of difficulty. Older people in all four groups have the most difficulty with stooping or bending.

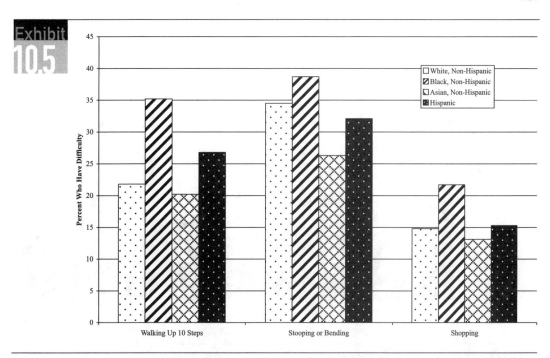

Percent of Adults Aged 65 and Above Who Had Some Difficulty With Physical Functions by Race and Ethnicity
Source: Schoenborn, Vickerie, and Powell-Griner, 2006.

Such data on the prevalence of functional limitations have implications for the everyday lives of older people. While most people find ways to compensate for gradual loss of function, there comes a time when people who live long enough will need some kind of assistance. Most people get the help they need from family and friends, for as long as possible. However, this informal assistance is only part of a complex and expanding system of long-term care. Thus, patterns of functional limitation in the older population have a direct bearing on the issue of long-term care—special services and assistance provided on an ongoing basis (either in nursing homes, in specially designed living units, or in an individual's own home) to people who need help with the activities of everyday life. We will return to the topic of long-term care in chapter 11.

Self-Assessment

Another more subjective measure of the health of the older population is **self-assessed (or self-rated) health status.** With this straightforward indicator of perceived health, people are asked to rate their own health as excellent, very good, good, fair, or poor. It is an informative measure. First, it is quite useful to know how people view their own health situation, since their views may influence their satisfaction and choices in other areas. Second, self-assessed health "is strongly associated with objective health status, such as physical exams and physician ratings" (Cohen & Van Nostrand, 1995, pp. 31–32). The fact that self-assessment is so closely connected with ratings by physicians is surprising to some people, but clearly older adults have a sense of how their bodies are working that goes beyond diagnoses or daily tasks.

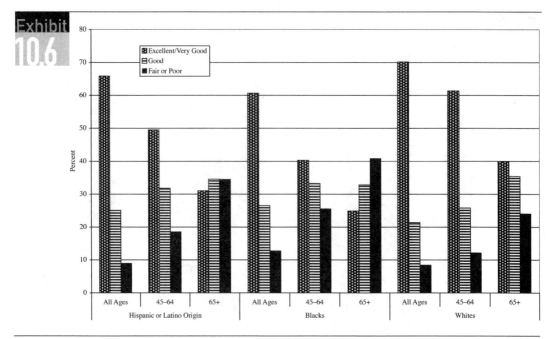

Self-Assessed Health Status by Race and Age in the United States, 2001
Source: Barnes, Adams, and Schiller, 2003.

Exhibit 10.6 displays variations in self-assessed health by age, race, and Hispanic origin. The majority of all older people in all groups rate their health as excellent, very good, or good. The proportion of people who rate their health as fair or poor goes up significantly with age, but the majority of those 65 and over still rate their health positively. There is a significant race/ethnicity pattern, suggesting that Whites have higher self-rated health than Blacks or Hispanics.

How does self-assessed health align with the prevalence of chronic conditions? Among the population age 75 and older, more than 50% have arthritis, 36% have heart disease, and 50% have hypertension (Schoenborn, Vickerie, & Powell-Griner, 2006). The majority of people over age 75 have at least one chronic condition. Given the high prevalence of major chronic conditions, how can older people rate their health as good, very good, or excellent?

Some researchers have suggested that older people rate their health positively because expectations about health change with age, and because people tend to compare themselves with age peers (Cockerham, 1998). This explanation implies that people make mental adjustments in the reference point against which they judge their own health, so that they see their health as better than they had expected for their age or better than others they know. An alternative explanation suggests that chronic conditions develop gradually, so that older people are able to adapt to and compensate for their health conditions. Many of their health problems have minimal impact on their everyday functioning. "Physical decrements can be accommodated within their customary lifestyle, so that good health is a reality" (Atchley, 1997, p. 86). According to this view, positive self-assessments of health are not the result of altered expectations, but are an accurate representation of the ability to perform daily activities.

Beyond the fairly high percentages of older people who rate their health as good to excellent and the growth with age in those indicating their health to be fair or poor, Exhibit 10.6 reveals significant differences among Blacks, Whites, and Hispanics on self-assessed health. Blacks and persons of Hispanic origin are much more likely than Whites to rate their health as fair or poor at every age, and much less likely to see their health as very good or excellent. These poorer self-assessments are not surprising, given the higher levels of illness and mortality among older Blacks compared to older Whites. They may also reflect cultural differences in defining categories such as good or poor.

Mortality

A final indicator of health status—or the ultimate lack of health—is mortality. **Mortality rates** reveal who dies, of what causes, and when (at what ages). One important way to compare mortality rates across time or across groups within the population is by looking at **death rates**. Rates of death tell us how many people per 100,000 in a particular group died in a particular year. Not surprisingly, death rates go up significantly with age. Exhibit 10.7 shows this trend. In the United States in 2002, the death rate for people between the ages of 15 and 24 was 81 per 100,000 people in that age group; the rate goes up gradually and then steeply increases for people ages 65 to 74.

But like most of the health measures discussed here, there is significant variation in mortality among the older population. Among people who are 65 and older, men have higher rates of death for heart disease, cancer, and lower respiratory disease; women have

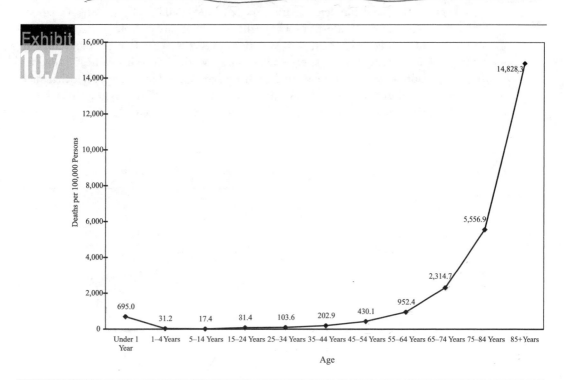

Exhibit 10.7

Death Rates by Age in the United States, 2002

Data Source: Kochanek, Murphy, Anderson, and Scott, 2004.

higher mortality rates for cerebrovascular disease (stroke) and Alzheimer's disease. For most of the causes on which comparisons can be made, Blacks have higher death rates than Whites, and Whites have higher rates of death than persons of Hispanic origin (Anderson & Smith, 2005). In 2002, for example, 605 of every 100,000 Black men ages 55 to 64 died of heart disease; for Black men 65 and older, that rate was more than 1,897 per 100,000.

Looking beyond general rates of mortality, we can consider causes of death. Exhibit 10.8 lists the leading causes of death by gender, race, and age for the United States in 2002. Heart disease and cancer are the two leading causes of death for all gender and race groups ages 55 and over. Diabetes, stroke, and chronic respiratory diseases, such as emphysema, are also leading causes for the age groups shown in this table. There is more variability by gender and race among the less common causes of death. Pneumonia and influenza ranks higher as a cause of death for older groups than for younger people. Alzheimer's disease is the fifth leading cause of death for White women 65 years and older, but it is not among the top ten for Black men at all. Some striking differences are not captured in this table, because the data are on the top 10 causes of death for the entire older population. Because there is variability, sometimes a leading cause for a subgroup will not be one of the overall top 10. For example, for Black men between the ages of 55 and 64, HIV is the eighth leading cause of death. For White men in the same age group, suicide is the eighth leading cause of death.

Additional dramatic differences in mortality patterns, with serious implications for society, are found in the younger population (not included in Exhibit 10.8). For Black and White men between the ages of 20 and 24, the three *leading* causes of death are accidents, suicide, and homicide (Anderson & Smith, 2005). The striking variations in leading causes of death illustrate that health and illness are complex outcomes of social forces, including social inequality, variations in access to health care resources, lifestyles, and, for some groups, immersion in a violent world. The cause of death rankings have implications for health policy and health promotion efforts, suggesting that such programs be tailored to meet the most pressing health needs of different groups. However, the largest *number* of deaths in a given year occur to White males, because Whites

Cause	Total Population	White Women 55–64	65+	Black Women 55–64	65+	White Men 55–64	65+	Black Men 55–64	65+
Heart disease	1	2	1	2	1	2	1	2	1
Cancer	2	1	2	1	2	1	2	1	2
Cerebrovascular disease	3	4	3	4	3	6	4	3	3
Chronic lower respiratory disease	4	3	4	6	7	3	3	6	4
Accidents and injuries	5	6	8	8	-	4	8	5	9
Diabetes	6	5	7	3	4	5	6	4	5
Pneumonia and influenza	7	10	6	10	6	9	5	-	7
Alzheimer's disease	8	-	5	-	9	-	7	-	-
Nephritis	9	9	9	5	5	-	9	7	6
Septicemia	10	8	10	7	8	10	10	10	8

Cause of Death Rankings by Age, Race, and Sex in the United States, 2002
Data Source: Anderson and Smith, 2005.

are the most numerous group in the United States and males are more likely to die than females. Therefore, the experiences of White males have tended to set the agenda for public health efforts, including research, treatment, and prevention.

It is clear that illness and the timing of death are not evenly distributed across the population, either within a society or around the globe. For children in developing countries without sufficient food and clean water and without adequate health care, conditions related to malnutrition and contaminated water and food are major causes of premature death (Bender & Smith, 1997). This unequal distribution of illness and early death is another example of the impact of social, economic, and historical context on the lives of humans. The following section, explores some of the individual, interpersonal, and cultural dimensions of mortality.

The Social Context of Mortality: Death and Dying

How, when, and where we die, and how we deal with death are further examples of social construction. While death is a physical event, it carries with it much social and cultural meaning, warranting our attention. Looking at the death rituals of any non-Western culture, or at our own culture in different historical periods, illustrates how differently we deal with death in the United States today than people have in other times and places. In India, for example, the body is wrapped in white, laid on a board, carried through the streets while mourners chant and toss flowers, and then taken to be cremated (Dube, 1963).

In earlier times in the United States the approach to death was quite different than it is today. Helton (1997) provides an account of how death was handled in rural Kentucky during the early decades of the last century. Both family and community had central roles in carrying out funeral practices. Women prepared the body, cleaned house, and prepared food; men dug the graves and made the caskets. Body preparation included washing and dressing the body and trying to make the body look as good as possible by putting coins on the eyes to keep them shut and covering the face of the corpse with a washcloth soaked in baking soda to help preserve the color of the skin. Helton's description of the traditions and rituals in early 20th-century rural Kentucky—where the body was handled by the family, and the entire community participated in the planning and the experience of the funeral—is in direct contrast with the majority experience of death in the United States today. Our impersonal and business-like approach to death has evolved to the point that we now have drive-through funeral homes.

The majority of deaths in the United States occur in hospitals or nursing homes; only about 20% of people die at home (Edmonson, 1997). The place of death tells us something about our attitudes and approaches to death. Death has become highly medicalized and professionalized. Sustaining life and preventing death for as long as possible is a hallmark of the tremendous advances in our medical technology. However, our success at prolonging life has been accompanied by a reluctance to deal with death—as a physical reality or as an ethical and emotional reality. The emergence of end-of-life ethical debates among politicians and health providers about euthanasia, physician-assisted suicide, and Dr. Jack Kevorkian's guilt or innocence reflects the fact that our technological ability to keep people alive has outpaced the development of clear societal values about humane death.

Just as we have come to rely on the medical system to prevent death, we have come to rely on other professionals to deal with death once it occurs. The funeral industry has become firmly established in the American way of death, offering products and services including funeral planning, casket selection, and body preparation. Turning these matters over to practitioners in the funeral industry is consistent with our professionalized and segregated approach to death.

Moller (1996) provides a thorough analysis of the ways in which social and historical context shape the rituals, meanings, and experiences of death. He argues that in the United States, "the movement away from ritual and community to bureaucratic management and medical treatment of dying patients is consistent with broader patterns of social life" (p. 25). In particular, he discusses bureaucratization—having rules and regulations about everything—and technological approaches to all kinds of problem-solving, including dealing with death and dying. Death is dealt with in a very prescribed and impersonal way, with laws and regulations guiding how to handle the body and how to file the necessary paperwork.

Similarly, expectations about grief and mourning—that these expressions will be limited as to time and place—reflect a societal emphasis on minimizing disruption and getting back to work and everyday routines. Many companies have policies about how long people can stay home from their jobs when there is a death in the family, even specifying what degree of kinship is required before any time off is allowed. We also have informal norms about appropriate expressions of grief and about how long people should be in mourning, which vary significantly among religious and cultural groups.

When people return to regular routines following the loss of a loved one, they are expected to control their emotions and get on with their lives. Crying and discussing the loss are not acceptable except with close friends and family. While we would be sympathetic if a colleague began openly grieving during a meeting or a class, it would make most of us very uncomfortable. These rules about how long or under what social circumstances grieving can legitimately go on, where and how it can happen, and who can legitimately grieve reflect a unique set of cultural values.

Doka (1989) offers the idea of **disenfranchised grief** to help explain the ways in which experiences surrounding death are socially constructed. He suggests that when a person experiences a sense of loss but does not have a socially acknowledged role or relationship with the deceased, the "rights" to grief are not recognized and thus the grief is disen-franchised (Doka, 1989). Clearly, the lack of social support and the lack of opportunity to participate in sanctioned, open mourning can make this process much more difficult. Homosexual relationships, divorced spouses, and assisted deaths defined as merciful (such as with advanced Alzheimer's disease) all can give rise to this disenfranchised grief (Doka, 1989). For example, the partner in a same-sex couple that is not accepted by the family might be excluded from participating in the funeral and related activities. The degree to which the loss for that person is acknowledged is crucial. People who are in relationships that are not sanctioned, in roles that are not clear, or in situations where the death is not recognized are likely to experience disenfranchised grief. The legitimization of grief and mourning on the basis of sanctioned and recognized personal relationships to the deceased is another example of the individualism that marks our culture. Clearly, death is not a collective or community experience in our society, but is highly restricted.

There is an extensive literature in both academic journals and the popular press about how people experience and adapt to loss. One of the best known approaches to under-standing death and dying is the work of Elizabeth Kubler-Ross, who identified five stages that dying patients go through: denial, anger, bargaining, depression, and acceptance (Kubler-Ross, 1969). This model has also been applied to the experience of bereaved persons. Kubler-Ross developed her model out of her conversations with dying people.

Clearly the model has validity; it summarizes the experiences of many people and helps both dying people and their loved ones to understand their experiences. The approach has been critiqued, however, for implying that there is a universal trajectory through the phases and for potentially imposing linear stages as the only appropriate way to deal with the intensely personal and complex phenomenon of dealing with death (Moller, 1996).

Perhaps in response to the imposition of a single "right" way to experience death and grief, and certainly in response to the medicalized, technological, impersonal, and individualized way of death in the United States today, some countervailing trends are emerging. The growing visibility and popularity of **hospice** care is probably the best example. Hospice emphasizes care, not cure; it uses liberal pain management to keep the person comfortable and takes a holistic approach to the dying person and his or her family and loved ones, including everyone in the experience and knowing the dying person as a whole person, not just as a medical patient. In addition, the ongoing debates about euthanasia (literally meaning "good death"), quality of life for the dying person, and control over the circumstances of one's own death suggest that we are trying to develop norms and values that will balance our awesome technological capacity to sustain life.

Mental Health and Aging

The foregoing discussion of health status has focused on physical health and mortality. The mental health status of the older population is an equally important issue. Parallel to the different ways in which physical health can be defined and measured, mental health also has different meanings. It can refer to emotional well-being in our everyday lives. But like physical health, most often the term is referenced negatively, to mental illness, mental conditions and illnesses that are a departure from health. Mental illness includes cognitive, emotional, and behavioral problems, including Alzheimer's disease, depression, and anxiety disorders. A thorough discussion of the comparative prevalence of mental disorders among older people, and of their causes, consequences, and treatment is beyond the scope of this book. However, a description of the overall mental health status of the older population will fill in our picture of the health of older people.

Using the broadest definition, about 15% of older people in the community and 25% of nursing-home residents suffer from depression (Fogel, Gottlieb, & Furino, 1990). Schizophrenia affects less than 1% of the older population living in the community, but about one-third of the residents of nursing homes and state hospitals (Fogel et al., 1990). About 1 in 20 older people in the community have anxiety disorders (Burns & Taube, 1990).

As with physical aspects of health, there is variation among groups in the prevalence of various mental conditions. Depression, for example, was found to be more common among Hispanic and Black older people than among Whites (Dunlop, Song, Lyons, Mannheim, & Chang, 2003). However, most of the racial/ethnic differences in depression disappeared when the researchers also examined group differences in education, health insurance coverage, income, and physical health status. So it may not be so much the race/ethnic group as the other factors (like income or health insurance) that are connected both to these categories and to depression. In all groups, having functional limitation in physical health is the strongest predictor of having major depression, more than doubling the odds of experiencing depression (Dunlop et al., 2003). Another recent study showed that depression is related to education such that people with lower education have higher rates of depression. This difference grows even more pronounced with age (Miech & Shanahan, 2000). Education is linked to social advantage, especially economic advantage. The same disadvantage of low education in determining physical health and freedom from disability in later life affects mental health as well.

In general, rates of mental conditions are much higher among nursing-home residents than among community-dwelling older people. About 12% of older people living in the community have diagnosed mental illnesses, while 65% of the nursing-home population is estimated to have some mental disorder. Cognitive disorders such as Alzheimer's disease account for 73% of all mental diagnoses in nursing homes, and are very likely the reason that they are in the nursing home in the first place (Burns & Taube, 1990). In addition, nursing home populations are much older than the older population overall.

Cognitive impairment refers to the loss of mental capacity for higher-level mental functioning; memory loss, confusion, disorientation, and loss of ability to care for oneself are some of the symptoms of cognitive impairment, often referred to as **dementia**. The most common cause of severe cognitive impairment is Alzheimer's disease. Fogel and his colleagues (1990) suggest that about 5% of the population 65 years and older have severe cognitive impairment. This proportion increases to about 20% for the population aged 80 and older. Cognitive impairments such as Alzheimer's disease are gradual, progressive deteriorations. In the early stages, people with Alzheimer's dis-

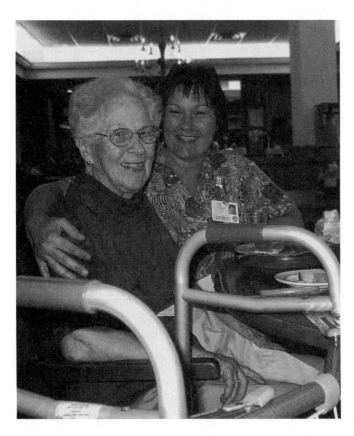

Positive mental health is an important aspect of one's overall health at all ages. (Credit: E. J. Hanna)

ease are very often cared for at home by family members. "For each demented patient in a nursing home, there are two to three more in the community with equal levels of impairment who are cared for by some combination of family, friends, and paid caretakers" (Fogel et al., 1990, p. 4). There are many consequences of, and issues related to, family caregiving for Alzheimer's victims. Some of these issues are presented in chapter 6.

The burdens of family care for cognitively impaired older people can lead to mental and physical health problems for the caregiver. "Some studies have suggested that more than half of family caretakers of demented patients may suffer from a diagnosable depression at some time during the course of care" (Fogel et al., 1990, p. 4). This latter point—that family caregiving for cognitively impaired older people may cause mental health problems for the caregiver—echoes some of the well-known literature about caregiving in general. Many caregivers enter their own old age with health and financial deficits. This situation is another example of the social production of health and illness. Since we have a service delivery system that provides few good options for caring for people with Alzheimer's disease, family caregiving is the foundation of that care system. Family care also reflects social values about families' taking care of each other and about the government's not interfering with the primacy of the family unit.

Estimates of the prevalence of other mental health problems vary, depending on whether the estimate includes all or some of the following: diagnosed conditions (for which individuals have been seen by health care professionals), diagnosable conditions (serious enough to be diagnosed if they are seen by physicians), and symptoms of conditions such as depression or psychological distress (they have signs of the disease but not at the clinically diagnosable threshold). Many people of all ages have conditions that remain undiagnosed for many reasons, so typically mental health conditions, which carry more stigma than physical health problems, suffer from especially high rates of undercounting.

Explaining Gender and Race Variation in Health

On all of the measures of health we have reviewed, there are significant differences by race and gender. We have alluded to the various explanations for these differences. For both gender and race, the explanations for patterns of health difference fall into two main categories: biological and social/behavioral. Here we will look more systematically at some of those explanations.

Summing up the dynamics of gender differences in health and mortality, Verbrugge (1990) suggests that risks are "added up over time, and occasionally subtracted. They are derived from a biological foundation ... and from the overlay of lifetime exposures" (p. 185). By lifetime exposures, Verbrugge means the accumulation of experiences and risks that affect health and mortality. Nathanson (1990) further illustrates these two dimensions of the gender gap by pointing out that, while females outlive males in nearly all species, the nature and extent of the difference in human life expectancy vary across time and across cultures. That the differential persists across contexts provides some support for a biological basis for longer lives among females; its variation across historical and cultural context reinforces its social basis.

In chapter 3, we discussed some of the biological bases for the female advantage in longevity, including the protective effects of estrogen. We also discussed the different health behaviors of males and females in our society. One of these differences is awareness of, and seeking help for, health problems. Women are more likely to attend to changes in their bodies (in part perhaps because of the emphasis placed on appearance and weight, and partly because of attention to changes that routinely happen during the menstrual cycle and maternity) and to visit physicians more regularly. One of the results of women's more frequent contact with health care providers is that they get diagnosed and diagnosed sooner than men for many health conditions. A related result is earlier treatment of health problems, which helps to explain women's greater longevity. Although this pattern of women's earlier and more frequent help seeking does not hold for all health problems, it is an important social factor in the gender difference in health and mortality.

Life-style risk factors for which men and women have been differently socialized also have an impact on risk for developing illness. For men, these behaviors include smoking, alcohol consumption, hazardous occupations, and driving fast; for women, stress related to competing demands on their time (e.g., work and family pressures) and feeling stressed are two socially produced health risks. Gender differences in health in later life are thus a product of the cumulative effects of biology, life-style, and behavior; the latter two effects are strongly influenced by social forces.

Race differences in health are similarly created by a combination of biological and social forces. "Some conditions such as hypertension and sickle cell anemia have a genetic basis, but living conditions associated with poverty influence the onset and course of most physical health problems" (Cockerham, 1998, p. 52). The impact of biology on race differences in health is primarily limited to the genetic component of select diseases and conditions. The social forces that influence racial variation in health patterns are, as in the case of gender differences, socioeconomic and cultural. In the United States there is a strong relationship between race and socioeconomic status, and there is a strong relationship between socioeconomic status and a range of health variables, including prevalence of chronic conditions, obesity, lack of preventive health care, and early mortality. The historic link between race and poverty has meant that Blacks have poorer lifelong access to health care than Whites, greater health risks from hazardous jobs, poorer nutrition, and poorer prenatal care. The impacts of inadequate prenatal care are lifelong.

Race and ethnicity can also operate through cultural factors that shape health behaviors related to diet, exercise, and willingness to seek the advice of a health care professional. Earlier discussion in this chapter suggested the impact of culture and life-style on health. An excellent example is the case of the Pima Indians. This group experienced almost no diabetes until, as a result of forced life-style changes, they began to eat more processed foods high in simple sugars and fats and to lead more sedentary lives. Today almost half of all adult Pimas aged 35 and older have adult-onset diabetes (Alessio, 2001). The high rate of diabetes among these Native Americans clearly cannot be attributed to a biological predisposition. Another illustration of the cultural (versus biological) explanation of racial and ethnic variation in health: Africans do not have rates of stroke or hypertension nearly as high as Blacks in the United States.

SUMMARY

Throughout this chapter we have considered how the health status of older people is a product of lifelong forces—genetics, behaviors, life-styles, and access to a particular kind of health care system. At the risk of oversimplification, we can reduce this array

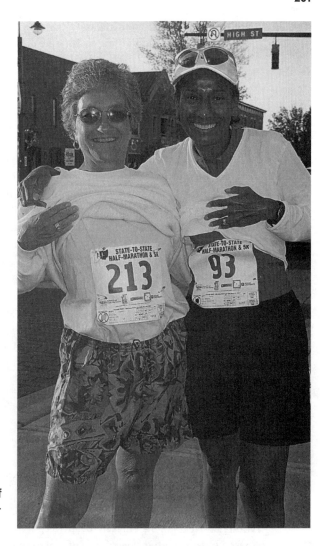

Healthy aging is a blend of a number of social factors, including heredity, diet, lifestyle, and exercise. (Credit: E. J. Hanna)

of factors affecting health to two primary categories: individual and societal. Individual influences include the decisions people make (about diet, exercise, and smoking, for example) as well as one's genetic heritage. These individual factors interact with societal forces including our health care system (which will be discussed in the next chapter) and social characteristics such as education, income, gender, and race/ethnicity. For example, older people with higher income have lower rates of many conditions, partly because of their lifelong access to health care. Women have longer life expectancies, partly because of the way they are socialized—to seek medical help and to minimize unhealthy behaviors. The variations in health status by these social characteristics point to the importance of social forces in shaping health. The emphasis placed on the social context of health is related to the social construction of health. This is the premise that health and illness are the result of many social arrangements, including gender socialization and socioeconomic variations in access to health care.

Interestingly, age by itself is not as powerful an influence on health as some of these other factors. Although some diseases are age-related, for many conditions people do not simply arrive at later life and develop a common set of diseases. There is incredible diversity among individuals in how healthy they are at age 30, age 70, or (for those who survive) age 102. While health is not entirely under individual control, there are decisions that individuals make that shape their health in the future.

The complicated interrelationships among individual and social forces in affecting an older person's health will continue to play out in fascinating and important ways. The health of aging individuals in the future will be a product of the same forces and of changes that are taking place in our nation's approach to health. There is an increasing emphasis on preventive health and on the role that individuals can take in their own health. There are some optimistic trends in understanding long-range health outcomes, including the potential for delayed disability and expanding life expectancy. Momentous research from the human genome project will contribute to our understanding of the ways in which biology contributes to health. In stark contrast, however, recent skyrocketing rates of obesity in our society will influence future cohorts who have spent much of their lives eating more and exercising less than current older adults. Recent research suggests that obesity increases an individual's chance of disability, but does not reduce life expectancy; thus obesity may result in normal life expectancy, but more years spent in disability (Reynolds, Saito, & Crimmins, 2005). This sobering prospect should encourage us to take stock of the individual and social forces that shape our individual health and the health of our older population.

WEB WISE

National Center for Health Statistics
http://www.cdc.gov/nchs

The National Center for Health Statistics (NCHS) is a part of the Centers for Disease Control and Prevention, United States Department of Health and Human Services. This Web site provides background information about NCHS, its products (publications and catalogs), current health-related news releases, and answers to frequently asked health-related questions. Information on NCHS data systems and national health surveys are offered. This site also presents various vital and health statistics, organized in tables from NCHS's warehouse. In addition, an opportunity to search chosen topics (older adults) as well as a list of other sites for health-related information and resources are available.

Profile of Older Americans: 2004
http://www.aoa.gov/prof/transportation/research/profile.asp

The Profile of Older Americans, compiled by the Administration on Aging, contains current statistics on older Americans in several key subject areas (future population growth, marital status, living arrangements, racial and ethnic composition, geographic distribution, income, poverty, housing, employment, education, and health/health care/disability). There are narrative sections as well as charts. In addition, this page contains access to special topics and profiles from earlier years.

Health and Retirement Study/AHEAD Study (also in chapter 2)

http://hrsonline.isr.umich.edu

This is the Web site for the Health and Retirement Study, a major national panel study of the lives of older Americans. The Health and Retirement Study includes the original HRS study (data collection in 1992, 1994, and 1996) and the AHEAD study (data collections in 1993 and 1995). These studies were merged in 1998 and now represent the U.S. population over age 50 in 1998. Two new cohorts were added in 1998: the Children of the Depression (1924–1930 birth cohorts) and the War Babies (1942–1947 birth cohorts). More detailed background information on study design, sampling techniques, content, and response rates is available on the Background Information page.

Columbia/HCA Health Care Corporation: Mental Illness in the Elderly

www.columbia.net

This site was prepared by psychiatrist Robert V. Blanche and provides information on mental illness in the older population. The site includes a brief discussion of the barriers on assisting older persons with psychiatric illnesses and offers information on depression, manic depression, dementia, anxiety disorders, and specialized treatment for older adults.

Community Health Status Indicators

http://www.communityhealth.hrsa.gov

This site, funded the federal government's Health Resources and Services Administration, provides data on demographic, health, and economic characteristics of every county in the United States and some comparative information with "peer" counties.

KEY TERMS

chronic condition	functional ability	prevalence rates
cognitive impairment	functional limitation	self-assessed (or self-
death rates	hospice	rated) health status
dementia	medical model	successful aging
disenfranchised grief	mortality rates	

QUESTIONS FOR THOUGHT AND DISCUSSION

1. Picture two older people you know, one who is very healthy and active and one who is in poor health and quite frail. Can you explain why they are so different? What life circumstances, individual choices, or random events helped to influence their health today?

2. Consider the ways in which individual choices and behaviors affect health and the ways in which social and cultural conditions play a role. Can you give an example of an individual health behavior that is not influenced by social and cultural factors?

3. The human genome project has the potential to change the way we understand aging, health, and disease. Are there any ethical questions that are raised by the wealth of information we might have about the role of genetics in our lives?

4. What health condition (including both physical and cognitive problems) do you think older people worry about the most? Why would it be of such concern?

Anti-Aging: Cosmetics and Aesthetics

Contributed by Mike Payne

"Vanity of vanities, all is vanity." It's hard to believe that observation came from the Old Testament (Ecclesiastics 1:2), thousands of years before the manufacture of facial creams, skin tucks, hair restoration, and liposuction. If they could only see us now.

Fittingly, the term *vanity* serves as a double entendre, with special application for aging. The word *vain* may be interpreted as excessive pride and preoccupation with one's appearance; the phrase *in vain* suggests the futility of battling the finiteness of human endeavors on Earth.

What could be more ultimately vain, and in vain, than the human struggle against time and age? Not much. But, currently, as Hollywood and Madison Avenue universally assert, there seems to be little that is more important—or as lucrative. The American Society for Aesthetic Plastic Surgery (ASAPS) estimates that surgical and nonsurgical (e.g., BOTOX® injections) procedures in the United States increased by 44% from 2003 to 2004, adding up to a total of 11.9 million in a year (Sacramento Bee, 2006).

Surgical procedures, almost all aimed at a more youthful appearance, climbed by 17%, while nonsurgical procedures rose 51% from the previous year. ASAPS puts Americans' overall spending on cosmetic procedures in 2004 at $12.5 billion. Liposuction led the way of the most preferred procedures (478,251). Eyelid surgery and facelifts, the procedures most directly related to a younger appearance, numbered 290,343 and 157,061, respectively. Among both surgical and nonsurgical treatments, BOTOX® injections (2.9 million) were by far the most favored (ASAPS, 2006).

But the money handed over for medical procedures in 2004 was almost doubled by the amount Americans spent on anti-aging products and remedies (such as anti-wrinkle creams, anti-oxidants, and vitamins) in the same year—roughly $20.2 billion. Annual growth in these products is projected at nearly 9%. At this rate, the anti-aging market will likely climb to a $30 billion industry by the year 2009 (Fredonia Group, 2006). Some estimates put that figure much higher.

Interestingly, though, it is health maintenance products—most notably those relating to memory improvement, sharper vision, and sexual health—and not cosmetics related to a younger appearance—that are expected to constitute the bulk of the gains in the years to come. Perhaps all is not vanity after all.

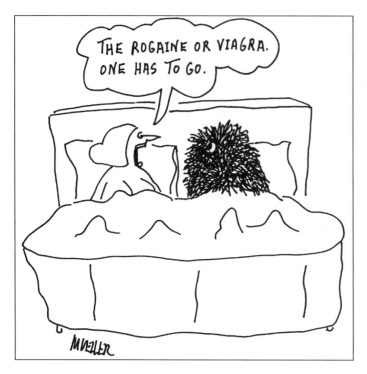

THE ROGAINE OR VIAGRA. ONE HAS TO GO.

MUELLER

Americans are increasingly interested in not only looking younger, but feeling younger as well. The past 30 years have brought an increasing emphasis on physical health and put a spotlight on the "use it or lose it" approach to keeping both body and mind in sound condition as the years go by. As our average life span has risen from 47 to 77 years in the last century, we have become more aware of how much life—and the deeper, broader appreciation of it that often comes with age—holds for people still blessed with good health well after the traditional time of retirement.

While a rapidly growing number of Americans are living to age 100 and beyond (from roughly 50,000 in 2000 to a projected 1 million by 2050 (Krach & Velkoff, 1999), the outer limit of the human life span has remained essentially constant for the past 100,000 years—at roughly 120 years (Hayflick, 2000–2001). However, maybe because collagen and airbrushing can't make a centenarian look 30, and all the antioxidants in the world won't make him or her feel it, most of us don't appear eager to reach those outer limits. An AARP study from the late 1990s found that only 27% of Americans surveyed hoped to live 100 years (Rostein, 1999).

But it might be just for the time being that 100 years of living brings with it undisguisable wrinkles, poor health, and a fading memory. Who knows what science may achieve in one of our final earthly frontiers—the human body. Some doctors and scientists in the field of aging expect to see humans routinely living beyond 120 years before the 21st century is over (Rostein, 1999).

Others, like Leonard Hayflick, Professor of Anatomy at the University of California, San Francisco, view the aging process and human life span as a predictable correlate of the brain-weight/body-weight ratio in primates, so that a sudden jump in the human life span would be unnatural and improbable (Hayflick, 2000–2001). Such life extension might also be undesirable, given the numerous social and ethical dilemmas an abrupt lengthening of the life span could unleash. For example, would only the wealthy, those now able to afford BOTOX®, facelifts and hair transplants, be able to afford the costly treatments leading to longer life? What would the new retirement age be if most people live to 130? How long would people stay in school? How many couples would celebrate their 100th wedding anniversaries?

Just this small sample of questions can seem daunting; certainly the technological and social challenges of significantly extending life expectancy are enormous and perhaps even overwhelming. But, we might take advice from some other scholars in the field who warn against being "gerontological Luddites," opponents of scientific change, when it comes to life extension (Moody, 2000–2001). The complexity of life extension and anti-aging are summed up nicely by Cole and Thomson (2000–2001):

> Anti-aging is fueled by many elements: ancient yearnings for immortality; contemporary possibilities in genetic and clinical research; widespread fear of decline, dependency, and death; a consumer culture eager to exploit this fear; and legitimate clinical care and self-help aimed at improving the quality of later life. (pp. 6–7)

It is important to question the underlying message of the many aspects of the anti-aging movement. Promoting healthy long life is quite different from fighting aging. We would be wise to question who benefits from anti-aging medicine and products, and what the burgeoning multibillion dollar industry implies about growing older in our society.

Aging and the Health Care System

A person's chances for illness and successful recovery are very much the result of specifiable social arrangements ... products of deliberate policy choices. In large part, illness, death, health, and well-being are socially produced. (Freund & McGuire, 1999, p. 3)

I he "specifiable social arrangements" mentioned in the quote above refer to a health care system—what services are provided, to whom, where; how those services are paid for is another crucial element of our health care system. Health care is a large and fast-growing segment of the U.S. economy. In a comparison of the percentage of gross domestic product (GDP) spent on health care in 30 countries, the United States ranked first (Reinhardt, Hussey, & Anderson, 2004). In 2004, the United States spent 16% of its GDP for health care and had the highest rate of per capita health care expenses; this proportion is projected to reach 20% by the year 2014 (National Coalition on Health Care, 2006). A number of factors help to explain this rank, including the advanced medical technology of the United States; an aging population; cultural preferences for the very best (and often most expensive) care available; a medical model approach to solving health problems after they occur (which is discussed more thoroughly below); relatively high administrative costs for providing insurance and managing health services; and fee-for-service reimbursement, which has dominated the payment system for health care in the United States.

In **fee-for-service** (FFS) systems of care, doctors, hospitals, and other health care providers are reimbursed for all of the services they provide; the more they do, the more they are reimbursed. Because Americans tend to value the idea that everything medically possible is being done for them, their expectations as health care consumers reinforce the financial incentive for providers to do as much as possible. Spiraling health care costs result in part from this circular relationship among fee-for-service reimbursement, technological advances, and demands for the best possible treatment. Such a system encourages innovation, encourages consumer demand for high-tech services, and encourages providers to deliver costly services. The fee-for-service model is gradually, and to a limited extent, being replaced by a **prospective payment system,** in which standards set ahead of time determine what costs will be reimbursed for the treatment of a given condition. This kind of payment system encourages more limited use of health care resources, especially expensive, high-technology care.

The high-tech, medical-model system of health care in the United States is a poor fit to the needs of the older population. The most common conditions that older people have do not lend themselves to high-tech cures—or to cures at all, for that matter. The surgical or chemical treatments that are the foundation of the U.S. approach to fixing health problems simply are not appropriate for ongoing, chronic conditions such as diabetes, arthritis, and heart disease. A system of care that is especially responsive to the health situations of older people would focus on the broader definitions of health, not just the absence of disease. Managing rather than curing a condition, and maintaining or enhancing an individual's ability to function in everyday life, would be the major goals of a health care system matched to the needs of the older population. Instead, the health system in the United States is oriented toward "curing" illnesses, is biased toward care provided in institutions such as hospitals and **nursing homes,** and is financed in a very fragmented and uneven fashion.

The Medical Model of Health Care

Much of the approach to the provision and analysis of health care in the United States is derived from a **medical model** of health and illness. This model of health and health care focuses heavily on the diagnosis and treatment of disease within specific systems of the human body. As discussed in chapter 10, when we summarize the health status of an individual or group, we tend to report the most common conditions or illnesses, the most common causes of death, and the success of various treatments for ill health. These statistics reflect the medical model emphasis. Although a focus on disease is certainly a central dimension of health, some important assumptions and limitations underlie this view of health.

First, the medical model implies that **health** is simply the absence of disease: If you are not sick, you are healthy. However, broader definitions of health include positive dimensions such as physical, psychological, and social well-being and the ability to function in, and perform the tasks associated with, everyday life. So health is not just the absence of something negative (disease), but rather the presence of positive mental and physical conditions.

Second, the medical model is founded on some assumptions that limit the perspective. Freund and McGuire (1999) identify several key aspects of the medical model. **Mind-body dualism** is the assumption that there is a clear separation between physical functioning and psychological, spiritual, behavioral, and emotional dimensions of the person. One outcome of this view is a focus on disease as a physical process, with little attention to the complex interplay between the physical and the social, emotional, and spiritual aspects of existence. **Reductionism,** which is based on mind-body dualism, is the tendency to reduce any illness to a disorder of the physiological systems of the body of the afflicted individual. With a reductionistic view of health and illness, no attention is given to the social context (e.g., stress or poverty) that affects social, psychological, and emotional states, which in turn have a great impact on physical health. A very obvious example would be a diagnosis of malnutrition as the absence of essential nutrients and caloric intake. Obviously, to understand why someone is malnourished and what might be done to correct the situation requires a much fuller understanding of the social, economic, and psychological condition of that person. Finally, the medical model rests on the **doctrine of specific etiology,** which searches for a specific cause for disease and tends to ignore contextual factors such as nutrition and stress.

These three assumptions of the medical model (mind-body dualism, physical reductionism, and the doctrine of specific etiology), as well as its limited definition of health as the absence of disease, all have a strong impact on many aspects of the health care system and our health behaviors. The skills, training, and decisions made by physicians, the expectations of health care consumers, and what health care insurance programs will pay for are all based on the medical model.

The implications of the medical model on health and illness are well illustrated by the "discovery" of diseases. Examples of discovered diseases from history include drapetomania, which caused slaves to run away from their masters; revolution, an irrational opposition to the rule of the English monarchy; and onanism (otherwise known as masturbation), which allegedly caused stunted growth, impaired mental capacity, and a variety of other symptoms including headaches, appetite problems, cowardice, and weakness in the back (Freund & McGuire, 1995). The deep-rooted focus of the medical model on physical processes fostered the naming of troubling behaviors as diseases. Our distance from the historical and social contexts that gave rise to the identification of these conditions allows us to see both the profound impact of social forces and, by extension, the limitations of the medical model.

The way in which menopause is commonly defined and treated in American society—as a medical condition—is another manifestation of the medical model. Current views about menopause have roots in some interesting, startling, and reductionistic ideas about women's health. The primary assumption underlying the treatment of menopause as a disease is that a woman's reproductive organs define her essence. Giving an extremely clear example of physical reductionism, a late 19th-century physician stated that the uterus is the "controlling organ in the female body; as if the almighty, in creating the female sex, had taken the uterus and built up a woman around it" (Ehrenreich & English, 1990, p. 277). The uterus and the ovaries were thought to be the source of any abnormality, from irritability to insanity.

This reductionism helped to pave the way for the medicalization of menopause. **Medicalization** is "the process of legitimating medical control over an area of life, typically by asserting the primacy of a medical interpretation of that area" (Freund & McGuire, 1995, p. 201). In the case of menopause, medicalization means that we focus on physical symptoms and biochemical processes, focus on these symptoms as unpleasant and uncomfortable, and transform the natural process of menopause into an estrogen deficiency disease. Defining menopause as a disease has several important implications. First, identifying something as a disease implies a course of treatment. In the case of menopause, the prescribed treatment is hormone replacement therapy (HRT), which is quite controversial. Artificial hormones reduce hot flashes, vaginal dryness, and other symptoms of menopause, but have been implicated in increased incidence of breast cancer. Recent research has found that HRT provides benefits that have nothing to do with menopausal symptoms—lower rates of heart disease and osteoporosis.

While the medical controversy over the advantages and disadvantages of HRT continues, a second concern about the medicalization of menopause persists. Many scholars see "treatment" for menopause as a mechanism of social control, perpetuating the ideology of women as sexual or reproductive objects and as passive participants in managing their own health. "The locus of solution then becomes the doctor-patient interaction in which the physician is active, instrumental, and authoritative and the patient is passive and dependent" (McCrea, 1983, p. 113).

Finally, focusing on menopause as a disease requiring physician intervention, gives less attention to the subjective interpretations and meanings women give to their own experiences. Many women report very positive reactions to this phase of life, including a sense of physical and psychological freedom. Giving greater voice to the subjective social and psychological experiences of women going through menopause would provide a counterbalance to the medical model approach.

Analyzing this approach further, Estes and Binney (1991) suggest that the tendency to medicalize normal physical processes has resulted in the "biomedicalization of aging." They assert that society has constructed aging as a medical problem, and numerous areas of professional practice (including a huge health care industry, policy efforts, and research agendas) have arisen to deal with this medical challenge. The growth of the aging "industry" (including increasing numbers of professionals involved in dealing with the medical problems of aging, and expanding opportunities for economic gains) is accompanied by an increasing social and psychological investment in the medicalization of aging.

In a provocative challenge to the medical model, McKinlay and McKinlay (1990) suggest that traditional "medical care is generally unrelated to the health of populations." They cite data on mortality trends following the introduction of major medical interventions, such as vaccines for polio, smallpox, and flu and treatments for pneumonia and typhoid. They conclude that "at most 3.5 percent of the total decline in mortality since 1900 could be ascribed to medical measures" introduced for the eight infectious diseases they considered (p. 21). Social factors such as improved nutrition, a rise in real income, and improved sanitation played a more significant role in improving the health of the American population than did the medical measures for treatment or prevention of disease. Although no one would argue against the value of medical measures at the individual level, McKinlay and McKinlay draw attention to the contextual factors involved in population health and the limitations of the medical model.

One alternative to a purely medical model is the **biopsychosocial model of health**. This approach, offered to clinical practitioners such as physicians, emphasizes a multidisciplinary and holistic view of health care, acknowledging that "complex problems of health and illness are inherently multidimensional in nature" (Schwartz, 1982, p. 1040), requiring bridges among disciplines, redefinitions of health, and a general paradigm shift within medicine. While focusing somewhat narrowly on clinical processes of diagnosis and treatment, the biopsychosocial model represents an important alternative to the unidimensional, mechanistic views of health and illness of the medical model. Interestingly, this model of care sounds very much like the approach used by **geriatricians** (physicians who take additional training in caring for the health needs of older

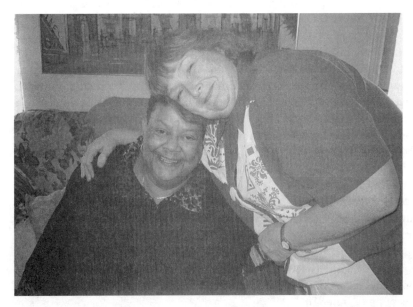

Geriatric medicine is distinguished by a holistic approach to understanding the interactions between aging, autonomy, mental health and disease. (Credit: E. J. Hanna)

people). Geriatric medicine is distinguished by specialized training in conditions that affect older people; a holistic approach to understanding the interactions among aging, disease, mental health, and independence; and a focus on coordinated, interdisciplinary care that involves families and other caregivers important in the lives of older patients (AGS/ADGAP, 2005). Even though such an approach to health care for aging people seems like a better fit than the traditional medical model, the United States faces a severe shortage of physicians trained in the principles of geriatric medicine. There are currently fewer than 7,000 certified geriatricians in the United States; the discrepancy between available and needed geriatricians is expected to reach 36,000 by 2030 (AGS Core Writing Group, 2005).

Elements of the Health Care System

Chapter 10 described the health status of older individuals as a product of many factors, including genetics, life-style, and health behaviors. The structure of the health care system is another important influence on health status. The availability of health care services, and the factors that influence when and how people utilize those services, are important determinants of health outcomes.

One of the most comprehensive and often-cited frameworks for understanding health behavior and outcomes is the Andersen model, which specifies these social influences on individual health behaviors (see Andersen, 1995, for a discussion of the evolution of this model). The Andersen model incorporates individual characteristics including age, gender, and race that influence personal health practices, such as seeking health care and using preventive health care measures. Andersen and colleagues also include income and availability of insurance coverage as primary examples of enabling resources—factors that give an individual the economic freedom to seek health care.

The Andersen model also emphasizes the role played by the health care system. That system interacts with population characteristics to help shape health behaviors and outcomes for individuals and groups. This effect is easiest to see in the case of the enabling resources. Compare a society that provides universal health care access to a country such as the United States, in which access to health care is based on ability to pay (usually because of insurance coverage and/or personally having enough money). Where access is based on ability to pay, some groups will not receive the same amount or kind of health care as those with the necessary economic resources. These disadvantaged groups will have lower levels of health care utilization and poorer health outcomes than groups with better access. Van der Maas (1988) discusses the public health implications of the impact of a health care system on population characteristics, health behaviors, and health outcomes.

> Under the prevailing government policies, most Western societies tend to produce increasing social inequalities, including access to health care. These developments may lead to a further increase in the health gap between high and low socioeconomic strata, and this may in turn seriously limit our efforts to improve general health levels and longevity. (p. 111)

For older people, lifelong inequities in access to health care result in variations in health status, as discussed in chapter 10.

The way the U.S. health care system operates—who has access to health care, under what conditions—has a powerful influence on the health status of older individuals. The U.S. health care system has been characterized as "high tech, limited access" (Lassey, Lassey, & Jinks, 1997). Those who have access have very good technologically advanced care, while those lacking insurance or financial resources experience serious gaps in health care. In addition, the effects of health care access and preventive care throughout all stages of life can significantly influence the health status of people as they move into and through the later stages of their lives.

Access and Utilization

It was mentioned at the beginning of this chapter that the United States ranks first in the amount of money (GDP per capita) spent on health care. However, a growing number of people do not have access to this well-supported system. A growing number of U.S. citizens have no health insurance and thus have very restricted access to health care. In 2004, 45.8 million Americans were uninsured, a significant increase compared to only 4 years prior when 39.8 million had no coverage (Center on Budget and Policy Priorities, 2005). Many of the uninsured are employed or are children of workers; in eight states, 20% or more of working adults do not have coverage (Robert Wood Johnson Foundation, 2005).

Older adults are less likely to be without medical insurance thanks to Medicare, which is discussed later in this chapter. However, individuals who enter their Medicare-eligible phase after years of no health insurance are likely to have some accumulated health deficits. National data show that high percentages of people without health insurance forego medical care and prescriptions, are less likely than those with insurance to have a usual source of health care, and face large out-of-pocket expenditures for the care they do receive. Missed opportunities to receive health screenings and early interventions in diseases can have substantial consequences for health and functioning

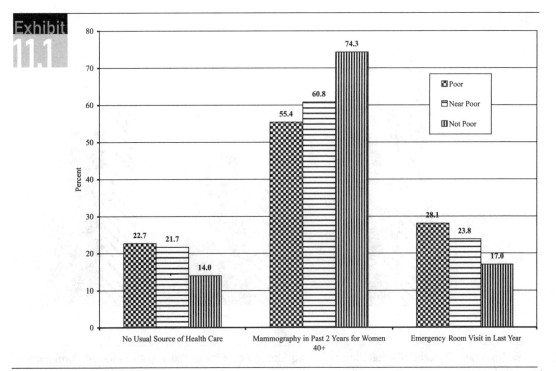

Health Care Access by Poverty Status in the United States, 2002–2003
Source: U.S. Dept of Health and Human Services, 2005

once people achieve Medicare eligibility. Exhibit 11.1 illustrates differences in utilization of health care by poverty status by adults in the United States. Poor and near poor people were less likely to have a usual source of health care, but more likely to have used the emergency room in the last year (probably in part because they had no usual source of heath care). Poor women were much less likely than non-poor women to have had a mammogram in the past two years. These differences in health care use can have lifelong consequences.

Even though virtually all older people have the benefit of Medicare coverage, differences in health care access persist throughout the life course, perhaps because of lifelong patterns of health care use. For example, poor older people were significantly less likely than non-poor older people to have gone to the dentist in the last year (37.1% compared to 67.8%) (U.S. Department of Health and Human Services, 2005). Poor dental care has been linked to other health problems, broadening the impact of poor care in this area.

Another illustration of unequal health care access and its implications comes from infant mortality data. Even though this example seems far removed from issues of aging, it is a powerful illustration of health care access, which has lifelong consequences for those who survive. In the United States, babies born to Black mothers are more than twice as likely as babies born to White mothers to die before the age of 1. In 2003, the U.S. infant morality rate overall was 6.9 per 1,000. For White infants, the rate was 5.72 compared to 14.01 for Black infants (Hoyert, Heron, Murphy, & Kung, 2006).

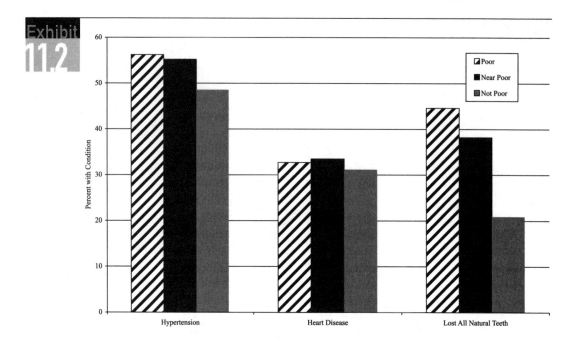

Annual Average Percent of Adults in the United States Age 65 and Older With Selected Conditions by Poverty Status, 2000–2003

Source: Schoenborn, Vickerie, and Powell-Griner, 2006

Low birth weight is the biggest risk factor for infant mortality. Although birth weight is related to individual factors such as the age of the mother and her health habits, the most powerful influence on birth weight is the adequacy of prenatal care, including education about nutrition, smoking, and alcohol consumption. Access to adequate prenatal care is linked to income and the availability of services in the mother's geographic area. Income and availability of services, in turn, are linked to race and ethnicity. In this way, an intensely personal outcome—the life or death of one's infant—is linked to larger social forces such as social inequality. The connections among health outcomes (infant mortality), individual health behaviors (mother's nutrition), and macro-level societal forces (unequal access to prenatal care) operate throughout our lives.

For older adults, variations in health status are at least partly attributable to lifelong differential access to health care. Exhibit 11.2 shows variations in some health conditions by income. Income in later life can be used as a rough proxy for lifelong health care access and utilization. Older people who are poor or near poor have higher rates of hypertension, and much higher rates of dental problems, than do older people who are not poor. Rates of heart disease do not show much difference by poverty status, probably because some of the other factors discussed in chapter 10 (such as gender and race) play a greater role than lifelong health care access.

Even for older people who do have good access to care, the structure of the current health care system presents some significant challenges. The system is fragmented and confusing. Acute care for short-term conditions that can be treated and resolved quickly

Political Economy of Health Care Access

The **political economy of aging** is a critical perspective that draws attention to the ways in which economic and political forces shape the policies, services, and experiences of an aging population. In particular, the political economy framework looks to the U.S. economic structure—capitalism—as an ideological and political force in shaping policies and services for older people. Estes (1999) suggests that a critical look at aging requires an examination of "the dilemmas and contradictions in maintaining both a market economy and democracy—that is, jointly advancing public interest in a democracy and private profit through capitalism"(p. 29). Profit motives and universal protection of the rights of citizens are not always compatible.

This perspective often draws strong reactions, because it calls into question the very foundations of American society. However, it does provide a very important lens through which to look at some of the inequality in the U.S. health care system. The United States does not have a universal health care system that would guarantee some degree of access to every citizen; the fact that more than 45 million people have no health insurance and the evidence provided throughout this chapter and in chapter 10 on differential health care access and outcomes among the older population provide clear illustration of the of the lack of universal access to health care. In the United States, health care is seen as a privilege rather than a right of citizenship. That privilege is earned through certain kinds of employment or through reaching age 65.

The political economy perspective proposes that our lack of universal health serves the economic purposes of those who profit from the current arrangement. In contrast, those who take issue with the political economists argue that the opportunity to make a profit from health care has driven the United States to be the best, most technologically advanced health care system in the world. In response, a critical theorist might argue that there are actually two health care systems—the best in the world for those who have access to it and one of the worst for those who cannot get minimum health care.

One of the most provocative challenges to our thinking about health care came from a 1987 book titled *Setting Limits: Medical Goals in an Aging Society.* Author Daniel Callahan argued that medical care should be rationed, especially expensive life-extending treatments, in order to spread health care resources among the greatest number of people. In a rationing system of this sort, older people would be unlikely to receive advanced and costly medical care, because the long-term benefits of such treatments for society and for the patient are limited. Callahan's work sparked extensive debate on a variety of fronts. One source of opposition came from those who were understandably concerned about the ageism implicit in a rationed health care system; others argued that rationing would produce a two-tiered system, one for people who can pay their own way and receive the best care possible, and another system for those who would only have access to services based on the rationed system. Political economists argue that we already have a two-tiered system of health care, but that the rationing is based on social class and race. Further, it is not an explicitly designed or openly discussed system of rationing.

Callahan's proposal calls for an explicit formulation of principles to be used in rationing health care. Since age would become a factor likely to limit access for older people, few gerontologists would support such a proposal. However, political economists of aging might see value in bringing to light the implicit rationing that already takes place. Acknowledging that we have a two-tiered system is a necessary, if small, step toward declaring health care as a right of citizenship, rather than a privilege. Whatever direction we decide to take as a nation, exploration of the tensions between market-driven advances in and universal access is an essential first step.

is provided in one kind of location (doctors' offices and hospitals), while long-term care for ongoing chronic conditions and disabilities is provided in another (nursing homes, assisted living facilities, or an older person's home). There is inadequate linkage among acute and long-term care services; older people often have to navigate the difference systems of care on their own or with the help of family and friends. The fragmented system reflects, in part, the way that health care for older people is financed.

Financing of Health Care for Older Americans

In the past several decades there has been a significant change in funding for health care for older Americans. In 1960, the system relied mostly on direct patient out-of-pocket payments. In 1960, just before Medicare legislation was passed, the government's share of the health care bill came to only 25 percent, including federal, state, and local sources. The remaining 75 percent of the nation's health care expenditures were paid for by private insurance or **out-of-pocket** (paid for by individuals). The story has changed considerably. The health care system now relies heavily on third-party private and government insurance programs. The transition occurred largely because of two important public policies for the financing of health care: Medicare and Medicaid.

    Medicare and **Medicaid** are the major payers of the government's share of health care, which amounted to 44.4% of the total in 2004. Individuals covered 15.1% out-of-pocket, and private insurance paid for 36% of the bill (Kaiser Family Foundation, 2006). Exhibit 11.3 shows these distributions for 1994 and 2004. The public and private proportions remained virtually the same, but Medicaid paid a slightly higher share of the public costs in 2004, and private health insurance paid slightly more in 2004 than in 1994. Public sources still account for about 44%, and private sources about 56% of the total health care bill.

Medicare

Medicare is federal health insurance for people 65 and older; it also covers some younger disabled people, but older adults constitute the bulk of its clientele. The legislation

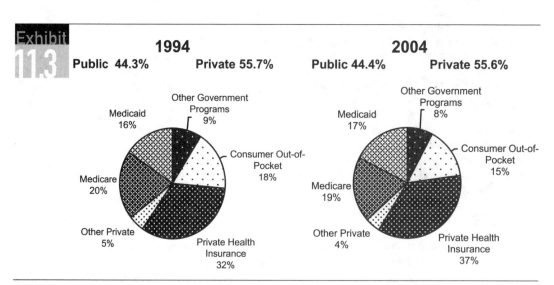

Exhibit 11.3

1994 — Public 44.3%   Private 55.7%

- Medicaid 16%
- Other Government Programs 9%
- Medicare 20%
- Consumer Out-of-Pocket 18%
- Other Private 5%
- Private Health Insurance 32%

2004 — Public 44.4%   Private 55.6%

- Medicaid 17%
- Other Government Programs 8%
- Medicare 19%
- Consumer Out-of-Pocket 15%
- Other Private 4%
- Private Health Insurance 37%

U.S. Distribution of Health Expenditure by Source of Payment, 1994 and 2004
Source: Kaiser Family Foundation, 2006.

establishing Medicare passed in 1965, after decades of debate and concerns over whether it was the beginning of the slippery slope toward socialized medicine. This issue is especially problematic, given that it goes against American norms and values regarding independence and self-reliance. Medicare is virtually universal for the older population, with about 97% of those over 65 insured by the Medicare program.

Since there are limits to what services are covered and how much of the cost remains with the individual, it is useful to have a brief summary of the program. Medicare has two sections: Part A and Part B. Part A, sometimes called hospital insurance, covers room, board, and nursing services in the hospital; it also covers up to 100 days of skilled nursing home care in a Medicare-approved facility, provided that certain conditions (such as a 3-day prior stay in a hospital) are met. Part A also covers hospice services and, to a very limited extent, home health care. There are co-payments (a certain percentage that the insured must pay) and deductibles (an amount that the insured must pay before Medicare pays any part of the charges). The yearly deductible for hospitalization was $952 in 2006. There is no co-payment required of a Medicare recipient for the first 60 days in the hospital. But, if someone stayed in the hospital for 61 to 90 days, they were charged $238 a day in 2006.

Part B, sometimes called supplementary medical insurance, covers doctors' fees, outpatient hospital treatment, lab services, and some limited home health care. For doctors' fees and special therapies, there is a deductible ($124 in 2006); Medicare then pays 80% of an approved amount and the insured is responsible for paying the remainder. Part B is optional and carries with it a monthly premium. In 2005, the cost to the consumer was $66.60 per month (Centers for Medicare and Medicaid Services, 2006). In short, while Medicare is a major component of paying for health and hospital care for older adults in the United States, it certainly does not remove the cost of health care as a significant item in the household budget.

Medicare has been a very successful program, providing nearly universal access to hospital care and reducing the cost of routine health care services for all older people. The major successes of the program include increased access to high-quality medical care, equality of treatment, and high levels of satisfaction reported by beneficiaries (Lave, 1996). There are challenges to the program as well. From the perspective of policymakers and budget analysts, the major concern with Medicare is the cost of the program. Medicare program payments were estimated at $325 billion for 2005, accounting for 13% of the federal budget (Kaiser Family Foundation, 2005). More importantly, the Medicare fund currently faces short-term and long-term financial problems.

Other problems with Medicare include its acute-care focus and the lack of coverage for long-term care and for home-based health care. In addition, the co-payments, deductibles, and gaps in Medicare coverage mean that many older people need to purchase **gap-filler insurance**. These private insurance policies, designed to cover the charges not covered by Medicare, are purchased by individuals or made available through employers. In 2003, nearly 63% of the older population had some form of private health insurance policy to address gaps and co-payments as well as aspects of care not covered by Medicare. The advantage of such extra coverage provided by private insurance is not spread equally among all groups within the older population, as Exhibits 11.4 and 11.5 illustrate. The first chart shows that, among those age 65 and older, non-Hispanic Whites are the most likely to have private health insurance, and Hispanics are the least likely. Some of this differential is explained by employer-provided insurance programs. Whites are much more likely to receive employer-funded private insurance than are any other group. Poverty status, which is related to both race/ethnicity and employment opportunities over the life course, also has a strong relationship with having private insurance in later life, as shown in Exhibit 11.5.

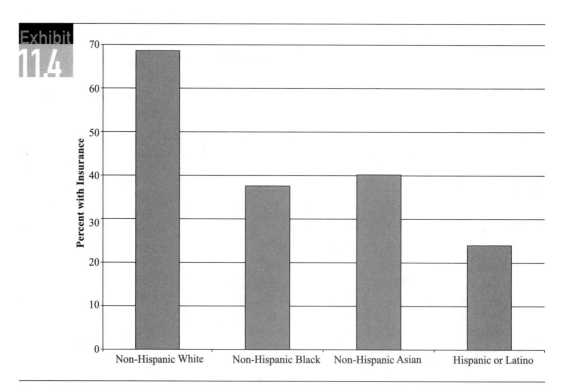

Exhibit 11.4

Percent of Adults in the United States Age 65 and Older with Private Insurance, by Race and Ethnicity, 2003
Data Source: Department of Health and Human Services, 2005.

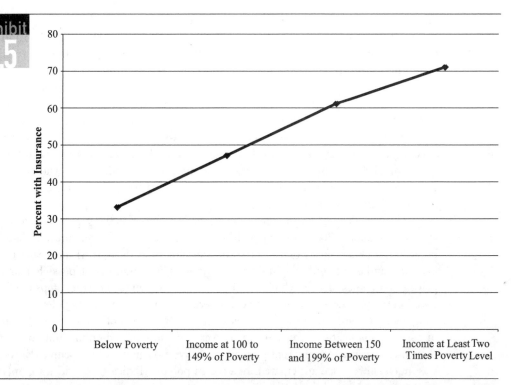

Percent of Adults in the United States Age 65 and Older With Private Insurance, by Poverty Status, 2003
Data Source: Department of Health and Human Services, 2005.

Individuals at or near the poverty level do not have sufficient disposable income to be able to afford gap-filling policies.

The need for gap-filler insurance has resulted in an ever-increasing array of choices. Many insurance companies offer such policies (generically referred to as **Medigap** policies). Medicare offers its own options under the umbrella of Medicare Advantage. Designed to offer benefits similar to private Medigap policies, the Medicare Advantage plans include managed care and preferred provider organization plans, which rely on a network of physicians and hospitals to provide greater coverage for reasonable costs (Centers for Medicare and Medicaid Services, 2006).

While Medicare is a significant benefit to older people, rising health care costs and gaps in coverage mean that individuals have high out-of-pocket costs. The average older person paid $3,455 in 2003 for health care; this amount represented 22% of the average older person's income (Caplan & Brangan, 2004). In addition, the program covers primarily acute care, not long-term care, which is the greatest health care need of the older population in general.

Medicare Part D

Prescription drugs are another major health care cost for older people. Not uncommon are stories about older people who cut pills in half or who skip doses in order to make the medicine last longer. Some media coverage even featured low-income older people who did not fill their prescriptions because they could not afford both medicine and groceries or heat for their homes. Prescription drugs are one of the fastest growing components of national health care spending, increasing more than four-fold between 1990 and 2003 (Kaiser Family Foundation, 2005). In an effort to help older people with their prescription drug costs, Congress recently signed into law the Medicare Prescription Drug Improvement and Modernization Act of 2003, commonly known as Medicare Part D.

As with any major policy change, implementation has been challenging. As a result of the compromises necessary to make the coverage reasonable and the costs of the program manageable, the legislation became a confusing mix of protection for those with very high or low drug expenses, but a gap in the pharmaceutical coverage for those whose medication costs are not particularly high or low. Individuals who already had drug coverage through private or employer-based programs may decide not to enroll in Medicare Part D at all.

Medicare Part D enrollment opened in November 2005, and coverage became available in January 2006. Implementation of the program has posed unusual challenges, because the beneficiaries of the program (and/or their designees) must sort through extensive and often confusing information about a large number of possible plans from private companies, decide which plan to choose, and then take further steps to officially enroll in the program. Extensive media coverage has portrayed the high levels of confusion among consumers trying to understand the provisions of the law and the nuances of complex medication program alternatives. The burden and opportunity of selecting their own coverage is apparently weighing heavily on many older people. Enrollment was much slower than anticipated. In a recent poll of Medicare beneficiaries, only 31% of the respondents had a favorable impression of the prescription drug program, and 61% said that they did not understand the program well or at all (Kaiser Family Foundation, 2005).

Medicaid

Originally conceived as insurance for the acute health care needs of welfare recipients, Medicaid now plays a crucial role in financing health care for older people, especially long-term care in nursing homes. Jointly funded by states and the federal government, and administered by the states, Medicaid was created as the primary health insurance program for low-income individuals and families. Medicaid has always been available for low-income older people, but over the past few decades two important shifts have taken place. First, an increasing proportion of Medicaid expenditures have gone for health care for older people. Second, an increasing proportion of those expenditures for older people have gone to long-term care rather than acute care. In 2001, older people represented about 11% of the Medicaid beneficiary population, but 24% of Medicaid expenditures went to services for older people (Flowers, Gross, Kuo, & Sinclair, 2005). Medicaid benefits for older people are spent primarily on long-term care in nursing homes. Of the money that Medicaid spent on long-term care in 2004, 51% went to nursing homes (Kassner, 2006).

How did this shift occur so that Medicaid is now a major payer of nursing home care for older people? From the beginning, Medicaid coverage included nursing facility services. Older people who needed fairly extensive assistance with activities of daily living resorted to Medicaid-financed nursing-home placement because they lacked other options. Most people with long-term care needs do not have the financial resources to stay at home and pay for long-term services out of their own pockets for very long. Since Medicaid originally covered long-term care only in institutions, older people who came to the end of their own and family financial resources often faced the dilemma of not being able to afford home care and not having access to government assistance unless they went to a nursing home.

For decades Medicaid provided almost no financing of community-based services, such as home health care or support in activities of daily living. That situation is changing, with the proliferation of **Medicaid waiver programs**. These programs allow states to waive certain restrictions that typically would apply to the delivery of services; specifically, waiver programs allow Medicaid dollars to be spent on home and community-based care, rather than institution-based (nursing home) care. Waiver coverage is limited to those older people who both qualify financially for Medicaid and who are impaired enough to be eligible for nursing-home placement. Since average nursing homes cost $5,000 per month in 2005 (Kassner, 2006), and community-based services, on average, less than one-half of that, the waiver programs are a potential source of cost savings. In addition, most people prefer to receive long-term care services in their own homes rather than in institutions (Kane, Kane, & Ladd, 1998). Yet the availability of openings in state Medicaid waiver programs are often limited, so that this alternative still is not broadly available in all states to those who might wish to use it.

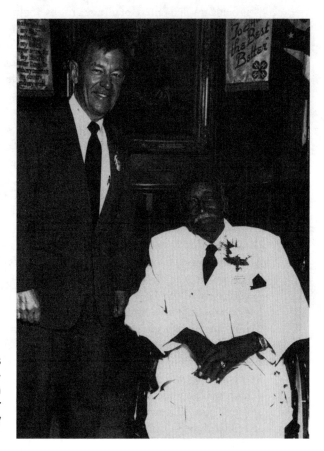

Senator George Voinovich (R-Ohio) was instrumental in vastly expanding Ohio's in-home service Medicaid-waiver program (PASSPORT) when he served as governor in the 1990s. (Credit: Mike Payne, courtesy of the Ohio Department of Aging)

The potential for using waivers for home and community-based care to save money is of great interest to state and federal agencies. Since Medicaid is jointly funded by states and the federal government, there is great concern at many levels about the growth of Medicaid expenditures at both levels of government. In 1980, Medicaid state and federal spending totaled about $25.5 billion; by 2004, the total was $288 billion, growth far beyond that related to the significant inflation of health care costs. Between 1980 and 2000, Medicaid's expenditure growth rate averaged about 11.2% annually. The current Medicaid price tag, dramatic rates of growth, and the looming demand that baby boomers will place on the health care system combine to suggest that innovations and reform are necessary (Ku & Guyer, 2001).

In summary, Medicare and Medicaid provide the foundation for the financing of health care for older Americans. Because of the restrictions on what these programs will pay for, they also play an important role in shaping how and where health care is delivered to older adults. The acute-care (i.e., hospital) and institutional (nursing home) biases in these programs has produced a delivery system that is not particularly responsive to the needs or preferences of the older population. The emergence of the Medicaid waiver programs signals a significant attempt to restructure the financing and delivery of some health care services to better fit the demands of an aging population.

Managed Care

Managed care is an increasingly common approach to the provision of health care that is being implemented for all age groups, including older adults. The Medicare Advantage program described earlier is based on the principles of managed care. This model is very different from the traditional fee-for-service approach to health care. Under fee-for-service, health care decisions are made by physicians; the insurer is billed for the diagnostic procedures, preventive or maintenance services, and treatments the physician has provided to the client. Financing and decisions about the delivery of health care are kept separate in this model.

In managed care, financing and delivery are linked. A single organization, which employs physicians and other health care professionals, takes on both financial and clinical decision making and risks. For Medicare recipients who choose to enroll in managed care, the managed care organization—sometimes called a **health maintenance organization** or **HMO**—receives a predetermined monthly amount to provide the care required for that older person (known as the capitation amount). If the client receives no services that month, or if the client receives extensive services that month, the HMO still gets the same flat fee for that client. The implications of this approach for quality of care for older (and younger) people are the cause of some concern. There is an obvious incentive to do less in the way of screenings, procedures, prevention, and treatment under a managed care system, since the business can profit from whatever funds remain from the capitation amount. In contrast, a fee-for-service system provides no barriers and perhaps an incentive to provide more health care to garner additional dollars. Under managed care, the same organization that pays for the care also employs the doctor who decides about the care. While a physician's code of ethics and standards for professional practice still dictate that she do what is best for the patient, there are new constraints on the decision-making processes—and those constraints relate directly to the costs of care.

The challenge for an HMO, as for almost any enterprise, is to balance quality of care with cost controls. Two major features of managed care are designed to look after that balance: gatekeeping and quality review. **Gatekeeping** is the process whereby a primary care physician coordinates the care a client will receive, providing some of that care directly and selectively authorizing additional services (e.g., lab tests or referrals to specialists) according to the guidelines of the HMO. The role of the gatekeeper is to provide necessary care at the lowest cost, and to avoid providing unnecessary care. **Quality review** is a process that monitors the adequacy of care provided under an HMO; information from client satisfaction surveys, complaints, and data on the health outcomes for managed care clients form the basis for quality review. An inadequate quality review might require that an HMO reconsider its guidelines or work with its doctors to adapt their decisions to improve quality.

Older Americans are signing up for managed care in increasing numbers. In 1992, only 6.2% of Medicare recipients were enrolled in managed care organizations; by 2003 that proportion had increased to 9.5%—almost 1 in 10 older adults (Health Care Financing Administration, 1992; U.S. Department of Health and Human Services, 2005). Why would an older person choose to join an HMO, with its built-in incentives to restrict services? The primary advantage of Medicare managed care is that it does away with the need for gap-filler insurance, because it has very low or no premiums and significantly expanded benefits. For example, prescription drugs were not covered under Medicare until 2006, but most managed care organizations have provided such a benefit as part of a managed care program. The major disadvantages are the loss of choice and control over which physicians and which specialized services a client can seek and the concern about the incentives to limit the kind and extent of care provided. The strong preferences of many people (including those over 65) to make such choices means that the great majority of older adults remain outside of managed care, a circumstance that may continue to shift with new cohorts reaching 65 having already experienced managed care as part of their employer health plans.

How do older people fare under managed care in comparison to traditional fee-for-service Medicare programs? To answer this crucial question effectively, we would need to be able to compare people with precisely the same health conditions receiving care under the two different models. Such outcome studies are just beginning to emerge, so the evidence is not complete by any means. So far, there is little evidence of a difference in the health status of HMO versus FFS clients. However, one key study (Ware, Bayliss, Rogers, & Kosinski, 1996) found that 68% of HMO patients who were both poor and elderly experienced a decline in health over the 4-year study period, compared to only 27% of similar patients enrolled in FFS plans. Studies such as this suggest caution with regard to outcomes for the most vulnerable older adults.

Whether managed care will be an effective and appropriate means of providing high-quality health care to the older population remains to be seen. The success of such programs in saving money, the outcome that is most pertinent to state and federal government, also has yet to be clearly demonstrated. In the meantime, more and more older people are joining Medicare managed care organizations and are conducting a real-world experiment in health care delivery.

Long-Term Care in the United States

One of the most important issues regarding health care for older people is long-term care. **Long-term care** is the system of services provided to assist people with long-term medical problems and limitations in their ability to complete the tasks of everyday life. It is fundamentally different from acute care in its focus. Rather than curing illnesses, long-term care is focused on managing chronic health conditions such as severe arthritis or lung and heart disease and cognitive conditions such as dementia, and maintaining function for as long as possible. Long-term care provides people with assistance in the activities of daily living (ADLs) and instrumental activities of daily living (IADLs) that were briefly mentioned in the preceding chapter. Help with bathing, dressing, meal preparation, and transportation are some examples of the assistance that long-term care provides. Some people also require medical care from the long-term care system, including administration of medications that might be forgotten by someone with dementia or medical treatments of various types. The diverse needs of older people for long-term care are met by a fragmented, complex array of programs and services that those needing long-term care must attempt to navigate (Kane, Kane, & Ladd, 1998).

The long-term care system includes a range of services (such as home care, adult day services, and home-delivered meals), locations where services are provided (such as senior centers, assisted living facilities), consumers (including older adults and disabled or seriously ill people of all ages), and payers (governmental, insurance, and personal/family funds). As discussed above, some types of long-term care assistance are paid for with public dollars; in other instances insurance or personal funds are required to cover the costs of care, sometimes extending over several years. However, as discussed in chapter 6, the vast majority of the day-to-day assistance that older people get is provided by family and friends in an informal system of support, without pay.

Programs within the long-term care system can also vary with respect to the duration of care, the intensity of medical or other treatment during care, and the goals for physical or cognitive functioning outcomes. Although nursing homes are sometimes thought to be synonymous with long-term care, these services can be provided in a range of settings—from an individual's own home to a specially designed congregate setting (such as assisted living), or in a more medically focused institution such as a nursing home. Some long-term care programs are designed to provide services to clients indefinitely for chronic or degenerative conditions from which recovery is not expected, while others might be set up as a shorter-term solution to an immediate crisis, such as rehabilitation after major surgery. Finally, long-term care can be designed to improve an individual's functioning, to provide services to compensate for losses in functioning, or to prevent further decline in functioning; some systems claim all three of these goals (Kane & Kane, 1987, pp. 7–8). Such long-term care situations might include rehabilitation after a hip fracture or stroke.

This diversity of services and programs that fall under the umbrella of long-term care thus includes paid and unpaid care, services provided in a person's home, services provided in specially designed housing, and services provided in a nursing home. In general, people in nursing homes have the highest level of need for assistance, followed by those in community housing with services, as shown in Exhibit 11.6. We will briefly discuss each of these components of the long-term care system. Individuals living in the community on their own have the lowest level of need for assistance, on average.

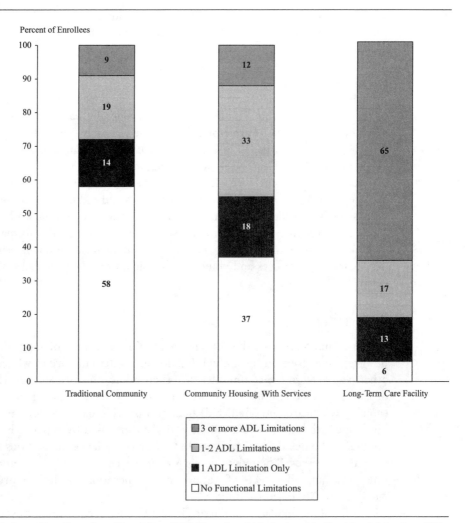

Percent of Enrollees

Traditional Community   Community Housing With Services   Long-Term Care Facility

■ 3 or more ADL Limitations
▨ 1-2 ADL Limitations
■ 1 ADL Limitation Only
□ No Functional Limitations

Percentage of Medicare Enrollees Age 65 and Over With Functional Limitations, by Residential Setting, 2002
Note: ADL=activities of daily living
Source: Federal Interagency Forum on Aging-Related Statistics, 2004.

Unpaid Long-Term Care

As noted in chapter 6, the vast majority of the day-to-day non-medical help that older people receive comes from family and friends. The unpaid help that is provided by family members and friends can range from relatively infrequent help with a few activities and needs, such shopping and transportation, to a nearly constant level of daily assistance with more complicated personal needs (such as bathing, getting in and out of bed, and eating) and medical treatments, including medications and wound care. A great many people are involved in providing these services. An estimated 21% of the U.S. population provides unpaid care to family and friends over age 18 (not all of whom are older people); the economic value of the care donated by family and friends has been estimated at $257 billion annually (Pandya, 2005). This astounding figure challenges us to think about how long-term care should be provided and paid for. Obviously those who pay for health care services (private insurers and various levels of government via Medicare and Medicaid) prefer that families continue this substantial contribution toward long-term care of their members.

Clearly, donated care is the economic, social, and personal foundation for the current system of long-term care. Families and friends generally want to continue to provide as much help as they possibly can for as long as they possibly can, and caregiving has many rewards. However, extended intensive family caregiving can take a toll, as discussed in chapter 6. In addition, caregivers who are employed (for example, an adult child providing care to a frail parent) face added costs. The working caregiver forfeits an estimated average of $660,000 over a lifetime in lost wages and reduced Social Security benefits because of missed days of work, unpaid leave, and reduction in work hours (Metlife Mature Market Institute, 2001). Because of the importance of informal caregiving to older people and to the long-term care system, increasing attention is being given to the development of services and employment policies that help to shore up the informal networks of support.

Nursing Homes

Nursing homes are a significant part of the formal system of long-term care today; however, they grew out of a much less formal system of care in which families took other people from the community into their homes for care and services. This form of care expanded and became more formalized when additional sources of funding (notably Medicare and Medicaid) began to provide payment for care. Today nursing homes are highly regulated and strictly controlled by states, which oversee the number of homes that are built and monitor compliance of facilities with state and federal guidelines. The federal government has national standards and strict guidelines regarding all aspects of nursing home operation for any facility that receives Medicare or Medicaid funding.

Much of the regulation of nursing homes has come about through cyclical discoveries over decades of serious problems in some nursing homes—including abuse, inadequate nutrition or facilities, or insufficient medical treatment. As a consequence of the negative coverage that ranges from committees of the U.S. Senate to local media outlets, most Americans carry negative attitudes regarding nursing homes. Incredible amounts of resources are expended to try to avoid negative events through tight regulation, regular inspections, and training requirements of staff.

More recently, nursing homes have changed their orientation from caring for seriously ill or demented older adults and disabled people of all ages to include more active rehabilitation and short-stay visits. One recent study of all nursing home residents in Ohio found that 57% stayed for 3 months or less; the majority of these people were in the nursing home to receive rehabilitative services (Mehdizadeh, Nelson & Applebaum, 2006). Some nursing homes also offer short stays so that family caregivers can have some respite to deal with their own health issues, take a break for a vacation or other reason from their nearly constant responsibility to oversee care. Nursing homes are serving an increasingly diverse range of needs, from short-stay rehab, short-stay respite, to long stay; they are no longer simply the "last home for the aged" (Leiberman & Tobin, 1976).

The population living in nursing homes has over the past decades become more sick and impaired than they were previously. Part of the reason for this is that nursing homes have focused on being the providers of long-stay, medically supported care—including care to the end of life. While many people go home again after a short-stay or rehabilitation visit, long-stay nursing home patients are often there until they die. The second reason is that nursing homes have, in the past 20 years, faced real constraints and competition. First, states have been interested in keeping people out of nursing homes, both because it is what people prefer and because home care (and family care in particular) cost the state much less in their Medicaid budgets. The second reason is that nursing homes, once the only alternative to family care, are now faced with more competition from the burgeoning assisted living sector and from home- and community-based services.

To further strengthen their reputations and their quality of care in a newly competitive environment, some nursing home providers are rethinking the way that nursing homes are run, including the physical environment, the amount of personal attention and other aspects of care. This culture change movement is interested in bringing person-centered care and an improved quality of everyday life to those in nursing homes through a variety of innovations, such as allowing pets in the nursing home to giving individuals with dementia more choice over how they spend their time to designing new physical living spaces.

Assisted Living

One major, new player in the long-term care sector is **assisted living**, which is generally considered to be a less medical setting, often featuring private efficient apartments decorated with one's own belongings within a building that looks more like a hotel in some cases than a hospital. The philosophy of assisted living focuses on providing privacy, autonomy, and personal attention within a setting where services to support activities of daily living are also available (Zimmerman et al., 2005). Much of the early development of assisted living was done by those in the hotel industry, who knew relatively little about the care needs of older adults who might live there. Since most people prefer to remain in their own homes, individuals or couples choosing to move to assisted living do so because living at home is no longer possible due to some health or cognitive problems. So rather than just being a "cruise ship on land" that provides housing, housekeeping, and meals, developers quickly learned that residents may require supervision in taking their medications, monitoring for falls, and assistance in dressing and bathing (Morgan, Gruber-Baldini, & Magaziner, 2001).

Assisted living is distinct from the nursing home environment in that most of the cost is paid for privately, by the residents or their families. A small percentage is paid for through Medicaid waivers or through long-term care insurance. Therefore, much of assisted living is not available to low-income individuals, who cannot afford the monthly fees and instead still must choose between home and nursing home.

As more time passes, the resident population of assisted living settings, which seldom provide extensive health care services as part of their environments, is becoming older and facing more health challenges. This forces decisions about whether to bring more services into assisted living or whether residents must move to a higher level of care, typically a nursing home. Some assisted living facilities include specialized units to care for those with dementia, including a larger staff and locked doors (Sloane et al., 2005). As these progressions continue, some contend that assisted living environments are becoming more like nursing homes without the same level of regulation. In response to negative events that have taken place in assisted living, all states have moved in the direction of regulating assisted living in a modified version of nursing home regulations (Mollica & Johnson-Lamarche, 2005). Nonetheless, their favorability compared to nursing homes remains fairly strong.

Community-Based Long-Term Care

This phrase describes assistance with daily activities that is provided in people's homes by community-based agencies (rather than nursing-home services). Options for home care (sometimes called **community-based care**) began to expand in the 1970s. This expansion occurred because of the convergence of three factors: the sometimes inappropriate placement of individuals in nursing homes, the high costs of nursing home care, and the preferences of the older population to stay home as long as possible. Even though home care was hotly debated at first (with strong opposition coming from the nursing home industry expressing concern that care provided in a person's home cannot be regulated as well as care provided in an institution), this form of service delivery has increased steadily over the past three decades. As discussed in an earlier section of this chapter, waivers helped states to include home care as an option for their long-term care systems.

One of the recent innovations in community-based care is called **consumer direction**. The philosophy of consumer direction holds that consumers have the right and the ability to assess their own needs, determine how best to have those needs met, and evaluate the quality of the services they receive. Consumers choose and hire their workers, decide how and when services will be delivered, and provide feedback about how well the services are working. In practice, the most fully developed model of self-direction is embodied in Cash and Counseling. In this model, consumers are the legal employer of record—hiring and supervising their own workers and managing their own services. Supports are in place to assist consumers with the paperwork involved in hiring and paying workers and with the development and monitoring of a purchasing plan, but the consumer is in charge. Currently 15 states have Cash and Counseling programs in various stages of implementation (Cash and Counseling, 2006). Based on the early successes and widespread diffusion of participant-directed service delivery models (Foster, Brown, Phillips, Schore, & Carlson, 2003; Kunkel & Nelson, 2005), it is clear that consumer direction is becoming part of the long-term care landscape. Consumer direction brings to long-term services greater flexibility, expanded options, and greater responsiveness to individual preferences. As a model of service delivery, consumer direction reinforces growing commitment to participant voice and choice in long-term care (Kunkel & Wellin, 2006).

Continuing Care Retirement Communities

A final option within long-term care is a **CCRC,** or continuing care retirement community. In this arrangement, housing and service options are combined and offered on a single campus. These communities typically offer independent living units (cottages, apartments, or houses), assisted living units, and a health care facility or nursing home. There is a steep entry fee to move into the community, and monthly charges that vary depending on where in the community the individual resides. In exchange for the entry fee and monthly charges, residents receive the promise of care that is tailored to their changing needs, all provided by the CCRC. Because of the high cost of CCRCs, this option is not available to all older people (Nelson, 2002).

Financing Formal Long-Term Care

Methods of paying for long-tem care are fragmented, much like the system itself. A small amount of institutional and community-based long-term care is paid for by Medicare. Most assisted living is paid for privately and thus is restricted to those with higher incomes. A large portion of nursing home care is paid for by Medicaid for older people who are poor or who become poor after they have used up their personal financial resources. A small (but growing) portion of home care is paid for by Medicaid, for people who are poor enough to qualify. Through Medicare and Medicaid, the federal government is the largest purchaser of long-term care services. Local programs, such as those funded by county tax levies or state subsidies, are becoming more common, but federal sources are still the primary payers of long-term care. Exhibit 11.7 shows the proportion of long-term care funded by various sources.

One alternative to expand the capacity for individuals to support whatever long-term care needs they may face is long-term care insurance. It is widely discussed but not adopted by many people. These policies provide coverage for individuals who require long-term

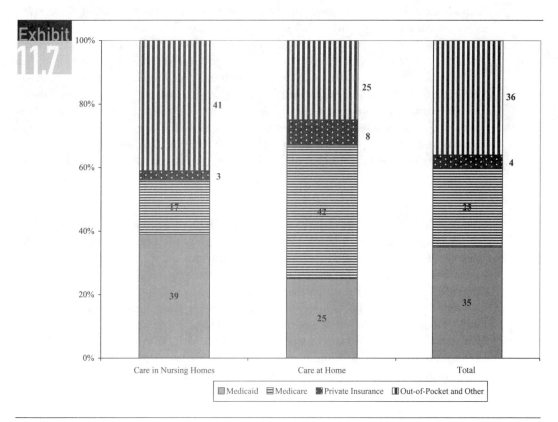

Long-Term Care Expenditures for Aged Americans by Source of Payment, 2004
Data Source: Congressional Budget Office, 2004.

care services later in life, often including alternatives to enable them to receive care at home if that is medically feasible. The low adoption rate of long-term care insurance is probably linked to a general societal distaste for thinking about issues such as severe illness and end-of-life issues. We would rather gamble that we won't need long-term care than contemplate that possibility. In addition, the policies can be costly, so that many people cannot afford to insure themselves against the prospect of a nursing home stay in their future.

Long-Term Care System Redesign

The preceding discussion of the financing and delivery of long-term care reveals that the United States does not have a very coherent long-term care system. We lack a neat continuum of care, and gaps and inequities are abundant. Where and how care should be delivered (in nursing homes or in the community, by family members or by paid professionals) and how it should be financed (by the government, by individuals and their families, or by some combination) are questions on which there is no agreement. Rather, long-term care represents a "paradigm by default … it arose out of unintended consequences, short-term solutions, and unexamined discrepancies between societal values and common practices" (Applebaum & Kunkel, 1995, p. 28). Medicaid has become a major payer of long-term care in nursing homes, not because that was the original intent of the legislation, but because it could be made to fit the growing need for financing long-term care. Most older people strongly prefer to remain in their own homes, but the current government financing system strongly supports nursing-home care.

Because the current system of care does not reflect a carefully crafted vision and plan for the provision of long-term services, considerable effort is being devoted to redesigning the system. The Centers for Medicare and Medicaid Services supports projects that consider innovative alternatives for service delivery, achieve better balance among institutional and community-based programs, and more effectively align options to consumer preference. The emergence of new options for long-term care—including government-financed, community-based long-term care and the development of assisted living—are harbingers of change in the long-term care system.

SUMMARY

The medical model has given rise to a system of health care not well suited to the needs of an aging population; it emphasizes acute care when the greatest need among older people is for long-term care for chronic health problems and functional limitations. The financing of health care for older people is fragmented, uneven, and biased toward care provided in an institution rather than in the community or in people's homes.

Another ideological challenge facing society in the near future is coming to terms with the question of whether health care is a right of citizenship (much as education and clean drinking water are) or a privilege (tied primarily to employment or economic resources). More than 45 million Americans currently have no health coverage; apparently many consider health care a privilege rather than a universal right. Relying on employers to fund health insurance increasingly is problematic, as companies try to cut costs by reducing benefits. Health insurance costs are being shifted to workers. Concerns about how to design, finance, and provide health care to the older population are part of these larger societal issues.

Even if we can agree that a coherently financed, integrated, and accessible system of health care is the goal, the fundamental problem of how to pay for it remains. The cost of providing health care to an aging population has proved to be an enormous stumbling block in moving toward a better-designed system of care. The large portion of the federal budget currently spent on Medicare is the starting point for projections of an untenable financial burden posed by health care costs of the baby boom generation. However, one should use a critical eye in considering the problems in the health care system and their potential solutions. Certainly the growing numbers of older people play a part in increasing health care costs to the nation. But the fees charged for health care services have increased also. Blaming older people for rising health care costs is an example of what Robertson (1991) calls **apocalyptic demography**—"the social construction of catastrophe by suggesting that an increasing aging population will place unbearable demands on the health care system" (p. 144). Robertson goes on to suggest that the health care system focuses on the aging population as a growth market and responds by medicalizing many aspects of aging—creating diseases such as menopause or sexual dysfunction or aging itself (as described in the essay on anti-aging), offering treatments for them, and receiving reimbursement for providing those services. This process—provider-induced increased demand for health care services for older people—and not the size of the older population may play the more significant role in increased health care costs. The ubiquity of advertising for drugs of all sorts, and the instant demand for Viagra® when it hit the market, suggest that induced demand is a reality. If that is the case, the solution to the crisis in health care financing may lie in reconsidering what aspects of aging really require medical treatment and limiting the fees charged for health care services.

The crisis in financing is one of the major issues facing the U.S. health care system. The resolution of this crisis—as well as debates about what care should be provided to whom, under what circumstances, and by whom—will depend on basic values about access to health care and who is responsible. The importance placed on individual responsibility, self-reliance, and independence have stood in the way of major health care reform. Government responsibility is sometimes seen as damaging to private initiative, family responsibility, and independence. However, the current fragmented and underfinanced system of long-term care for older adults is a good example of the need for a system with more integrity. Difficult decisions face us in the very near future, as we prepare for the aging of the baby boomers.

WEB WISE

Centers for Medicare & Medicaid Services
http://www.cms.hhs.gov

The Centers for Medicare & Medicaid Services (CMS) is a federal agency within the U.S. Department of Health and Human Services responsible for Medicare and Medicaid. The site provides a description of the agency, information for consumers and professionals on Medicare and Medicaid, and managed care plans related to both programs. Data on national health care expenditures, individuals covered by Medicare and Medicaid, and health care service utilization are also provided.

Kaiser Family Foundation: Medicare

http://www.kff.org/medicare/index.cfm

The Kaiser Family Foundation site contains a page focusing on Medicare, including policy issues, changes in the program, understanding how it works, and recent policy-based analyses. The site is useful for both understanding some of the complex issues of the program and supporting individuals in understanding their rights as participants in Medicare.

International Longevity Center

http://www.ilcusa.org

The International Longevity Center-USA (ILC-USA) is a not-for-profit, nonpartisan research, policy, and education organization whose mission is to help societies address the issues of population aging and longevity in positive and constructive ways and to highlight older people's productivity and contributions to their families and to society. The ILC is involved in projects and provides publications and links related to the extension of life and enhancing the quality of these added years. Some issues mentioned are improving health care delivery, sleep and aging, and palliative care, among many others.

AARP Policy & Research

http://www.aarp.org/research

AARP Policy & Research features authoritative information on issues affecting the 50 and over population, including housing, economics, and caregiving. This expanding collection of research publications, speeches, legal briefs, and opinion pieces seeks to provide deeper insight and fresh perspectives to opinion leaders, scholars, and other professionals. Health care topics include Medicare, wellness, and long-term care.

KEY TERMS

apocalyptic demography
assisted living
biopsychosocial model of health
CCRC
community-based care
consumer direction
doctrine of specific etiology
fee–for–service
gap–filler insurance

gatekeeping
geriatrician
health
health maintenance organization (HMO)
long-term care
managed care
Medicaid
Medicaid waiver program
medical model
Medicalization

Medicare
Medigap
mind-body dualism
nursing homes
out-of-pocket
political economy of aging
prospective payment system
quality review
reductionism

QUESTIONS FOR THOUGHT AND DISCUSSION

1. What do you think are the most important policy issues facing our aging nation? What are the most important health policy issues in older people's lives? What are the greatest challenges to our health care system?

2. Have you talked with older friends or family members about Medicare Part D? What is their view of the program? Are they enrolled in the program? How do these experiences mesh with what you may be reading or hearing in the news?

3. Look in your local telephone directory for physicians who specialize in geriatrics. Are there many of them compared to other specialties? Do you know an older person who sees a geriatrician? How does geriatric medicine better fit the needs of an older person than more traditional approaches?

4. Health care for our aging society includes wellness, acute care, and long-term care. Which topics receive the most attention among your family and friends? Which of these topics seems to be receiving the most attention at the state and federal policy levels?

Public policy reflects and reinforces
the "life chances" associated with
each person's social location within
the class, status, and political structures that comprise society. The lives
of each succeeding generation are
similarly shaped by the extent to
which social policy maintains or re-
distributes those life chances. (Estes,
1991, p. 20)

I n the realm of politics, members
of the older population are both
participants in and the subject
of debate. The roles of older persons in politics extend from being voters and advocates for
programs such as Medicare and Social Security to holding high electoral office. As a subject of political debate, the aging of the population focuses our attention on the socialties
among age cohorts as well as the interests that divide them. We have already begun to discuss social
policies (and the debates surrounding them) having to do with retirement and income maintenance.
Here we continue and expand those discussions, focusing more directly on politics and the place of the
older population in the political system.

Age-Based Government Policies

The Old-Age Welfare State

For the vast stretch of recorded history, older people (in relatively small numbers, since
life expectancy was short) were the responsibility of their families or themselves. Governments and leaders took no special note of the elderly as a category, often grouping the
disadvantaged, frail, or ill of other ages together with needy elders (recall the discussion

of the British Poor Laws in chapter 9) (Quadagno, 1982). Only relatively recently, primarily during the 20th century, have governments assumed any specific responsibility toward their older citizens by developing programs and laws focusing on the older age group. During the same time period, old age has been identified as a unique and distinctive time of life, deserving of special attention and support.

Robert Binstock (1991a) describes American public policy in the middle of the 20th century (from the 1930s through the 1970s) as **compassionate ageism.** By ageism Binstock means "the attribution of the same characteristics, status, and just deserts to a heterogeneous group that has been artificially homogenized, packaged, labeled, and marked as 'the aged'" (p. 326). Compassionate ageism stereotyped older people as poor, lonely, neglected, in ill health, and inadequately housed. Although founded on stereotypes, Binstock argues that the approach was compassionate, intended to help those "deserving and needy" older people who were unable to provide adequately for themselves (Binstock, 1991b; Quadagno, 1982). These stereotypes set the stage for policymakers to categorize older persons and to develop income, housing, and health policies to remedy their collective plight (Jacobs, 1990). Thus, governments in the United States and in many other nations developed policies to address the problems that were believed to afflict the elderly in their societies. Political support was based on the view that the problems of the old were not their fault and that the needs followed years of contribution to society (i.e., that they were deserving). Thus it came to be accepted as appropriate for society to provide help collectively, rather than rely on individuals or their families to meet all needs (Binstock, 1991a). Exhibit 12.1 outlines the timing of selected social policy developments in the United States, with those during the era of compassionate ageism shaded, many of which are discussed in this book.

This definition of the aged as a distinct and especially deserving population has prompted policies to be enacted that would otherwise face potent political opposition.

Exhibit 12.1

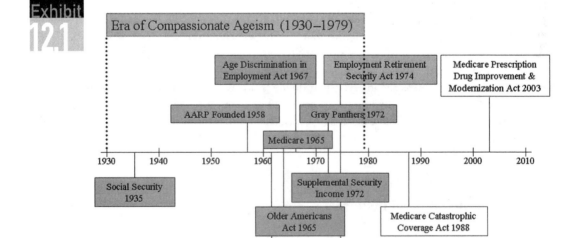

Time Line of Selected U.S. Aging Policies

For example, despite vigorous resistance in the United States to any national health insurance program throughout the 20th century, just such a program targeted to the elderly (Medicare) was passed by Congress in 1965. Programs and services for the elderly proliferated from the 1930s through the 1960s, and the popularity of helping older people rated alongside "old-fashioned family values" as campaign issues.

Initiatives to assist older adults reached a peak of activity in the 1960s as part of Lyndon B. Johnson's Great Society (Estes, 1979). The deservedness of the older population in the 1960s, including high rates of poverty and poor health and housing, was unquestioned. Programs to help expanded rapidly (Binstock, 1991b). Legislation passed during that time led to an array of programs, services, and agencies at state and federal levels that has been called the **old-age welfare state** (Binstock, 1991a; Myles, 1983). The old-age welfare state had a clear purpose to address the serious problems presumed to be common in the older adult population. Programs today still evidence this legacy.

Although we can talk about this network of programs as a whole, its development was fragmented, leading to gaps and overlaps, such as those discussed in chapter 11 relating to health care. Programs were established on a piecemeal basis, with no single agency or group responsible for the well-being of the older population. "Existing social policies for older people include a vast array of fragmented, complicated but important agencies, services and benefits" (Torres-Gil, 1992, p. 37). "The system involves numerous administrative mandates, each with funds and authority over specific areas. Often, one agency knows nothing of what the others are doing. No single, overarching policy or agency wields responsibility for coordinating services or developing policy direction" (Torres-Gil, 1992, p. 58).

In fact, Torres-Gil (1992) reports that there are programs related to the older population under the auspices of virtually every cabinet department serving the president. The largest concentration of programs is under the Department of Health and Human Services, including Social Security, Medicare, the Administration on Aging, and the National Institutes of Health (Torres-Gil, 1992). The largest program in terms of dollars of assistance each year is Social Security, described in chapters 8 and 9. Social Security, Medicare, and Medicaid together accounted for 47% of all dollars expended in the 2002 federal budget (*Senior Journal*, 2004).

The Older Americans Act

The **Older Americans Act (OAA)**, designed to be the focal point of federal government policy on aging, established the Administration on Aging, a unit of the Department of Health and Human Services, to oversee the well-being of adults over age 60 (Torres-Gil, 1992). Passed with broad support in 1965, the OAA mandated a wide array of programs intended to deal with a comprehensive list of issues facing older adults: enhancing employment options, improving long-term care, improving housing, and developing coordinated, comprehensive services to care for older adults with dependencies (Binstock, 1991b; McConnell & Beitler, 1991). The OAA, an age entitlement, was initially directed to assist all Americans aged 60 and over (Binstock, 1991a). The context for its passage in the era of compassionate ageism was a booming economy, in which public funds seemed plentiful, and a high degree of social consensus regarding the desirability of solving social problems through government programs (Binstock, 1991b).

The goals outlined in the OAA were lofty, but funding has never been sufficient (Binstock, 1991b). OAA programs have been hindered by a limited staff and budget over the past 40 years (Estes, 1979; Torres-Gil, 1992). Minimal initial funding for OAA was expanded in the early years, mostly as additional program responsibilities were added, but has shrunk since 1981 (Binstock, 1991b). Nonetheless, experts suggest that the Older Americans Act has had some successes.

> Its accomplishments, at the least, include (1) continuous and dynamic identification of needs of older persons; (2) creation and exemplification of strategies, programs, and services for meeting those needs; (3) provision of tangible and intangible help to innumerable older Americans; (4) development of a nationwide infrastructure for helping older persons, comprising 57 State Units on Aging, 670 Area Agencies on Aging, and about 25,000 associated service-providing agencies; and (5) recruitment and socialization of thousands of career professionals to the field of aging. (Binstock, 1991b, p. 11)

The programs offered under the auspices of the OAA have included senior citizen centers, nutrition programs, employment training initiatives, and a network of local and state agencies providing and coordinating services (Area Agencies on Aging). Successive commissioners of the Administration on Aging, faced with inadequate resources, have selected priorities for special attention during their administrations (Binstock, 1991b). As a result, the priorities under the OAA have shifted over time (Estes, 1979; Quirk, 1991). In the past 25 years, the OAA has moved significantly toward serving older adults in greatest need (low income, frail, and minority elders), moving away from its initial, broader age entitlement approach.

The Older Americans Act has also been a part of larger ideological debates regarding federal versus state versus individual responsibility to meet the needs of vulnerable populations of all types. Providing services at the state and local levels, the model utilized by the Administration on Aging, is viewed as preferable by many politicians (Torres-Gil, 1998). Although the Administration on Aging continues to provide services, it operates in a legislative limbo, without guidelines and with limited funding to meet its extensive original mandate.

The Aging Enterprise

Some have viewed the development of initiatives to assist older persons with an uncritical eye. In contrast, Estes (1979) has pointed out that programs and services for older persons can have some unanticipated consequences. The policies and programs established to ameliorate the problems of older adults have generated a system of agencies, service providers, and professionals that Estes refers to as the **aging enterprise**—"the congeries of programs, organizations, bureaucracies, interest groups, trade associations, providers, industries, and professionals that serve the aged in one capacity or another" (p. 2). Included are both government and private organizations, most of which have grown up since the introduction of major aging legislation in the 1960s—notably, Medicare and the Older Americans Act. Over time, Estes argues, the aging enterprise has become a force in itself, with a vested interest in sustaining the dependency of the older population. According to Estes, "the age segregated policies that fuel the aging enterprise are socially divisive 'solutions' that single out, stigmatize, and isolate the aged from the rest of society" (p. 2). She argues that the programs (and the people who implement them) reinforce stereotypic views of older people, foster dependency, and sustain a myopic "social problems" approach to dealing with what is today a highly diverse population of older adults to reinforce the need for their agencies and activities—and keep their jobs.

Many experts now question the viability of the old-age welfare state, as political ideologies have shifted and legislative control has moved into the hands of conservatives (Binstock, 1991a; Cole, 1995). Given these changes, limited funding and the changing demographic profile of the population, questions arise regarding whether the programs and policies that originally created the aging enterprise will survive, be modified away from the original intent, or be eliminated entirely.

Age and Need Entitlements

Most programs developed during the era of compassionate ageism share a basis in age entitlement. As described in chapter 9, in age entitlement programs individuals become eligible for benefits on the basis of chronological age. Usually the legislation includes age limits, such as the 40–70 age range in the Age Discrimination in Employment Act or the age 65 minimum currently in force for Medicare benefits (Quadagno, 1996). Age entitlement means that all individuals are eligible for assistance, with only proof of age required. Age entitlement programs are fairly simple to administer, because most people can establish their ages relatively easily.

Age entitlements are based on two somewhat contradictory goals: adequacy and equity.

> The adequacy goal seeks to protect those most needy by assuring a minimum standard of living and granting special benefits to the disadvantaged. The equity goal seeks to reward individualism and self-reliance by basing government benefits on the amount contributed individually during the working years. (Day, 1990, p. 121)

When one goal (either adequacy or equity) is met, the other necessarily cannot be fully met, challenging policymakers to weigh the two goals. The focus of age entitlement during the period of compassionate ageism was more on adequacy than equity. Current debates have turned attention more toward the equity goal.

Age entitlement contrasts with need entitlement—a system of providing benefits or services based on need, such as low income, poor health, or inadequate housing (Quadagno, 1996). Need entitlement results in fewer individuals receiving benefits (thus saving money), but requires more effort to establish who is (and who is not) eligible, raising administrative costs. Need entitlement programs, often referred to as welfare programs, have been subject to pressures in many countries to reduce funding when governmental budgets are tight (Hoskins, 1992). Because need-based programs designate their recipients as different from the rest of us, such programs are more politically vulnerable; they lack broad-based, bipartisan support from those not using (or expecting to need) their benefits. In fact, it is often said that "programs for the poor become poor programs." The social stigma and negative public opinion toward welfare benefits for unmarried mothers and their children, for example, indicate the vulnerability of public support for programs costing tax dollars but providing no direct benefits to those paying the bills (Kingson, 1994).

To reduce expenditures, conservative politicians have suggested changing some current age entitlement programs, such as Social Security and Medicare, to incorporate some targeting of benefits based on need (Quadagno, 1996). This push toward need entitlement is evident in the incremental changes that have already occurred in some age entitlement programs. The 1983 Social Security Reform Act started this trend by introducing taxation of Social Security benefits for higher-income older persons, in effect recapturing some benefit dollars going to those with economic security (Binstock, 1994). Similar changes have been built into other legislation, instituting sliding scales for taxes, deductibles, or targeted services based on the level of need of the older person. Thus, as Binstock (1994) reports, "a substantial trend of incremental changes has firmly established the practice of combining age and economic status as policy criteria in old-age benefit programs" (p. 728).

Since the late 1970s, when the era of compassionate ageism ended, both the stereotypes of the elderly and the political popularity of programs for them have changed dramatically. A growing conservative political trend, growing government deficits, and shrinking confidence that social programs could successfully resolve social problems all contributed to this transition (Torres-Gil, 1992). Views on using age as the basis for entitlements involve two related issues. The first issue is whether age is a good proxy for need for services and benefits. The circumstances of older persons in the early 1960s were that many of them were poor, inadequately housed, unable to afford medical care, and discriminated against in employment. In other words, by directing social policy interventions at this age group, Congress was fairly certain to hit most of those in need of assistance, and only a few who weren't, while keeping administration of the programs simple and inexpensive. So, during the era when many of the programs were established, age was a fairly good proxy for need.

Ironically, it is the success of these same programs in alleviating problems such as poverty and poor health that brings about lower percentages of the older population living in dire need. This improving situation *in the aggregate* makes the public and political support of policies to assist the elderly more tenuous (Hudson, 1996). Aggregate improvement does not mean that any individual's circumstances have improved over time. As living conditions for the population over 65 have become more varied, age becomes a less adequate proxy for need. The change is reflected in the political rhetoric, which has shifted the stereotype of older Americans from the "deserving elderly" to "greedy geezers" (Binstock, 1995; Ekerdt, 1998). Under the new stereotype, the older population is seen as mostly affluent and as a significant political force, voting in self-interested ways to protect their age entitlements (Binstock, 1991a; Hudson, 1996). Although ageism has survived, according to Binstock and others, the compassion has evaporated. The new stereotype of affluent, healthy, and politically savvy elders has undermined the prior political clout of advocacy groups and engendered resistance from some political interest groups (Torres-Gil, 1992).

The second issue has to do with the American cultural norm of individualism, and whether the government should be responsible for helping individuals in need. Whether and how to maintain a safety net for older persons who are poor or infirm are questions that reflect the schism between conservative and liberal ideologies regarding the role of government and the responsibility of individuals for their own well-being. The **liberal agenda,** championed during the ascendance of compassionate ageism, focused on government programs to address problems appearing in old age. The role assumed by government since the middle part of the 20th century has since been challenged by the **conservative agenda,** which argues that individual responsibility should be the norm, thereby reducing the role of government in the lives of individuals. This battle over old-age entitlements is actually one about core political ideologies, with strong advocacy on both sides. The U.S. policy dilemmas today arise from divided political opinion within the country on both the meaning and the implications of old age and on the role of government with regard to the welfare of older adults (Ekerdt, 1998; Torres-Gil, 1992)—a debate that will not be easily settled.

Aging and Politics

Age Norms and Rules for Political Participation

The U.S. Constitution includes formal age minimums for holding high federal office. Candidates must be at least 35 years old to run for the presidency, 30 to run for the Senate, and 25 to run for the House of Representatives (Office of the Federal Register, 1995). Presumably these rules were instituted in the belief that sufficient maturity and experience are necessary to fulfill these offices. Many states also have laws defining the minimum age for those seeking to hold public office. States vary in whether they specify lower limits on age for governors, members of the legislature, or other offices. For example, the most commonly specified minimum age for governor is 30 (in 34 states), with three states allowing anyone over 18 to run and six states having no age specified (Council of State Governments, 1994). Other offices, such as attorney general or lieutenant governor, less often have specific age limits, but almost all states have minimum ages for members of their legislatures. The most common is age 21 (in 22 states), with 14 other states specifying age 18 and 7 more states selecting ages 24 or 25 (Council of State Governments, 1994). None of these laws, state or federal, imposes a maximum age for officeholders, a point to which we will return shortly.

Socially constructed age norms guide the timing of events in political careers, just as they do in families and in other occupations. For the ambitious politician, these norms include progress through adulthood from local or regional office to state and possibly national office. Generally the pattern involves expansion of responsibilities with maturation and demonstrated ability, but the timing of political careers can vary widely. As an example, Exhibit 12.2 shows the distribution of ages at which individuals have entered the highest elective office, president of the United States. The range is quite broad, from the youngest entrant (Theodore Roosevelt) to the oldest (Ronald Reagan). The modal age for entry is in the mid- to late 50s. Examining the trend over time shows no pattern of age change over time. Starting with Teddy Roosevelt, the first president of the 20th century, the ages ranged from his low of 43 to 52, 57, 56, 51, 55 and 61; at the end of that century and the start of the 21st century, we had presidents aged 61, 53, 70, 65, 47, and 55 (the current incumbent). Among all who have held the

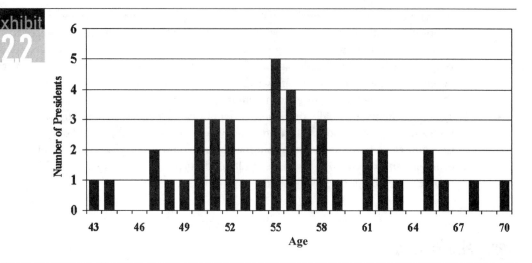

Exhibit 12.2

Ages of U.S. Presidents Entering Office

office of the president, most are well past the constitutional minimum age of 35, but only five entered office past age 65.

Besides the formal rules that set legal age minimums, informal norms regarding age and office-holding sometimes become apparent. The media often make note of instances in which individuals are violating implicit age norms by seeking public office at inappropriately young or advanced ages. Stories highlight newly elected members entering the House of Representatives at "only age 27," town mayors elected at 18, or veteran office-holders seeking reelection. In 1996, when Robert Dole, age 73, ran for president, he faced some of the same concerns regarding his age, focusing on the health and vigor necessary for the office. The late Senator Strom Thurmond was 92 when he successfully sought reelection in 1996 to a term that would take him to age 98. Critics questioned his capacity to complete the highly demanding duties of office (Grove, 1996). The candidates in both the 2000 and 2004 presidential races were robust 50-somethings. Whether extremes of age actually hurt a candidate at the voting booth is unclear. The fact that the issue is raised suggests an implicit age norm for being either too young or too old to become president or hold other high office. Reactions to extremes of age, in either direction, point out that our informal norms approve of individuals in the 50–60 age range as most appropriate for high office in the United States.

Aging, Period, and Cohort Effects on Political Behavior

Political behavior includes voting, participating in political activities, and running for office. One major topic of debate in the political life of any aging society should be whether the changes related to aging, period effects, or the flow of cohorts through society influence any of these political behaviors. An extension of this debate has to do with the issue of political power among the aged. As populations in many countries age, is there a likelihood that the older population will take over the political process and control the direction taken by the government? The issue is important because political control determines who fashions the policies of any government. If younger people are politically active in large numbers, politicians in democratic societies will be responsive to their interests and agendas. If, on the other hand, older persons dominate the ballot box, the political agenda could take a different path. Do aging, period, or cohort really make a difference in how people engage in politics and vote? What are the overall dynamics of these three forces in how individuals and groups (based on age, gender, race, or socioeconomic status) interact with and react to the political institutions of society?

Period effects seem likely to be especially potent in the political domain. People of all ages are influenced by social and political events that shape their attitudes toward government and specific public policies. It is therefore not surprising that major period events, such as the Watergate scandal in the 1970s or the Iraq war of the early 21st century have had significant effects on attitudes toward government and toward political parties across all age groups (Kahn & Mason, 1987). But such events may also influence people's orientations toward politics, and their attitudes and confidence in the political institutions that govern them, selectively on the basis of age (Peterson & Somit, 1994). Did young adults during Watergate, for example, experience a larger and more enduring reduction in their confidence concerning government than did older cohorts, who had experienced the solidarity of World War II? According to Jacobs (1990), such cohort effects do occur. "Distinct political and economic experiences may separate generations and have lasting impact" (p. 350).

Answering our questions about the effects of age on political activity and orientation engages the theoretical debate on the relative influence of aging and cohort experience. As discussed in earlier chapters, Mannheim hypothesized that, during a formative period in late adolescence and early adulthood, core attitudes and orientations (including political ideas) are set, changing little with advancing age (Alwin & Krosnick, 1991; Silverstein, Angelelli, & Parrott, 2001). If Mannheim's hypothesis is true, young people's political attitudes are shaped by political socialization within their families and by the political attitudes of the times in which they mature. Further, political behaviors and orientations in society would change slowly, as succeeding cohorts with differing attitudes move through the age structure of society (Alwin & Krosnick, 1991). If, however, events (period effects) can modify political attitudes and behaviors at any age, then Mannheim's view would not be supported, and political change could occur at a more rapid pace. If we find evidence that attitudes and political behaviors change dramatically, then Mannheim was wrong about the importance of cohorts.

Fortunately, politics is an area with a fairly long history of data collection, enabling us to examine how age groups voted, affiliated themselves with political parties, and participated in other ways in the political system. Using these data resources, we can develop fairly sound answers to our questions about age, period, and cohort.

Voting and Activism: The Potential for Old-Age Political Power

There is a long tradition of political involvement and activism among older adults in the United States.

> Since the Townsend Movement of the 1930s, senior citizens have strongly influenced public policies and political decisions. Their political activism pressured Franklin

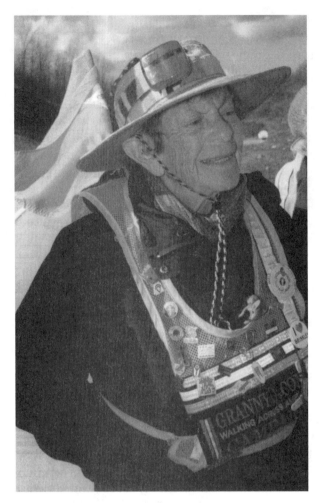

Political participation in the later years may take many forms beyond voting. At age 90, Doris Haddock (aka Granny D) finished her 3,200-mile walk across the country, from Pasadena, California, to Washington, DC, to advocate for campaign finance reform. (Credit: Mike Payne, courtesy of the Ohio Department of Aging)

Roosevelt to pass Social Security, and their alliance with President John Kennedy, labor unions, and the Democratic Party helped establish Medicare and Medicaid. (Torres-Gil, 1992, p. 75)

Political activism can take many forms, from voting or volunteering in campaigns to contributing to political causes, running for office, or simply following political issues in great detail in the media. Research data going back to the 1940s suggest that young adults are consistently less likely to be politically active by contacting their elected representatives or belonging to political organizations than are members of older age groups (Foner, 1973). Individuals also demonstrate more interest in political campaigns and public affairs debates as they grow older (Torres-Gil, 1992). Torres-Gil argues that both high voting rates and membership in advocacy organizations continue to empower older citizens politically.

One of the most consistent findings in the study of political behavior among the older population is their high rates of participation through voting (Foner, 1973; Jacobs,

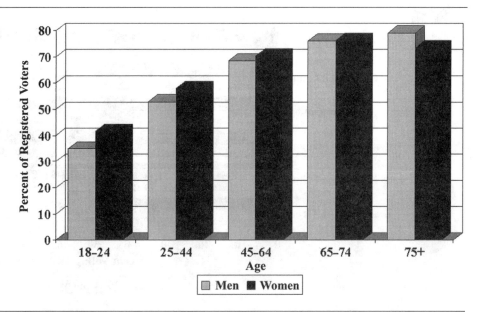

Voter Registration by Age and Sex
Source: Hobbs and Damon, 2006

1990). The percentage of eligible voters who cast ballots has been higher among older voters for several decades, suggesting a potential aging effect in this type of political behavior. First, there are fewer younger people registered to vote. Second, fewer of those young adults who are registered cast ballots on election day. The percentage of adults who are registered to vote rises consistently as age increases, with a clear progression upward until age 75 and older (see Exhibit 12.3). The age gap in voting has grown over time, mostly as a result of declining voting among young adults (Torres-Gil, 1992).

Several explanations have been offered for why younger people vote less often. They may have less political experience, feel lower party attachment, and relocate more often across boundaries of political jurisdictions, requiring re-registration to be eligible to vote (Foner, 1973). Strate and his associates (1989) suggest that age is related to voting behavior through a variety of forces that increase social integration with advancing age, up to the oldest age groups in which social integration declines. According to Strate's **civic development hypothesis,** young people are neither well socialized into the political process nor do they have the strong connections with family, community, and employment (the social integration) that foster voting among more mature adults (Strate, Parish, Elder, & Ford, 1989).

Studying the effects of aging on behaviors such as voting is complicated by factors that are related to both. For example, Exhibit 12.4 shows that, among men and women age 65 to 74, those with the most education are more likely to vote. So we cannot simply group people by age and have all of our answers. Many experts predict that the political activism of the older population will increase further with the rising educational levels

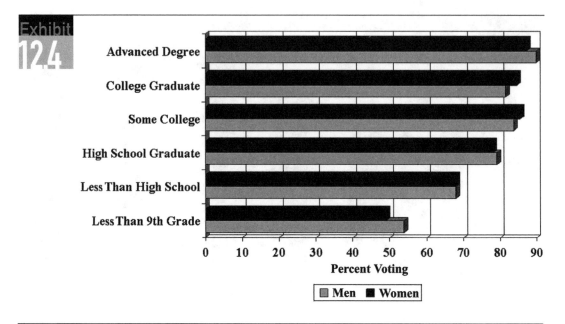

2002 Election Voting of 65- to 74-Year-Olds by Education and Sex
Source: Hobbs and Damon, 2006

and generational experience with political activism of baby boomers entering later life (Peterson & Somit, 1994; Rosenbaum & Button, 1992). Among younger cohorts, women outpace men in voter registration (see Exhibit 12.3); this situation is reversed in the cohorts beyond age 75, perhaps as a result of cohort experiences (recall the Nineteenth Amendment women voters from chapter 2). Thus, voting among older women—the majority of the older population—will likely become more common as current cohorts move through the life course.

Individuals from higher socioeconomic status (SES) backgrounds tend to vote more regularly than their less advantaged counterparts (Peterson & Somit, 1994; Wallace, Williamson, Lung, & Powell, 1991). They also tend to live longer (Rogot, Sorlie, & Johnson, 1992), meaning that as age increases, the composition of the older population shifts more toward higher-SES individuals (Riley, 1987). So, if voting rates increase with age, it may be that part of this increase is due to the cohort composition effect discussed in chapter 2. Selective mortality may leave a higher percentage of civically involved individuals alive and healthy enough to participate to advanced old age.

As you are already well aware, the size of the older population (both in absolute terms and as a percentage of the population) is growing. Through high voter turnout, the population over age 65 wields proportionally more influence than their actual percentage of the population. In short, if current patterns hold, the older population will likely continue to exercise political influence in the future. Candidates and issue campaigns—those focused on passing referendums, voter initiatives, or the recent campaign regarding changes to Social Security—already recognize this potential voter power as they seek favor with older voters (Torres-Gil, 1992; Wallace et al., 1991). Candidates often visit senior centers and develop sound bites on issues that appeal to older voters, who are more likely to watch the news than are younger voters. They discuss capturing groups, such as soccer moms and older adults as though they are homogeneous in their interests and political behavior (Jacobs & Burns, 2005). The remaining question is whether the pool of older voters ever has or ever will act as a voting bloc?

For cohorts or age groups to act according to age-based or generational interests requires some degree of **age identification**—whereby individuals label themselves as part of an age group or generation. Age identification has been studied for some time, and the findings are consistent that majorities of study participants who are chronologically over 65 do not identify themselves as older adults, selecting instead the label of middle-aged (Day, 1990). If individuals reject being labeled as part of the older population, it is less likely that they will join age-based organizations or vote (or make other political choices) based on age (Day, 1990). Instead, they may use other identifications (gender, religion, region, social class, or party) that seem to have greater relevance and have been used throughout their lives to make political choices.

Analysis of the 2004 election shows that older adults were not distinctive in their choices in the polling booth (Campbell, 2005). Campbell suggests that attitudes toward particular issues, such as the recent Medicare drug benefit, were less important than party in voter choice, so that voters age 60 and over acted much like the rest of the electorate, rather than like a voting bloc (Jacobs & Burns, 2005). Although age identification among those over 65 has not coalesced, some predict that it will grow in the future, based in part on greater longevity; Torres-Gil (1992) refers to the baby boomers as the "most age-segregated generation of the century" (p. 129) and hints at the potential for strong age identification among its cohorts. Certainly we might wonder whether the baby boomers, identified throughout their lives as a distinct (albeit highly heterogeneous) generation, will be more likely to act politically in later life on this basis of experience as an age-identified group (Morgan, 1998).

A related concern in aging societies is the possibility of **gerontocracy**—a society ruled by the elderly. Some nations today could be considered gerontocracies. In the decades after its Communist revolution, for example, China saw the age of its governmental leadership, drawn from the revolutionary cohorts, steadily increase. Now that the last members of that group are dying, however, new and more youthful leadership from the post-revolutionary cohorts has emerged. This has coincided with major recent changes in the focus of policies in China toward market economies, but making any sort of causal connection is risky.

When does a gerontocracy exist? One piece of evidence is the domination by older people of positions of power and authority in the political and economic realms. We have already looked at U.S. history, where the modal age of presidents at election is 55, hardly old (Kane, 1993). The seniority system in both houses of Congress means that members, as they accumulate years in office, gain power to head major committees and shape the legislative agenda. However, although members of the 108th Congress ranged in age from 30 to 86 years, the median age of all members was 54.9 (Amer, 2004)—again, not very old.

A second way to evaluate the possibility of a gerontocracy is to examine whether economic power and wealth are concentrated in the hands of older people. Exhibit 12.5 shows the age distribution of the Fortune 400 wealthiest individuals in 2004.

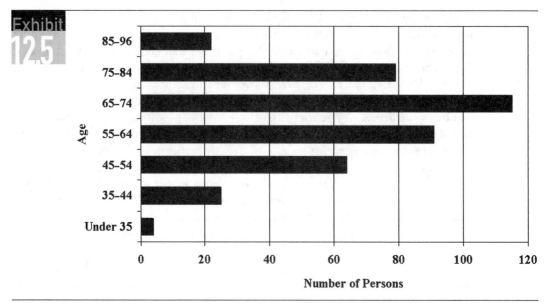

Age Distribution of Forbes Richest 400 Americans, 2004
Source: Forbes, 2005.

The distribution shows both self-made and inherited wealth (35 of 400 were listed as "inheritance") with some of the top names (Bill Gates) familiar to most of us. The exhibit shows relatively few wealthy individuals under age 35, with the highest concentrations in the 65–74 age range and a declining number at higher ages, in part due to mortality thinning the ranks. Almost half are under age 65, including many individuals who have made their own fortunes. In sum, neither political office-holding nor the resources of wealth are so concentrated in the hands of those over age 65 as to warrant concluding that a gerontocracy exists in the United States.

Attitudes and Party Affiliation

Sears (1983) defines two types of political attitudes or orientations. The first, symbolic attitudes, are items such as liberal or conservative orientation and party affiliation. Sears argues that such symbolic political attitudes are deeply rooted in an individual's sense of self and are less subject to the effects of short-term political events or change with aging. Following the Mannheim hypothesis, he believes that these attitudes are formed in youth and persist across the life course. Other, more specific attitudes—such as those toward the deficit, gun control, or particular initiatives or candidates—Sears contends are more subject to the influence of period effects or maturational changes. These attitudes are more likely to change with age and the passage of time.

The evidence on non-symbolic political attitudes is mixed. Using a life cycle approach, Alwin and Krosnick (1991) tested the Mannheim hypothesis, described earlier, with regard to changes in political attitudes among various age groups over time. Their study used two three-wave panel studies—one from the 1950s and one from the 1970s—with national samples of voting-age individuals. The analysis showed that the attitudes of mid-life and older adults were only slightly more stable across time than those of young adults, arguing against the Mannheim hypothesis at least for non-symbolic political attitudes. Both mid-life and older adults demonstrated changes in several political attitudes, albeit slightly less change than the young adults experienced. Detailed analysis of non-symbolic attitudes, however, failed to show systematic differences by age. In a more recent study, Silverstein and his colleagues (2001) examined attitudes regarding whether Social Security benefits should be increased, maintained, or decreased. They found that there was a general shift in this non-symbolic attitude over time, with the most dramatic shift happening among those approaching old age, who might have been expected to defend the system in self-interest. In addition, the youngest individuals studied were most swayed by the ideological shift questioning entitlements, such as Social Security, suggesting that cohort effects remain important.

One area of political attitudes that gets much public attention has to do with confidence in public institutions, including government. In a 2005 survey by the Gallup Organization, a national sample of adults was asked about their confidence in a number of entities, some of which are arrayed in Exhibit 12.6. Examining the results by age shows that the relative confidence in these organizations is more similar across age than it is different. All age groups are confident in the military, churches, and the presidency, with waning levels of confidence in criminal justice, Congress, and big business. In some cases younger and older adults agree more than those in the middle age groups, but in other cases adults under age 30 have views distinct from all other adults. Clearly, age does influence some attitudes more than others, and differences, where they exist, are moderate.

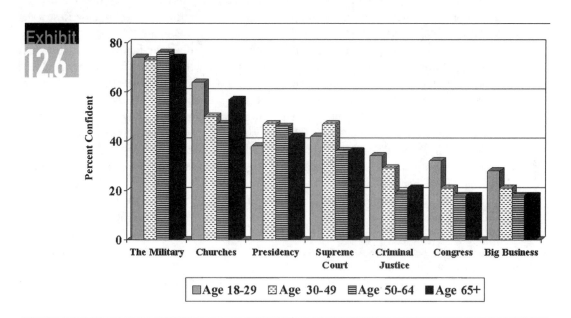

Exhibit 12.6

Confidence in Major Institutions by Age
Source: Gallup Poll, 2005

Turning back to symbolic political attitudes, early studies of the political attitudes of older persons proposed an **aging-conservatism hypothesis,** suggesting that people become more politically conservative as they age—a variation, perhaps, of the "old people are set in their ways" stereotype (Dobson, 1983). Research conducted in the late 1960s confirmed that older people espoused more conservative political views than did their younger counterparts. Such cross-sectional results, however, overlooked the complexity of aging, period, and cohort. Research conducted since the 1960s shows that liberal or conservative orientation, a symbolic attitude, does not change in systematic fashion with aging, supporting the Mannheim hypothesis. Instead, individuals maintain a fairly high level of continuity in their political orientations, with the intervention of period effects likely to have an impact on views across all age groups (Alwin & Krosnick, 1991). In fact, the political leanings of the older population have shifted over time such that older adults are more likely to report liberal orientations than are younger adults, including the younger portion of the baby boomers (Pew Research Center, 2003).

In a similar vein, aging was thought to affect political party affiliation, a related symbolic attitude. Cross-sectional data at that time established that as age increased, affiliation with the Republican party also increased. As an outgrowth of the aging-conservatism hypothesis, maturing individuals were thought to become more attuned to the Republican agenda. Careful analysis of cohorts, however, proved this conclusion to be mistaken. Although comparisons of the elections from 1946 to 1958 seemed to show higher percentages of Republicans among the oldest categories, when cohorts were followed across time Cutler (1969–1970) found that party affiliation did not change systematically with aging. That finding was reinforced starting in the 1980s, when older people began voting for the candidates of, and were more often affiliated with, the Democratic party in comparison to the young (Jacobs, 1990; Pew Research Center, 2003).

Instead of systematic age-related changes in party affiliation, family socialization toward political parties and the effects of major events (such as major victories or scandals) are more potent forces in shaping how, when, and whether individuals select a particular party or remain independent voters (Jacobs, 1990). In the study by Alwin and Krosnick (1991) discussed earlier, stability of party affiliation among various age groups over time was a particular focus. Since they followed various age groups over time in two separate decades, it became possible to test more directly the aging-versus-cohort issues regarding party affiliation. The results indicate that stability of party affiliation, unlike some other attitudes, increases slowly with age through most of adulthood, with a hint of decrease among those in the oldest groups (Alwin & Krosnick, 1991). The intensity of party identification also increases with age from rather weak to stronger through adulthood, but decreases slightly in the oldest group. People tend to keep their party affiliation as they age, with the intensity of partisanship increasing in the older groups—perhaps partly explaining higher voting rates.

The bulk of research fails to demonstrate that political party affiliation changes in systematic ways as individuals age. Yet the effects of cohort flow through age groups can bring about gradual change in the distribution of political affiliations and attitudes. Exhibit 12.7 shows the changes over 50 years in party affiliation, grouping those who identify themselves as strong or weak identifiers with Democratic

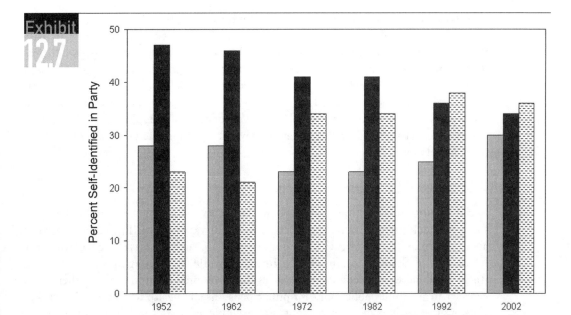

Party Identification, 1952–2002
Source: National Election Studies, 2004.

or Republican parties or independent, including those saying they lean toward one party or another (National Election Studies 2004). What is noteworthy is the over-all convergence among the three groups over time, largely as a result of decline in identification as a Democrat and growth of independents. Surprising, perhaps, is the relative stability of identification as Republican over time, resulting in almost equal party affiliation in recent elections (National Election Studies, 2004; Pew Research Center, 2003). This effect is not based primarily in individuals changing their party through the life course, but the changing composition of new cohorts entering the scene, as the fortunes of each party and its agenda shift over time. Political events, such as the 1973 Watergate scandal, the impeachment of Bill Clinton, and reactions to wars, economic trends, and other events shape how new-voter cohorts view politi-cal parties (Pew Research Center, 2003).

Working the Political System: Age-Based Advocacy

An interesting and diverse set of organizations advocate for and provide services to the older population. Most of the advocacy organizations for age-related issues developed after the advent of the major governmental programs to assist older people (Binstock, 1995), during the period of compassionate ageism. A few earlier movements, such as the Townsend movement that predated Social Security, were critical in the creation of these policies (Torres-Gil, 1992), but most of the major organizations of today have been created since the middle of the 20th century. Wallace and his colleagues (1991) argue that much of the influence that older adults have exerted has been through these organizations and via older individuals' participation in **power elites**—formal or informal groups that build policy and sway public opinion. Numerous age-based organizations have helped shape policies on the federal and state levels for many years. These groups are not organized and run only by older people, but often include and rely upon the work of younger people on behalf of the older population. This section describes select political battles engaging advocacy groups, the government, and the older population.

The Battle Over Social Security

Social Security was a political battleground before its passage in 1935 and has been the focus of much policy and partisan debate in its 70-year history. The current debates about reforming Social Security are not new, nor are such discussions occurring only in the United States (Hoskins, 1992). In the early 1990s, most aging societies of the world faced increasing economic pressures that prompted them to examine their fiscal capacity to meet their obligations for public pensions and health service entitlements to growing populations of older persons. For example, countries in Eastern Europe that have recently moved to capitalist economies have experienced both economic recession and dramatic political changes, rendering their former system of old-age income security inappropriate (Hoskins, 1992). They lack the resources to pay full pensions that are expected by older adults, resulting in negative political reactions toward the new regimes.

The United States has seen regular political and ideological battles over Social Security, including notable battles surrounding major changes to the program in 1977 and 1983. Prior to his election, Ronald Reagan proposed deep cuts to the program, which were formalized as part of his budget proposal in 1981. A tremendous public uproar followed, chastening the Reagan administration into steadfast support of Social Security (Jacobs, 1990). Like Reagan, other politicians have learned of the dangers of tampering with Social Security. Using the analogy of a subway system, Social Security has been called the third rail (the one carrying electrical current) of U.S. politics. Politicians quickly learn that if you touch it, you die. Social Security is a program with a very large and interested constituency, comprising not just those receiving benefits but also those expecting to receive benefits and those whose family members currently receive benefits (Day, 1993a), making it a high-risk target for change.

Following the abortive Reagan assault on Social Security, single-issue advocacy groups, such as Save Our Security and the National Committee to Preserve and Protect Social Security and Medicare, entered the battle over the future of the U.S. Social Security system, along with the political parties, a variety of think tank advocates, and the mainstream aging organizations (Day, 1990). After being reelected, President George W. Bush began a major push to change significant aspects of the program, including the addition of private accounts and reduction in the redistribution aspect of benefit calculation, despite the fact that Social Security ranked only at the middle of a list of issues of concern to the public (Blendon et al., 2005). After a prolonged publicity campaign, however, the effort seemed to lose steam in the face of strong campaigns from other groups, other events (the war in Iraq and Hurricane Katrina), and the continued belief by the public that there is no crisis (Blendon et al., 2005).

AARP and Capitol Hill

One of the major combatants in the recent debate over Social Security has been AARP, the new name for the organization that was founded in 1958 as the American Association for Retired Persons. AARP, which has expanded its mandate to include the vast numbers of baby boomers aged 50 and over, boasts 35 million members, a potentially formidable support group for any candidate or issue (Binstock, 1995). The organization has grown rapidly in the past few decades as the population has aged (Jacobs, 1990). Membership overrepresents White, middle-class individuals, many of whom would be considered among the "young old" (Day, 1990). Exploration of the AARP Web site shows active advocacy in multiple areas.

It is important to point out that memberships are initiated and maintained primarily for member benefits and discounts (e.g., travel and insurance discounts and a prescription plan), rather than for the political agenda that AARP pursues (Binstock, 1995). AARP employs a professional staff to provide member services and to sustain its reputation for political clout in Washington (Binstock, 1995).

There is some question as to whether AARP can deliver votes for particular candidates and whether its diverse membership supports all of the positions taken by the organization during policy battles in Washington (Binstock, 1991a). AARP has been accused of using what Binstock calls the **electoral bluff**. This bluff occurs when organizations of this size implicitly threaten to churn up major support for or against a candidate or proposal, pressuring legislators or policymakers for changes in AARP's desired direction (Binstock, 1991a). No one knows, in most cases, whether AARP can deliver on this bluff. Such large membership organizations wield much of their power through high levels of access to elected officials and policymakers, drawing legitimacy from their size when taking positions publicly and working through the media to make their views known. On Capitol Hill, AARP and its lobbyists vigorously advocate its priorities and on major issues affecting older adults.

The Case of Catastrophic Health Care Legislation

One of the noteworthy efforts to pass major legislation affecting the older population after the era of compassionate ageism shows how the political environment toward programs for the elderly has shifted. The Medicare Catastrophic Coverage Act of 1988 (MCCA) was intended to provide protection against impoverishment from major, costly illnesses by expanding Medicare benefits for the first time in many years (Street, 1993; Torres-Gil, 1992). The MCCA would have placed a cap on out-of-pocket medical expenses for Medicare beneficiaries, expanded coverage to include home health care, and protected the income and assets of the spouses of long-term nursing home patients receiving Medicaid (Torres-Gil, 1992). It did not address the situation of most concern to many older adults—the high cost of nursing home care (Wallace et al., 1991).

The legislation passed with strong bipartisan support in the Congress. The bill's rapid downfall, once it passed, was its financing system. Because the elderly were no longer considered by the public as being a "needy" category, funding had to be revenue neutral—covering its own costs (Holstein & Minkler, 1991). The financing included a surtax on older adults, based on income, so that the poorest would pay nothing and the wealthiest would pay about $800 per person per year (Street, 1993). In contrast to other age entitlements, in MCCA those more able to afford benefits subsidized those less able to pay. Once the bill had passed, a small but highly vocal opposition forced repeal of almost all of the bill's provisions within a year of its passage (Binstock, 1992; Torres-Gil, 1992). Interestingly, research (Day, 1993b) found that neither those who would have to pay the surtax nor those with supplemental insurance coverage (those least likely to benefit from the new coverage) were more likely to oppose the MCCA than other groups. This incident painted older persons as wanting government services but unwilling to pay for them, contributing ammunition to the emergent debate on generational equity, described later in this chapter (Street, 1993).

Crystal (1990) describes the passing and rescinding of the MCCA as a turning point in public policy on aging. The short life of the MCCA demonstrated the power of class politics versus age-based interests. It revealed a schism in the older constituency between the so-called "haves" (wealthier older persons, who were expected to pay for the services being added but were most likely to have private insurance to meet those needs) and the "have-nots" (those in need of services but not required to pay or able to afford private insurance). The affluent haves had already opted out of full dependence on the publicly funded Medicare system via private insurance, and many resented being called upon to finance benefits for others less fortunate (Crystal, 1990). This experience has generalized to make some policymakers cautious about proposing new entitlement programs in an era of public resistance to paying for them. This legislation and its repeal also divided the aging advocacy community in a way that had not happened before. According to Crystal (1990), the bill "divided many constituencies who previously have made common cause toward improving services to the elderly" (p. 23). Now advocacy organizations must confront the social class issues that divide the older population, and they can no longer make clear policy choices that assist "older people" as a category.

Some of the same themes emerged in the most recent change in legislation for Medicare Part D, which was described in the previous chapter. Political compromises were required to make the costs of the program manageable; the resulting legislation was a confusing mixture of protection for those with high or low drug expenses and a major gap for those whose medication costs are neither particularly high nor low. Its start-up represents another major test of public reaction to funding benefits for older persons.

Generational Politics: Conflict and Consensus

The Potential for Generational Conflict

Analysts disagree regarding the prospect of **intergenerational conflict** over the distribution of government resources (see Binstock, 1991a; Wynne, 1991). Some argue that such conflict will be inevitable if current policies and entitlements remain unchanged; others claim that cross-cutting allegiances pull people into groupings organized on bases other than age (Day, 1990). Although conflict between cohorts or generations is often discussed, scant evidence exists for it today or in the past.

This issue of political conflict between generations arose in the late 1960s during the era of youthful political activism by the oldest baby boomers during the Vietnam War. The issue boils down to whether the fundamental goals and interests of young and old are sufficiently different as to make them adversaries in the political arena. Under a scenario of age-based political conflict, groups would solidify for political action based on age identification. Young people might want more funding for college, while older adults might want more support for Medicare, for example. In times of scarce fiscal resources, the argument goes, the old and the young may splinter along age lines, with each group vying for its own political agenda. Evidence from exit polls during the 1996 presidential election suggests that Medicare, used as an issue by both sides in that campaign, was not effective in gaining such a response (Binstock, 1997). Wallace and his associates (1991) claim that when older adults have been mobilized to act on an issue, it has been more on the basis of economic interests than age.

The potential for age identification and age-based political action rests on the degree to which people hold narrow, self-interested views. For example, questions have often been raised about whether older adults vote in support of bond issues for schools, which affect neither themselves nor their grown children. Ecology advocates wonder whether older voters will care about (and vote to support) pollution-abatement programs to benefit future generations (Kneese & Cooper, 1993). Although there is some evidence of lower support for school bond issues among older adults (see Button, 1992), the evidence for this sort of generational schism is far from comprehensive, and voting on issues varies only slightly by age (Campbell, 2005).

Chapter 6 discussed reciprocity within the context of the family. It is also useful to consider reciprocity on a societal level, including across age cohorts. In this larger context, Social Security can be considered a form of reciprocity—support provided for the elderly in return for their contributions in earlier years to building both the economy and their successor cohorts (Wynne, 1991). Wynne argues for expansion of the concept of reciprocity within the larger society, encouraging civic involvement among young and old for the betterment of society. Under the macro-level version of reciprocity, the age strata of society can be seen to have mutual interests and goals, with exchange among them a natural occurrence (Kingson, Hirshorn, & Cornman, 1986). Generations are pulled together by this reciprocity, not pulled apart. Day's study (1990) concludes that "the lines that divide Americans on the issue of government benefits for the elderly are not generational, but economic and partisan" (p. 60).

Other research has focused on age-based voting patterns in Florida, the state with the largest percentage of people over age 65 as a result of elderly in-migration (Button & Rosenbaum, 1990). Florida is as ripe for political conflict based on age as any location in the United States. Evidence from the work of Button and Rosenbaum (1990) argues that the feared "gray peril" is an overstatement of the possible effect of a concentration of older voters. Florida government officials perceive, but can provide little concrete evidence of, resistance by the older population to increasing taxes or development of the local economy, changes that would not be in their self-interest (Rosenbaum &

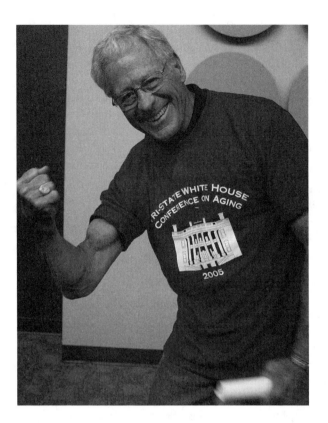

In times of scarce government resources, the young and old may flex muscles for their own specific agendas. (Credit: E. J. Hanna)

Button, 1992). These government officials did not see the older populations in their localities acting as a coherent bloc in terms of voting or supporting issues, because many traits also divided them. Local age-related strife has arisen over issues such as the location of congregate housing (nursing homes or retirement communities) and driving speed, with young and old mutually critical of each other's speed on local roads (Rosenbaum & Button, 1992). In other words, age-based politics were more expectation than reality.

The fact that the older population will be growing more racially and ethnically diverse as current cohorts age may further dilute the likelihood of an older adult voting bloc emerging (Torres-Gil, 1992). Torres-Gil projects that activism and organizations may become more focused and specialized, addressing the needs, for example, of disadvantaged older women rather than the economic issues of the elderly as a whole. Age, he argues, may be less compelling as an organizing force than as a common interest when the older population is so diverse. Given this focus on diversity and heterogeneity in the older population, it is useful to revisit a theory we have alluded to before, age stratification theory.

The Generational Equity Debate

Politicians and the media have paid attention to one specific aspect of generational conflict in recent years: the generational equity debate. The United States, like many other nations, transfers resources between individuals who are economically productive and

Age Stratification Theory

Age stratification theory posits that we divide the population into strata (or layers), which are ranked hierarchically. As in other stratification systems focusing on social class, race, or gender rather than age, the population is divided into groups; age stratification substitutes age as the criterion upon which individuals are divided. In age stratification, age is used to cluster groups of people together (into age strata or, in the term we have used most often, cohorts) and to differentiate among people on the basis of the age stratum to which they belong (Dowd, 1980). We can ask, for example, whether someone belongs to an age stratum in the teenage years or in "old old" age and, on that basis, make some educated guesses about the person. These guesses are based on the assumption that people in the same stratum have significant social characteristics in common and that members of different strata are different in critical ways. To visualize the idea of age strata, simply refer to the population pyramids presented in chapter 3. Age stratification systems are straightforward in a sense, because chronological age allows us to readily order individuals into groups and rank them hierarchically as having more or fewer accumulated years of life. In contrast, class stratification systems require considerable effort to define the boundaries and characteristics of strata and the placement of individuals within them. In age stratification, it is clear that someone who is 35 is older, and therefore in a different stratum, than someone who is 15. The question remains, however, whether the distinction between those two chronological ages is socially meaningful. And since age strata usually include several chronological ages (such as the 65–74 range used in Exhibit 12.2), the boundaries dividing strata may be ambiguous.

What about age stratification based on stages of the life course? If we attempt to develop stratification based on life-course stages, the strata become even less clear and distinct (O'Rand, 1990). What criteria must one meet, for example, to be considered an adult? Using life-course events, people might be considered adults when they marry, get a full-time job, leave their parents' home, have children, or some combination of these events (Hogan & Astone, 1986). It is much simpler, although not necessarily always equally meaningful, to use chronological age;

for voting purposes, for example, you are an adult when you become 18 years of age.

Age stratification theory goes beyond the recognition that societies divide their populations by age or into cohorts and examines how societies offer different rewards and opportunities to members of different age strata. According to Dowd (1981), "both age strata and social classes may be defined by their differential possession of valued resources and differential access to the means of acquiring these resources" (p. 158). People in the 35–40 age stratum as a rule hold more socially valued resources and are given more opportunities to augment those resources than someone who is 15 or 85. Age, like many other bases for stratification, serves as a basis of structured social inequality (Foner, 1973). Riley, Johnson, and Foner (1973) point to the opportunities for (or requirements placed on) individuals to be enrolled in educational institutions at certain ages and limited access to other activities (such as marrying, voting, or holding office) until a certain age has been achieved. Informal norms and sanctions that go with them also encourage people to "act their age," performing in ways that are consistent with the expectations associated with their location in the stratification system (Riley et al., 1973). The hierarchy of age stratification is not as easily grasped as the system of class stratification, however, because those higher in the age stratification system do not benefit as a group from greater resources than those in the middle, as they do with social class. Therefore, the concept of age stratification is less clear-cut from the perspective of social inequality (Cain, 1987).

Another element of age stratification that differentiates it from stratification by social class has to do with social mobility. **Social mobility** refers to the movement of an individual between levels of the stratification system. In stratification systems based on gender or race, such mobility is extremely limited; most people are stuck with their race and gender. In the case of social class, mobility between strata is quite possible—for example, when a young person from a poor background seeks an advanced education and achieves a high-level professional career, thereby moving to a higher social class. In age stratification, mobility through the age stratification system is automatic and unavoidable—you can't avoid growing older (Riley et al., 1973). In fact, according

(continued)

(continued)

to Riley, aging can be considered a type of social mobility. Simply by virtue of surviving, individuals and cohorts are upwardly mobile in the age stratification system; but upward age mobility, unlike upward social class mobility, does not necessarily mean an improvement in one's social and economic situation. In social class stratification, higher is better; in age stratification, older may or may not be better.

Although age stratification theory is formally introduced here, we have already used elements of age stratification theory throughout this book, especially in discussions of cohorts and their movement through the society. Dowd's explanation of exchange theory, described in chapter 6, also includes elements of age stratification; he argues that older persons have, by virtue of their location in the stratification system, less power and fewer resources, which disadvantages them in exchange relationships. Age stratification also has roots in modernization theory, described in chapter 3. Modernization theory examines the relative status of older age groups (compared with younger adults) in more and less developed societies, positing that as societies modernize, people in higher age strata lose the foundations that gave them power and prestige in less developed economies (O'Rand, 1990). Although modernization theory has been heavily criticized, it nonetheless directs attention to age stratification systems.

Age stratification theory is flexible, enabling us to look at movement of individuals through age-related roles and expectations on a micro level or focus attention on the flow of cohorts through social institutions on the macro level, adding the important element of inequality between strata (O'Rand, 1990). Age stratification theory focuses attention on the issues that age cohorts have in common—how society structures both opportunities and expectations based on the age of the individual, ignoring potentially important differences that exist among 20- or 70-year-olds. O'Rand (1990) points out that, in the 20th century, the state imposed more standardization on the lives of the youngest and oldest in society—for example, creating regulations requiring school attendance and institutionalizing retirement. In this way, governments define the civil rights and responsibilities of individuals in these age strata. You have doubtless felt the restrictions of age boundaries in your life—being considered too young or too old to participate in certain activities—and may have celebrated passing a milestone birthday as you experience mobility through the age stratification system.

To focus on age stratification in no way invalidates other systems of stratification. It is often informative to use multiple systems of stratification—for example, examining age strata and then, within age strata, looking at variations by gender, social class, or race to see how these systems augment or diminish opportunities and disadvantages for the individuals within their ranks. Stratification theory—using age, class, gender, or other criteria for establishing strata—encourages using the sociological imagination and taking a macro-social view of inequality of opportunity.

The fundamental question today for age stratification is its usefulness, given the growing fuzziness of boundaries and definitions of age strata (recall the discussion of retirement), the expectations for increasing diversity in the older population of the future (Torres-Gil, 1992), and the importance of other dimensions of stratification intersecting with age. Will age really matter more than social class, educational background, gender, or race and ethnicity in understanding the social placement and life chances available to individuals in various groups? The answer may be no, but as long as age-based restrictions on opportunities in society continue, there is some utility in using an age stratification framework to examine social and political issues.

those who are not (dependent children, disabled adults, and older persons). We often take these transfers for granted; we tax local property owners to finance public schools and tax wages to pay for Social Security and Medicare. The growth of the older population has prompted politicians, economists, and sociologists to examine the fundamental assumptions behind transfers (Cornman & Kingson, 1996). In the United States, families and state governments are responsible for much of the support of dependent children (the state provides public education), while the support provided to older people is managed more through public systems at the federal level (Achenbaum, 1992). The

U.S. system expends more federal dollars (but not necessarily state dollars) on programs for the older population than on programs for children.

It was not until the late 1970s that politicians and advocates for the elderly recognized the growing costs of benefits for older citizens. Hudson (1978) called this process the **graying of the federal budget** (see also Binstock, 1991a). This "graying" refers to the growing percentage of the federal budget each year allocated to entitlements for the older population, including the dollars spent on Medicare, Medicaid, and Social Security. Exhibit 12.8 shows the increase in the percentage of the federal budget allocated to these entitlements.

Alarms have sounded in some circles as the baby boom cohorts approach old age and life expectancy continues to increase. Demography, combined with the ongoing commitment to pay for these entitlements in future generations, have congealed into a broad debate on whether the economy can afford old-age entitlements (Cornman & Kingson, 1996), a debate with many assumptions that are seldom examined in detail. A major part of this debate has to do with the future financing of Social Security, Medicaid, and Medicare; these specific debates are described in greater detail in other chapters. Surprisingly, some countries with populations older than the United States' have not encountered public resistance to paying the costs of age entitlement programs (Myles, 1996).

Advocacy groups from the 1980s onward, responding to the entitlement alarm and to a broader political agenda, argued that we should look at age as a critical factor in understanding the linkage between politics and economics. Pointing to the improved economic well-being of the older population (the lower rate of poverty) and increasing rates of poverty among children, some posited a causal connection—that society

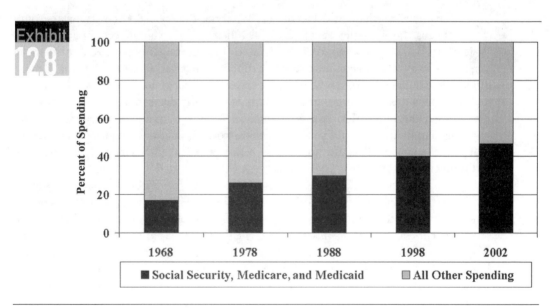

Exhibit 12.8

Percentage of Federal Spending Devoted to Entitlements
Source: U.S. Bureau of the Census, 1975, 1976, 1995; *Senior Journal,* 2005.

is allocating excessive resources to older people that would be better spent to support future cohorts (Minkler, 1991a; Quadagno, 1991). Several groups have advocated movement away from age entitlements to entitlement programs based on need by eliminating cost-of-living increases, raising the retirement age for Social Security, and using tax policies to encourage private old-age insurance (Quadagno, 1991).

Holstein (1995) points out that reducing entitlements for older people in no way guarantees that those resources would be redistributed to children. Quadagno's strongest complaint with the argument is its contention that increases in childhood poverty are caused by greater entitlements to the older population. During the time that child poverty has increased, other significant social changes (i.e., more single parents, changes in the labor market) have contributed to childhood poverty. Despite such critiques, there has been success in altering the nature of the debate about age entitlements from its prior focus on adequacy of benefits to issues of equity—specifically, intergenerational equity (Ekerdt, 1998; Quadagno, 1989).

At first glance, Exhibit 12.8 seems to provide support for this contention. The largest increase in entitlement spending occurred after the enactment of Medicare in 1965 and has slowed substantially in recent years (Quadagno, 1996). Yet using standard economic measures for the costs of programs, neither Social Security nor overall entitlements to the elderly have grown much in real terms since the early 1970s. Instead, as recent Congresses have cut spending in other areas (e.g., defense) and reduced taxes on individuals and corporations, old-age entitlements have become a larger percentage of overall spending, creating a false impression of dramatic growth in the dollars being spent (Quadagno, 1996). Quadagno concludes that the entitlements "crisis" has been socially constructed through careful rhetoric to advance a political agenda of reducing government programs, rather than emerging as a consensual social problem to be resolved.

Marmour, Mashaw, and Harvey (1990) argue that Social Security has become "a scapegoat for anxieties engendered by a distressingly volatile economic environment" (p. 127). Quadagno (1991) concludes that movement to a need entitlement system simply shifts economic support functions back to families and would most hurt those individuals who rely primarily on Social Security for income—those lacking private pensions from their employers. This group is disproportionately composed of women and minorities. As a consequence, she argues, many of these most disadvantaged individuals would need to continue working in low-wage jobs into advanced old age, having inadequate finances to retire on reduced Social Security benefits (Quadagno, 1991).

It is apparent that supporters of the generational equity debate have been quite effective in getting out its political message. Many popular magazines and other media now use the rhetoric of "greedy geezers" and sound the alarm regarding financing of entitlements in the future. In contrast, Achenbaum (1992) argues that it is necessary to make manifest the transgenerational benefits of programs such as Social Security to ensure their political survival for the future. Cornman and Kingson (1996) point out that we invest resources in children in anticipation of their future contributions to society and assist the elderly in reciprocity for their prior contributions, evening out the balance sheet over the life course. It is only if we freeze the picture at one point in time and define entitlements as a zero-sum game that the old and the young seem like drains on society.

By some measures, the programs of the old-age welfare state have been successful in dealing with the problems they were created to address. As chapter 9 discussed, overall poverty has been greatly reduced by the presence of Social Security benefits. The housing and health of the older population have improved, albeit only partly through the efforts of federal government programs (Quirk, 1991). Some aging advocates argue that these programs are now victims of their own success. Because the condition of the average older person has improved significantly in recent decades, there is less momentum to maintain the entitlements that have helped to bring about (and maintain) that success. In addition, there remain a substantial number of older persons, primarily widowed women, who are poor and receive little help from this safety net. It is a major failing of the old-age welfare system that it leaves behind some severe pockets of disadvantaged people (Binstock, 1991a).

While some researchers have spent considerable time forecasting conflict between the generations over entitlements and policies, others have begun to speculate about the possibility of intragenerational conflict (Day, 1993a) among members of the same generation or age group. Such conflict might be predicated on socioeconomic status, with many analysts predicting increasing distance in the future between the advantaged and disadvantaged elderly (Torres-Gil, 1992). It is already overly simplistic to discuss advocacy on behalf of "the elderly," because that population includes so many constituencies and interests. Such diversity may promote more intragenerational conflict in the future and serve as a hedge against formation of a voting bloc based on age.

SUMMARY

There is every reason to expect that the political experience of future cohorts will differ from those of contemporary cohorts of older Americans. For example, the concept of later life and the inclusiveness of an elderly constituency might change. People over age 65 who are employed, in good health, and with 30 or more years of future life expectancy might not consider themselves part of the interest group of older adults (Torres-Gil, 1992) and might behave accordingly.

Will old age continue its relevance as a focal category for social policy, or will cross-cutting issues such as social class, health, or race/ethnicity prove more politically powerful as the foci for societal intervention (Binstock, 1992)? Analysts disagree about the future of both advocacy and policy relative to old age. Torres-Gil (1992) expects a future of old-age politics that differs from what we have experienced in recent decades. He argues that social class will become the basis for government programs and that the strong advocacy network for old-age issues will self-destruct. Not everyone agrees, arguing that the baby boomers, by their sheer numbers and education, will be a political force to be reckoned with for many years (Cornman & Kingson, 1996). The pressure of the baby boomers has brought many of these policy discussions into sharp focus, even though the cohorts that immediately follow them will be much smaller in size. As policy is formulated, we need to ask whether the decisions make sense not only for the baby boomers, but also for the cohorts who will follow them into later life.

Torres-Gil (1992) predicts the growth of vertical alliances across cohorts or age strata—based on social class, race and ethnicity, or common interests—that would strongly divide age groups and minimize the potential for age-based alliances in support of policies. Some experts predict that transgenerational alliances (for example, an alliance between older people in frail health and younger disabled people) focused on specific issues such as health care, housing, or income may make the politics of age obsolete (Day, 1990). For example, in 1996 the House of Representatives passed legislation that would enhance criminal penalties for crimes of violence against both the elderly and children. Previous legislative approaches might have singled out one group or the other. Here, policy attention is given to both groups, based on the presumption of their shared vulnerability to crime.

If age becomes less salient as a criterion for policy, then it would be politically difficult to maintain current programs of age entitlements, and disadvantaged elders would find themselves vying with younger poor persons for the scarce resources that society provides those in need. Although concerns regarding "demography as destiny" have driven debates on age-based policies and entitlements in many aging societies, the issues are much more complex than just the dependency ratio. Political commitments and public attitudes, which have largely favored societal attention to the needs of older adults, are potent forces in shaping how collective resources are allocated. With regard to intergenerational politics and issues, Moody (1992) suggests the "political argument comes down to a matter of confidence and legitimization: a feeling that institutions of intergenerational transfer—whether Social Security or the public schools—can be counted on to do their job and remain reliable for successive cohorts" (p. 239).

WEB WISE

Administration on Aging/Older Americans Act
http://www.aoa.dhhs.gov/

One of the major pieces of legislation establishing the "aging network" was the Older Americans Act (OAA), found under the About AOA tab. The Administration on Aging, the governmental agency charged with fulfilling the mandate of the OAA, describes the legislation and how it has been implemented in the aging network and a range of programs. Information under the Professionals tab talks about the aging network, and a families and aging section provides caregiver information.

Senior Law
http://www.seniorlaw.com/index.htm

This site, which is maintained by attorneys Goldfarb & Abrandt specializing in senior law, provides information on legal/legislative updates in Medicare and Medicaid, a reference to articles on elder law topics, and other senior law information. Their "way cool sites" section includes topics reaching well beyond senior law.

National Election Study
http://www.umich.edu/~nes

This site includes data on the ongoing National Election Study, funded by the National Science Foundation and conducted by the University of Michigan. This set of studies examines various political behaviors and attitudes, including voter registration, voting, and confidence in the government and president. For the latest statistics on voting, this site holds a wealth of information.

KEY TERMS

age identification	compassionate ageism	liberal agenda
age stratification	conservative agenda	old–age welfare
aging-conservatism	electoral bluff	state
hypothesis	gerontocracy	Older Americans
aging enterprise	graying of the federal	Act (OAA)
civic development	budget	power elites
hypothesis	intergenerational conflict	social mobility

QUESTIONS FOR THOUGHT AND DISCUSSION

1. Period effects are thought to influence peoples' political party affiliation and their confidence in institutions, such as the government. Thinking through your life and through history, what are some of the events that you might expect to have a significant effect on these political views?

2. Think about or discuss with others the reasons people choose to vote or not to vote (including reasons not to register). What are the major themes that appear to be central for young adults compared to people of other ages? Can you identify any strategies that might accomplish what political parties have tried in recent decades—to get out the "youth vote?" What are the implications if few young people continue to vote in upcoming elections?

3. Generational equity proposes moving toward need-based entitlement for government benefits. What major programs would this influence? How would changes to need entitlement influence your neighbors, family, and friends?

4. Does it make sense to have minimum ages mandated for running for political offices? Would you suggest maximum ages for holding high office? If so, what age would you suggest and why would it be the relevant one to choose?

The Dynamics of Aging in Our Future

At the end of the 20th century, later life remains a season in search of its purposes. It is clear that the moral status of older people cannot rest simply on their entitlements, or their roles as abstract bearers of rights, or their image as dependent, passive recipients of treatment. But what do older people owe society? their families? themselves? (Cole, 1995, p. 342)

The preceding chapters have described the processes of aging and the social contexts that structure and give meaning to aging in society. But what will aging be like in the future? Will science fiction predictions of immortality become real? Advances in technology, efforts at health promotion, changes in our attitudes about aging, and changes in our age structures will all contribute to a new experience of aging, as will the new views and experiences of new cohorts reaching later life.

As examples of this new world of aging, in recent years a woman in her 60s gave birth to her first child with the assistance of a fertility clinic, and Senator John Glenn of Ohio—the first American to orbit the globe as an astronaut in the early 1960s—returned to space in his late 70s to study the effects of weightlessness on an aging body. Both these and the growing buzz about anti-aging breakthroughs and treatments push us to consider the future, as the aging of society becomes a factor in everyday life for all of us. Clearly we need to expand our ideas about what aging means and move beyond old stereotypes of age and the life course. Some scholars suggest that we will probably rethink many of our assumptions about aging and life stages as more of us survive to ages close to the century mark. This chapter examines some of what we know about the future and some of the speculations about the issues that we face in aging societies and an aging world.

Most of us easily conceptualize aging on an individual level—the physical and social changes that come as we move through various ages and stages of the life course. It is more difficult to grasp the complex implications of aging on a macro level, in a society characterized by high rates of social change where the general population is also growing older. Is aging an individual problem, to be addressed by personal choices (regarding employment, family, financial planning) and preventive behaviors (building a history of good nutrition and exercise and a strong network of social support), or is it a collective issue to be addressed by the larger society, through adaptation of social institutions and the provision of needed services and opportunities geared to an older population? Clearly the answer is both.

People age within a social context that dramatically influences them in many ways, both positive and negative. This socially constructed and culturally specific context not only defines the opportunities available to us based on age, but also the way we think of ourselves and others as young, middle-aged, or old. Our collective attitudes toward later life in the United States continue to be largely negative, despite the positive reports from older people regarding their well-being and satisfaction with life. The myths and stereotypes of ageism are perpetuated, giving way only slowly to a more realistic view of what the situation will be as we ourselves move into later life.

On the positive side, frailty, loss, and disadvantage do not define later life. Certainly older persons experience these problems, but the great majority of older adults live autonomously in the community, are financially independent, and, despite some health conditions, fend for themselves. Older adults make contributions to their families and communities on a daily basis. Recent evidence strongly suggests that many dimensions of the quality of life, from age of onset of disease and disability to economic well-being and social engagement, could improve in coming cohorts, in part through positive life-style choices of individuals (Rowe & Kahn, 1998). We are, in many cases, agents in shaping our aging selves through our decisions. Aging is not a spectator sport; our everyday choices will bear fruit over the long haul in terms of health, housing, economic status, and social networks. So a choice to exercise daily through adulthood significantly shifts the odds against early disability. Our choices, however, remain limited by tradition, expectations, policy, and social structures. They also are limited by external events, such as economic trends, wars, and natural disasters that can thwart the best-laid plans.

It is informative that older people do not see a picture of later life that is nearly as negative as the stereotypes portray. Exhibit 13.1 shows selected (the four highest and two lowest) responses to a national survey of adults (age 18 and over) regarding the problems faced by older adults. This chart shows the gap between what older adults report as problems for themselves (shown by the striped bars) compared to what respondents ages 18–64 and respondents 65 and over believe to be serious problems for older Americans in general. The most commonly reported serious problems reported by the older survey respondents were not having enough money to live on and fear of crime (21% and 19%, respectively). In contrast, 62% of 18- to 64-year-olds and 45% of adults over 65 think that not having enough money is a serious problem for older adults generally. Clearly the gap between public expectation and personal reality is great. Although the gaps between expectation and reality varied, reports from the older adults of problems they actually faced were consistently (and often significantly) lower than what the general population believes (Abramson & Silverstein, 2004). Eight of the 15 problems (e.g., no control over everyday life decisions, transportation, not enough to do to keep busy, not feeling needed, poor housing, not enough education) were reported by only 6–8% of older adults in the sample as being a serious problem for themselves. Many older adults, according to this study, appear not to find later life a stage of endless problems, worry, and decline.

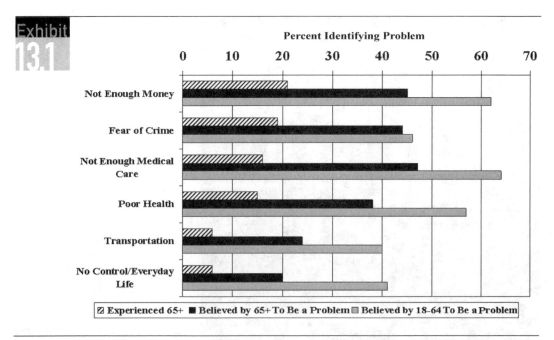

Expectation and Reality: Problems Reported Versus Problems Believed To Be Faced by Older Adults
Source: Abramson and Silverstein, 2004.

Those who are fortunate among us will approach later life with good health, strong family and friendship networks, a secure financial future, and opportunities to contribute to society in meaningful ways. It is undoubtedly true, however, that despite the changes we can anticipate in future cohorts of aging individuals, including all of our personal cohorts, some individuals and subgroups within the older population will still require assistance to meet daily needs. These individuals may experience poor health, inadequate housing or income, or other disadvantages as a result of the cumulative effects of a lifetime of poverty, disability, or educational disadvantage or through a single event, such as unexpected job loss, catastrophic health crises, or family disintegration. Diversity among older adults is expanding, not contracting, emphasizing our need to avoid generalities about older adults. Older adults are neither uniformly poor, unhealthy, and isolated; nor are they uniformly wealthy, self-serving, "greedy geezers." They reach extremes of advantage and disadvantage, but most reside somewhere in the middle.

Each society with an aging population is now making policy decisions regarding what types of support we are collectively willing and able to provide for older adults. These decisions reflect ideologies about whether disadvantaged elders are responsible for their own fates or whether society holds collective duty to provide support systems. If someone is poor in later life, we may be more sympathetic if the problem occurs because of a disabling workplace injury than if the person was a lifelong gambler. Policies being formulated today and viewpoints on the elderly go together. The media push since the 1980s to identify the elderly as well-to-do "greedy geezers" has implications for social policies that affect not just the wealthy elders but also those at the other end of the income

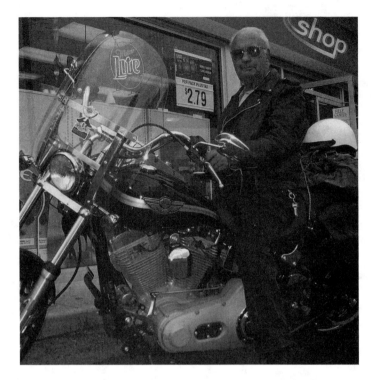

Contradictions to the stereotypes of aging are all around us. (Credit: E. J. Hanna)

spectrum (Ekerdt, 1998). If we make policy changes that restrict Social Security benefits based on an incorrect stereotype that older adults are wealthy, we undoubtedly harm the many individuals whose circumstances differ from that stereotype, especially those whose well-being pivots on benefits from that program.

In addition to our traditional systems of providing services and supports in health and income, private business and industry have been gearing up to provide for the needs of older adults able to pay for goods and services. The major boom over the past 20 years in independent senior housing and assisted living facilities (for those requiring more support) indicate efforts to meet a market demand for services to avoid nursing homes—at prices that vary from moderate to many thousands of dollars per month. Recently two physicians suggested, only half in jest, that older adults who need to avoid cleaning, cooking, and other heavy work simply go on endless cruises on ocean liners, since the costs and services would be comparable to those in a posh assisted living facility (Lindquist & Golub, 2004).

The remainder of this chapter summarizes some key points about understanding aging in this dynamic social context and describes trends for the future of aging in U.S. society. We also address some of the challenges that remain relevant to understanding aging in this new millennium.

Aging in a Changing Social World

Rethinking Old Age and the Life Course

In looking to the future it is important to recall that age and stages of the life course are social constructs that have been generated and given varied meaning in various times and places (Cornman & Kingson, 1996). Historically, life stages as we currently understand them did not always exist. In addition, not all cultures have distinguished childhood from adulthood, or adulthood from later life, in the ways that we do today (Aries, 1962; Cole, 1992). Being both socially constructed and culturally based, the stage of old age (or whatever term you prefer) is changeable. Chronological age presents many problems in making valid distinctions between individuals and groups. It is increasingly difficult to see meaningful physical, social, or psychological commonalities between those who have just reached age 65 and those approaching a century of life, but both groups are currently labeled as "old." We may, for example, raise the lower boundary of "old age" to age 75 or 80 or modify existing life stages (or add new ones) in ways that we cannot yet anticipate.

Do our existing life-course stages still fit the way that the life course is evolving? Will these stages remain meaningful in light of increasing life expectancy? In several ways the life course fits the current realities poorly. The addition of years at the end of life means an increasingly long period of socially undifferentiated adulthood, followed by an undifferentiated period of old age. As people spend more time in these phases of the life course, we may want to make finer distinctions. When most people died before what we call middle age today, it was less important to consider differences between 60-year-olds and centenarians.

The potential of new stages reinforces that we are utilizing some criteria (perhaps a combination of chronological age, physical characteristics, and social role engagement) to determine the boundaries of these stages. One recent indicator of movement in this area is discussions of delaying retirement benefits under Social Security to age 69, removing it further from the traditional chronological marker of 65 as the start of later life. And as longevity increases, does that mean that the boundary will move to 69 or beyond? We also find that researchers and practitioners are dissatisfied with "old age" as a stage, preferring to use terms such as "young old" and "old old," or distinguishing the "third age" of healthy post-retirement years from the "fourth age" reflecting a period of frailty and dependency (James & Wink, 2006; Laslett, 1991). While not formalized or widely used, the idea that there are different issues and opportunities for 70-year-olds and 100-year-olds increasingly calls for elaboration or reconsideration of our system of stages to reflect these differences.

On the other hand, research confirms that Americans continue to share general notions of age-appropriate timing of life events (Settersten & Hagestad, 1996a, 1996b; Zepelin, Sills, & Heath, 1986–1987). Some experts argue, however, that chronological age is becoming less relevant as a marker of human life and its connected social roles in adulthood (Zepelin, Sills, &

Brave New Whirl   by Scott-Allen Pierson

Heath, 1986–1987), suggesting that the life course no longer fits neatly into discrete stages. The Rileys argue that an age-integrated life course would provide better balance and greater flexibility for individuals to schedule events through time (Riley & Riley, 1994).

A second important question about the life course refers to a consistent theme throughout this book—the extent to which aging is constituted differently for various gender, class, race, and ethnic groups. Is there uniformity across diverse social groups in how they live out the life course and in the timing of major events? We have some clues, but further research is required for definitive answers (Settersten, 1999). The emphasis of research studies on White, middle-class men makes our understanding of other groups more tenuous. Differences in life expectancies across racial groups, for example, may result in drawing different chronological boundaries for being middle-aged or old. Higher rates of physical disability result in more early retirements among Blacks. If being retired places one in the category of old age, then disadvantaged Blacks may reach that benchmark chronologically sooner than others (Jackson & Gibson, 1985). Working-class individuals, whose careers plateau at earlier ages (and at a lower level) than those of middle-class workers, and whose families are usually started and grown at earlier ages, may engage in the social roles generally reserved for middle age (grandparenthood, for example) at earlier chronological ages than those in the middle class. From these few examples, it is clear that not all groups move through life-course stages in chronological lockstep. To the extent that these differences continue to exist or even expand, life-course stages may be less useful as a social concept for researchers or for us as participants in a more age-diverse society.

A third question about the life course can shed some light on future change. Do biological and psychological developments correspond meaningfully to the socially constructed stages of life? Perhaps not. Certainly physical development sometimes outpaces and at other times lags behind the social stages that we have developed. Puberty occurs long before society encourages marriage or reproduction, and retirement is mandated at ages when a majority of individuals are quite capable of continued productivity on the job. In addition, there are individuals whose health is impaired early in life through disease or accident, raising the question of whether they share social characteristics with the old old despite chronological age differences. Therefore, using physical traits or functional capacity to evaluate life stage or old age continues to be problematic.

Finally, how might we reorganize the stages of life to modify existing patterns? Who does the reorganizing, and how does it happen? The answers to these questions are more obscure. Consider the area of employment. Currently, roles are temporally structured in the life course in such a way that young adults face the pressures of attempting to succeed in jobs at the same time that they are bearing and parenting small children. Yet it is difficult to defer childbearing beyond the years of career building, especially for women. In addition, knowledge is now becoming obsolete more quickly, suggesting that restricting the timing of education to the span before initiating employment will be less useful over a 30- to 50-year career. Multiple careers, with individuals taking a mid-life sabbatical for updating their knowledge in a field or changing careers entirely, or simultaneous employment and education, could become more common. We already see evidence of more education taking place beyond the traditional ages of schooling (Hamil-Luker & Uhlenberg, 2002).

Implications of a Global Economy

The world is aging, but countries are aging at various speeds. Nations' population profiles are related to their levels of economic development, as well as a range of other social and cultural factors. Changes in the global economy, communications technology, and employment patterns affect aging in all parts of the world. The rapid aging of the Chinese population, as the country moves to control its population through the one-child policy, will have implications far beyond the borders of that country. As the world gets smaller, it is important to keep the larger world economy, and its many aging societies, in mind.

As some countries age more quickly, they face problems and opportunities in this larger economy. Will aging nations become more open to immigration to bolster the shrinking size of their labor forces for jobs not feasible to outsource, or will they be able to adapt via technology to a smaller work force? What would such migration mean for support of elderly kin in the countries losing the migrant workers? What impact might immigration have on the culture of the receiving country?

In the global economy, it is probably safe to bet that neither employment patterns nor retirement as we know it will survive without dramatic alterations. A majority of jobs will become more technological, requiring advanced education to be competitive in the marketplace. As health status and longevity improve worldwide, will older workers be prevented from retiring when they desire? Either governments or employers could alter their pension policies if the supply of or training of youthful workers entering the job market are insufficient to meet demand. How does retirement as a social event change its meaning for people who have primarily worked as independent contractors in the contingent labor force, constantly moving from job to job, or those who work at home, physically apart from a work setting?

The distinctions between the haves and the have-nots are growing, not shrinking, in many nations of the world. Studies of U.S. workers show declining rates of pension coverage, with the steepest declines among Hispanic and Black workers (Chen & Leavitt, 1997). Because disadvantages in early life stages with regard to education, jobs, health, and pensions have ramifications throughout the life course, it is too simplistic to presume that problems of a nation's underclass will disappear in the future or that most elders will be financially secure. For example, although more women are working full-time throughout most of their adult lives, the types of employment women hold (more in the service sector in the United States and in family businesses internationally) are less likely to offer pensions, indicating that perhaps their work will not have the same long-term payoff as a lifetime of work among men.

If pension coverage continues to decline, especially as contingent employment becomes more common, the financial security of more older people may be uncertain rather than a given. Even in countries where private pensions are widely available today, policymakers may need to revise benefits (both public and private) for their aging populations in the future. The future elderly will, if current trends continue, include some very advantaged and some very disadvantaged groups. Coping with that reality will continue to challenge societies in which those holding the advantages tend to make the policies.

Societies must also address issues of productive capacity as their populations age. Projections clearly identify a growing number of "young old" individuals under age 75 or 80, considered by some to be an "untapped resource" (Commonwealth Fund, 1993). Older adults already do a lot to support society, but some suggest they could do even more. Examining unpaid activities such as family caregiving, informal volunteer activities, and formal volunteer work, a 2002 estimate suggests that per person contributions by persons 55 and older (if paid) would be valued at $2,700 per year (Johnson & Schaner, 2005). If employment policies do not change to dramatically increase older adults' involvement in jobs, societies must examine how they can integrate those individuals into the society and effectively harness the skills, experience, and energy to improve their communities and nations. Could societies enhance norms of and opportunities for volunteerism so that healthy and willing retirees give a significant portion of their time to fighting poverty, illiteracy, teen pregnancy, environmental problems, or other social issues? Such norms, and the social policies supporting them, would have implications for income maintenance policies (would such work be paid or unpaid?), the marketplace for leisure activities (would purveyors of cruises and golf equipment suffer?), family life (would there be less support available from older to younger generations?), and other areas of social life.

Developing additional options for young old individuals not engaged in paid employment remains an unmet challenge in many aging societies. Nonetheless, research shows that adults over 55 make tremendous contributions to their families, their communities, and the nation through voluntary activity as well as paid employment (Bass, 1995). In addition, many are interested in contributing more, in either paid or unpaid work settings (Commonwealth Fund, 1993).

Changing Family Structure

Dramatic changes within families over the past several decades will play themselves out in future cohorts of elders. Within families, more women are employed full-time, making them less available as caregivers (Bianchi & Spain, 1996). In addition, lower fertility means that future cohorts will have fewer adult children as potential caregivers. Who will undertake caregiving for the childless or those with children geographically or emotionally distant from them? One answer is for the economy to respond with market alternatives (such as home health care services or supportive housing) to meet the needs of those unable to be fully independent. Yet such solutions require either public or private financing to ensure access for all citizens. When neither family nor society provides

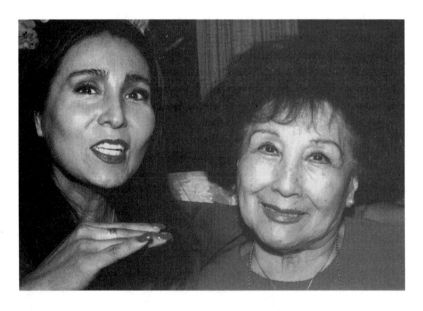

Although family ties remain strong, as women join the workforce in increasing numbers, fewer daughters are available to care for aging parents. (Credit: Mike Payne)

needed care, what type of negative fallout (such as insufficient care or premature deaths) is the society willing to accept?

We have yet to encounter the full ramifications of "serial monogamy" (sequential divorce and remarriage) on family relationships in later life. Its impact both on filial obligation toward noncustodial and step-parents, as well as on step- and half-sibling relationships, is far from clear. Will having eight or more full and step-grandparents be advantageous to a child, compared with having only four (Cherlin & Furstenberg, 1986)? On the one hand, we might be pessimistic that the family will relinquish its role of providing primary support to frail elders; on the other hand, the relationships that persist may be stronger than those engendered through only a sense of duty.

Some family relationships will last longer than they do today. A newspaper story chronicling the birthday of a 115-year-old woman in Maryland will soon not warrant special coverage as the number of centenarians grows. In the story, the mentally intact and physically healthy 115-year-old was visited daily by her 92-year-old daughter and less often by a 70-year-old grandson. Three generations of one family were receiving Social Security! All six generations of this family, including a 2-month-old great-great-great-granddaughter, were present for the woman's birthday celebration (Vitez, 1995). Although most of us will probably not achieve the century mark, having the potential for a century of fairly healthy life warrants a serious rethinking of how, and when in life, we do certain things.

Future Cohorts of Older People

What Can We Accurately Predict?

Predicting the future is a notoriously difficult (and risky) process, especially for those with some allegiance to the rules of science. Given the large number of unknown factors, what can we really say about the future and what the older population will be like in the year 2020 or 2050? It is perhaps easier than it seems, because the people who will be part of the over-65 population in those years are already born. We can examine these cohorts and identify ways in which they are similar to and different from current cohorts above the age of 30, 60, or 70. Based on these differences from their predecessors, we can speculate about how they may age differently. Let us first examine a few of the differences we can quantify and later speculate about other social changes and cohort experiences likely to make these cohorts very distinct from their predecessors as they age.

The federal government routinely makes projections of future sociodemographic characteristics for the purpose of planning. According to Easterlin (1996), "Projections of population in developed countries over the next half century consistently assume that the rate of childbearing will remain low, total population size will stabilize or decline, and the proportion of the older population will rise markedly" (p. 73). For instance, projections assume that there will not be another span of high fertility, such as occurred during the baby boom, nor will there be major breakthroughs that will significantly extend average life expectancy. Should these or other major changes occur, the projections will be off, either underestimating or overestimating the size or characteristics of future elderly. With that caveat in mind, let us examine what we are expecting to see in the next several decades.

Growth and Diversity

Throughout this book we have discussed the impact of the growing older population on society and on the lives of individuals. Just how significant is that growth? Exhibit 13.2 shows population trends (through 2000) and projections (beyond 2000) for those over 65. Several things are readily apparent from a quick examination of these trends. First, the growth in the population over age 65 will continue to be a major social phenomenon, with the size of the U.S. population over 65 more than doubling between 2000 and 2050. Second, the growth will be rapid for those between 75 and 84, but fastest among those above age 85, who will have grown from near invisibility as recently as the 1940s to nearly one-fourth of the over 65 population by 2050 if current assumptions hold true. In contrast, the size of the young old population (ages 65–74) is expected to grow quite slowly during this time period (Day, 1996; Hobbs & Damon, 1996).

The growth of the population over age 65 will not be matched by growth among the population aged 64 and under, according to population projections. Therefore, the median age of the society (the marker age with 50% of the population older and 50% younger) will also increase. History shows the effect of the birth rate on the median age, with the lowest point showing the effects of large numbers of children and teenagers just after the end of the baby boom. Exhibit 13.3 shows three projections for median age of the U.S. population to 2050, with the intermediate projection demonstrating an increase to around 38 years before a slight downturn. Keep in mind that the median age is shaped by both mortality and fertility (and sometimes by migration). The dotted lines indicate projections with either higher or lower fertility assumptions, which might

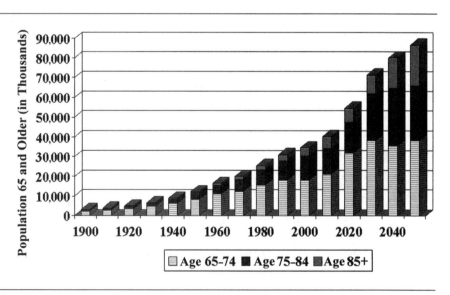

Middle Series Population Projections
Source: Day, 1996; Hobbs and Damon, 1996.

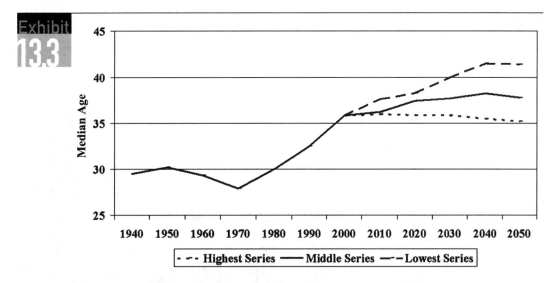

Projected Median Age of the U.S. Population to 2050 Under Varied Assumptions
Source: Day, 1996.

result in either an older society or a younger society, as indicated by the median age (Day, 1996).

Another way to look at these projections is in terms of the dependency ratio, as described in chapter 3. Exhibit 13.4 divides the dependent population into its two components, those under age 18 and those 65 and over. Clearly there have been dramatic historical changes in the overall dependency ratio during the 20th century, and we can expect continuing drama in the first 50 years of the 21st century. The level of

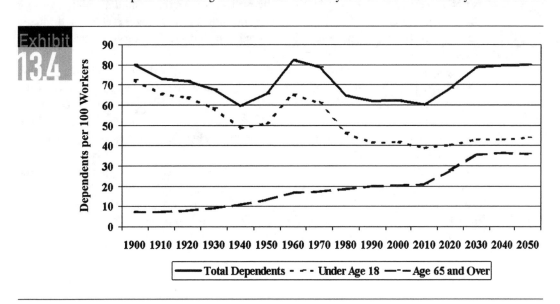

Dependency Ratios: 1900–2000 and Projections to 2050
Source: Day, 1996.

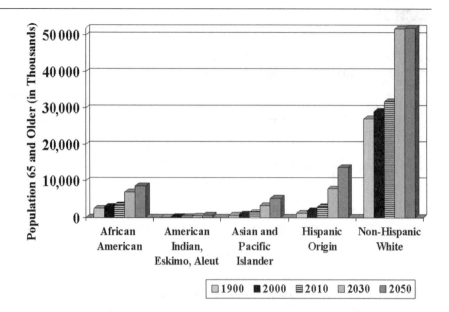

U.S. Population 65 and Older by Race/Ethnicity: 1900, 2000–2050
Source: Day, 1996.

dependency is expected to increase until about 2030, and then level off. This growth is largely accounted for by the growth in the population 65 and over, with relatively little change expected in the number of dependents under age 18. By 2050, children and older adults are almost even in their contribution to the total dependency ratio. Even with the growth of the older population, however, total dependency in the next several decades is not expected to exceed the levels of the peak years of childhood dependency during the baby boom era (see Exhibit 13.4). Barring unforeseen changes (such as a dramatic upturn in fertility rates, or a breakthrough reducing old age mortality), we can anticipate major, but not extreme, shifts in the dependency ratio.

One final area of population projection demonstrates the growing racial/ethnic diversity within the older population in the United States. Exhibit 13.5 compares the changes in the population 65 and over by race/ethnicity from 1990 to 2050 (Day, 1996). The American Indian, Eskimo, and Aleut group, while hard to see, reflects natural growth. The trend for some other groups (notably Hispanic and Asian/Pacific Islander and, to a lesser extent, Blacks) shows both natural growth (i.e., that driven by fertility and mortality changes) and the effects of immigration in driving a steeper growth in the numbers of older adults. Older Whites show a leveling-off around 2050, in contrast to other groups. In short, the composition of older adults in America will gradually come to reflect the diversity seen today among children and younger adults and the growing racial/ethnic diversity across the population in general.

Education

Education is an area of some complexity, requiring consideration of cohort differences and changing age norms to understand recent changes and future trends. Two related areas are worthy of examination. The first is that of the trends in educational attainment through high school and college among various birth cohorts. The second area is the growing trend toward education beyond traditional ages, sometimes referred to as adult or continuing education.

First, the education of successive cohorts has increased (U.S. Bureau of the Census, 2005a). Comparing younger cohorts with older cohorts, it is clear that more and more people are completing high school, attending some college, or completing college. Between 1960 and 2002 the proportion of high school graduates who were enrolled in college during the year following graduation increased from 45.1 percent to 65.2 percent (U.S. Bureau of the Census, 2005a). As a consequence of these long-term trends, the educational profile of the adult population is shifting as members of older, less educated cohorts die out, and younger, more educated cohorts move into adulthood and eventually later life. Exhibit 13.6 compares the educational attainment of the population over 65 in 1990 with projections for 2030 (Hobbs & Damon, 1996). The trend toward more education is apparent for both women and men, with increased percentages of both sexes expected to complete high school and college. Despite ongoing concerns about high dropout rates and the "cumulative disadvantage" potential of undereducated individuals, the older population overall will continue to grow more educated over the next several decades. Since more-educated individuals often fare better in later life, all else being equal (which it never is), the trend toward greater education is an encouraging one.

The second issue, education among individuals of non-normative ages, is one of growing interest to educators. Data on education have often reflected the out-of-date expectation that little additional education is likely to be sought beyond approximately age 25. Educational institutions have been age-segregated in the past, enrolling children and young adults. Increasingly since the 1970s, enrollments have grown dramatically for more "mature" students, including those returning to school after many years of involvement in work, family, or both. Also included in this trend, however, are those

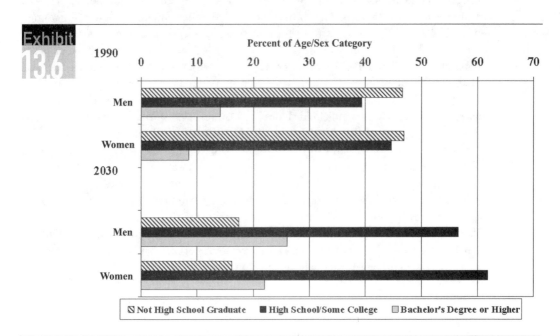

Educational Attainment of Men and Women 65 and Over: 1990, 2030
Source: Hobbs and Damon, 1996.

who are extending their education to the graduate or professional levels, where the extra years of training push completion to age 30 or beyond. From 1970 to 1994 the numbers of individuals enrolled in some type of schooling (mostly college) between ages 25 and 29 more than doubled, and the numbers for adults ages 30 through 34 grew threefold (U.S. Bureau of the Census, 1996a). A study of trends published in 2002 found increases in adult education rates for all ages continued during the 1990s, but the trends were strongest in older adults (Hamil-Luker & Uhlenberg, 2002). In 2001, 21% of adults over age 65, 38% of those 55–64, and 53% of those 45–54 had been enrolled in some sort of course for credit in the prior 12 months (U.S. Bureau of the Census, 2005a).

This trend portends a gradual transition of education to an age-integrated, rather than age-segregated, social institution (Riley & Riley, 1994). Of course, these cross-sectional snapshots of enrollment in specific years may mean that more adults are enrolled in school at one time or another throughout adulthood than indicated by the percentages. If education continues to become more integrated throughout adulthood, we may find it less relevant to distinguish among students of traditional ages and those augmenting their education in other stages of life—being a student may become an age-less role.

Sharing Lives and Households

Marital status, non-marital relationships, and living arrangements in later life are the product of a lifetime of opportunities and decisions, some not under the control of the individual. Will the outcome of these major life choices and events differ markedly for future cohorts? Major social changes have continued to sweep through the institution of the family, mirrored in sometimes dramatic changes in the lives of individuals of different cohorts. An example is marriage. In 1970, about 36% of women ages 20–24 and 11% of those 25–29 had never married; by 2003, the comparable figures for women were 75.4% and 40.3%, indicating both the possibility of delayed marriage (with ramifications for the later timing of other family events) or the increased likelihood of never marrying at all (Saluter, 1996; Hobbs & Damon, 1996). Men also experienced dramatic changes; 9% of men 30–34 had not married in 1970, compared with 33.1% in 2003. Exhibit 13.7 shows projections of the marital status of women over 65 through 2050, assuming that current trends hold (Hobbs & Damon, 1996). Among women, who constitute the majority of the older population (and whose marital fates differ substantially from those of men), we can expect a substantial increase in the percentage divorced, a slight increase in the percentage who remain single, and corresponding declines in the widowed population. The percentage of women over age 65 who are expected to be married remains remarkably stable across this time period (Hobbs & Damon, 1996).

These projections represent the current marital status of women 65 and over, not their marital histories. Given the continuing high levels of divorce, more individuals will approach later life having lived as single persons, perhaps having experienced one or more marriages or long-term relationships along the way. Since being stably married over many decades appears to provide certain advantages in later life, the smaller percentage of adults who will approach old age having experienced a continuous marriage, with its expectations of substantial mutual support and economic security, may have significant implications for issues such as caregiving. One neglected area is the potential for companionship and social support provided by non-marital couple relationships with either

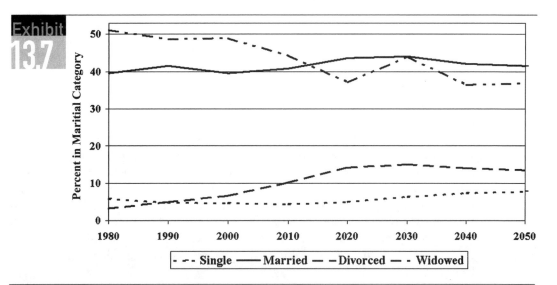

Trends in Marital Status for Women 65 and Over: 1980–2050
Source: Hobbs and Damon, 1996.

same- or opposite-sex partners (Kimmel, 1993). Researchers have generally paid attention to whether someone is married, but not to other, non-marital forms of partnering that may be meaningful and may be more openly practiced by future cohorts. Given the cohort experience of the baby boomers, it is likely that more will be in such non-marital relationships in the future.

In terms of living arrangements, households headed by someone over age 75 already constituted 11% of all U.S. households and will increase substantially by 2010, even before the baby boomers reach 75 starting in 2020 (U.S. Bureau of the Census, 2005a). One of the major trends regarding households is the increasing number and percentage of older adults living alone (Szinovacz & Ekerdt, 1996). Future developments in alternative forms of housing, however, may change where older people choose to live as they age. Alternatives such as continuing care retirement communities or active adult and co-housing developments, where independent elders have their own condo or apartment but may move to more supportive environments as needed, are becoming more commonly available to those who can afford them (Newcomer & Preston, 1994).

Political Participation

The area of politics and political participation is one in which we might strongly suspect that period effects will create differences in the behaviors and attitudes of cohorts. Once it was thought that aging led to political conservatism; today some speculate that aging leads to liberalism, because a higher percentage of older adults have voted for Democratic candidates in recent elections. How are major events, such as the Vietnam and Iraq wars, various political scandals from Watergate to Whitewater, and the swings that occur from domination by the Republicans to the Democrats and back again likely to influence these cohorts? Only sketchy information is available to try to answer such questions.

Data available on the party affiliation of older and younger cohorts and on the strength of their political attitudes suggest that if cohorts continue to maintain their affiliations throughout life, the older population will eventually swing back toward a more Republican concentration than is the case today. This swing will reflect the aging of the Reagan Republicans of the 1980s (U.S. Bureau of the Census, 1996a). It remains unclear, however, how younger cohorts to follow will distribute themselves across political parties.

A related issue has to do with the impact of the aging population on the profile of voters. Exhibit 13.8 shows the 1992 age structure of the voting population and projections for 2020, as the baby boomers begin to influence the over-65 vote. The chart clearly shows is a shift toward older age groups dominating the voting population as the larger cohorts swell the ranks of the population over 65. This projection is based on current low rates of voting among young adults; if those younger groups become more active, this profile could shift. However, if older adults ever congeal into a voting bloc, their potential impact in the years between 2030 and 2050 could be considerable.

Exhibit 13.8 also shows a shift on the lower half of the age distribution, with growing cohorts in the 25–44 age range compared to 1992. These reflect the "baby boom echo," children of the original baby boomers who themselves represent large numbers and large cohorts who will eventually follow their parents into old age, creating another wave of aging several decades later.

Speculations About Coming Cohorts

It is difficult to anticipate the nature and extent of changes in a number of areas, including health, disability, life expectancy, and the labor force. Although many experts believe in a biological limit to human survival of around 120 years, this figure is debated, as is

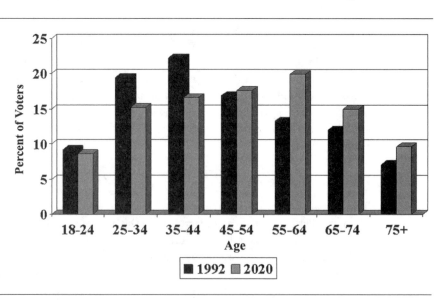

Percent Distribution of Voters by Age: 1992, 2020 (Projected)
Source: U.S. Bureau of the Census, 1992b.

the prospect that a major breakthrough in understanding the biological mechanisms of aging might enable an extension of average life expectancy. Such changes raise important ethical questions regarding access to potentially costly life-extending technologies that have, until only recently, been the subject of science fiction. Most biologists are not optimistic that a major breakthrough will be forthcoming in the near term; if it is, its social implications are potentially staggering. Who would be able to afford extensive medical procedures? Would a small but wealthy elite be able to double their lives as most people aged and died on timetables we see today?

Nor can we predict what small changes in health practices and preventive care will mean for health or longevity. For example, dietary changes from 1970 to 1994 included average 15% per-person decline in consumption of red meat, 20% reduction for distilled liquor and increases of 25% for fruits and 33% for the healthiest vegetables (U.S. Bureau of the Census, 1996a). Will widespread fluoridation of water, which began in the middle of the 20th century, mean that more elders retain their teeth and therefore get more satisfactory nutrition into their later years? Will the recent trends of drinking more water or smoking cigars have long-term effects? How have childhood immunizations for measles and flu shots for adults changed the outcomes for health and life expectancy? How will the movement toward management of AIDS shape mortality from that single cause of death? How will the countervailing trends toward more exercise and more sedentary jobs and leisure (watching television, surfing the Web) influence long-term health prospects? What will be the long-range outcomes for the growing percentage of overweight children and adults? The changes are so numerous that it is difficult to isolate the single effects of any one. Nonetheless, the cumulative effect of these changes will, without a doubt, influence life expectancy, well-being, and the types and ages of onset of illnesses.

The Risks of Prediction

Despite the predictions outlined here, there remains the potential for many unanticipated changes that will reshape current and future cohorts. It is difficult to speculate, for example, about how some changes we can see today will play out.

As an example of an unexpected issue, changes in recent decades have expanded life expectancy for individuals with developmental disabilities far beyond what had been the case just a few decades ago. As Ansello (2004) notes, "In less than 20 years, the median life expectancy for someone with Down's syndrome has nearly doubled, to almost 50 years" (p. 3). In earlier eras, parents typically outlived their developmentally disabled child and were often able to provide care. The policy and service communities were not prepared for the growing group of aging individuals with lifelong disabilities (Ansello, 2004), since policies and programs to deal with developmental disabilities (and some other types of disabilities) are entirely distinct from programs serving people as they age. As a consequence, some seemingly parallel programs exist, one set serving physically or developmentally disabled adults and another set focused on aging adults without prior experience of disability. Numerous analysts and commentators have pointed to the need to rethink this structure for providing services, and some experiments in collaboration are underway (Kane, 2004). Ironically, "For the disabilities system, aging is a success. For the aging network, [the occurrence of] disabilities is a failure" (Ansello, 2004, p. 4).

According to government statistics, most children use computers and many connect to the Internet at home, at percentages that are significantly higher than those for older adults (Administration on Aging, 2001). If utilizing such technologies is a cohort-based phenomenon, we might expect a gradual increase in the likelihood that older adults will be surfing the net, and we can contemplate ways to make use of that technology in providing services and even conducting research. Already pilot programs for "telemedicine" are enabling physicians to monitor the health markers of their patients at home, permitting early interventions and avoiding trips to the emergency room. On the other hand, if restrictions in pensions and Social Security benefits reduce the disposable incomes of older adults, fewer may be able to afford to keep up with cutting-edge technology or regularly access the Internet.

Although many changes are already upon us, we cannot anticipate what the next big thing will be that will reshape social life. Will some dramatic reorganization of family life or employment or politics make our understood ways of doing things, including growing older, no longer relevant? Will social attitudes about age and life stages change dramatically? Will a worldwide economic crisis mean that older people who are fit must continue to work and contribute to society? These possibilities are only a few of the endless alternatives. We cannot predict these kinds of changes—either positive or negative—nor can we always identify them as being the next big thing when they first appear. What is likely, however, given the pace of social and technological change in a global economy, is that major and currently unanticipated historical changes, generating period and cohort effects, will come.

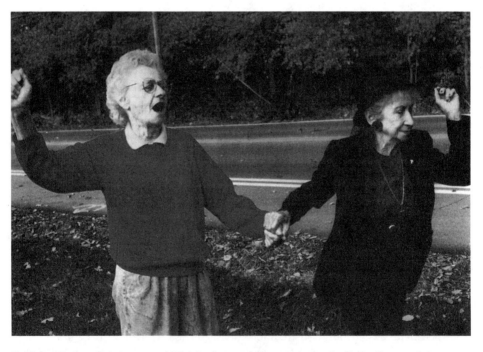

Social attitudes about age and life stages may change dramatically in the years to come. (Credit: Mike Payne, courtesy of the Ohio Department of Aging)

Challenges and Opportunities for the Field

Throughout this book we have outlined what we know about aging and, just as importantly, what we don't know about aging. The field is obviously still developing. In this section we discuss some of the issues facing the study of aging and some key opportunities for enhancing our understanding of this dynamic social process.

In order to organize the material in various chapters, we have drawn distinctions based on perspectives used to study aging, the level of analysis along the micro-macro continuum, and the subject matter under consideration. In preparing to conclude this book, one critical message to remember is that everything about aging is connected. Although we have divided material into categories for purposes of clarity in presentation, in the real world of aging societies and in the lives of aging individuals, everything is connected in complex and interactive ways that blur many of the distinctions we have drawn. Politics influences families; economics influence health; individual choices influence social change; and social trends reshape the life course (Settersten, 1999). Age, the life course, and how cohorts experience their particular shared movement through time are constantly experiencing dynamic changes that make aging truly a moving target.

Disciplinary Frameworks

Many people who look at older adults or changes related to aging take a disciplinary approach—they look at the issue of aging as a physician, a political scientist, or a biologist. Much of the material presented here has a social sciences frame of reference, using the concepts and the research methods most often applied by researchers trained in sociology, political science, psychology, economics, and history. Each of the many disciplines used to study aging has information and insights to help us understand the process of aging in all of its complexity. In fact, we doubt that anyone trained in the study of aging would argue for the usefulness of one discipline to the exclusion of all others in addressing the puzzle that is human aging in social context.

Applied aging research often occurs in an interdisciplinary fashion, with researchers from numerous disciplines—including history, epidemiology, economics, biochemistry, and physiology—coming together to address a question or policy issue. Even research that is more basic and less focused on solving problems often crosses boundaries of discipline in developing both theory and research techniques. A project might, for example, utilize theories from sociology, economics, and psychology and borrow research techniques applied in these or other disciplines to seek answers to the research question. This interdisciplinary approach strengthens, rather than weakens, the research process, because the physical, psychological, and social aspects of aging are all simultaneously interactive on the micro and macro levels. In fact, biologists, sociologists, psychologists, and those in other disciplines have a lot to teach each other about the process of aging for individuals, groups, organizations, and nations.

Micro-Macro Distinctions: Implications for Policy and Practice

Just as the distinctions among disciplines are instructive but somewhat arbitrary, micro-macro frames of reference actually represent a continuum. On numerous occasions we have identified questions or issues that can be thought of as having serious implications for policy or practice on both individual and societal levels. The example of longevity is a handy one. Any significant extension of human life expectancy would raise important micro-level dilemmas for aging individuals. How would the extended years of life be used? Would longer-lived humans demand more of a role for themselves in the later years than they do today? In the middle of this continuum, we might ask how increased life expectancy would influence family relationships, the world of employment, and other social groups and institutions. On a macro level, using the widest-angle lens possible, we would confront the issues of aging societies, which might need to restrict births in order to avoid overpopulation, and we would need to address changes in economic dependency in later years created by the current system of retirement.

When we point to questions on these various levels that researchers might want to tackle, it is important to emphasize that there are generally related questions for practice and policy. As the process of social aging changes, we examine whether policies based on chronological age have appropriate age limits (for example, is the age range of 40 to 70 appropriate for laws on age discrimination in employment, or should these cutoffs be altered?) and whether age criteria remain relevant to the issues the policies seek to address. For example, many programs (Older Americans Act services and even Social Security) have moved from eligibility based solely on age to a combination of age and need as the older population has grown more economically diverse. Practitioners, faced with growing demand for their services in an aging population, are attuned to these policy issues, because they will determine who is or is not eligible for services and, consequently, the practitioners' own job security.

As we examine social issues along the micro–macro continuum, it is important to consider all of the levels. Will the increasing rates of divorce among future cohorts of older adults mean any lessening informal support from kin, resulting in the need for more assistance from public programs? Will the preventive health behaviors of individuals in these same cohorts mean that the onset of disability will be delayed to later ages, reducing the burden on families and on the overall society? Will changes in Social Security policy that increase the retirement age result in impoverishment of older adults forced by ill health to retire before they can receive full benefits? The changes on one level reverberate in the others, and we encourage consideration of how changes at both the individual level and the societal level of the micro–macro continuum are intricately connected.

On the micro level of the individual, connections between these domains are fairly easy to see. As individuals move through the life course, the family shapes their initial socioeconomic status, thereby influencing their life chances and opportunities for education and occupation. Early health care and habits, taught by the family, will have long-range repercussions on health and disability into advanced old age. Attitudes taught by the family are also likely to shape political orientation and party selection. Throughout adulthood, work, economic status, and health are likely to have mutual influences; persons in poor health cannot be as competitive in work, and those who are poorer or work in less advantaged jobs are less likely to have health care coverage. For women especially, work may influence their involvement in family life, and their family responsibilities shape their likelihood of working full-time.

As the life-course perspective reminds us, the behaviors undertaken and choices made in early and mid-life have clear effects on the later-life well-being of individuals.

Today's working poor, for example, are less likely to have pensions, good health, or complete choice about when to retire, resulting in their continued vulnerability into later life (Meyer & Greenwood, 1997). Seldom do those who are economically marginal at earlier stages find themselves in a financially comfortable old age; generally those in excellent health or poor health find those statuses the starting point for whatever changes they experience in self-sufficiency and health with advancing age. Those intervening among physically frail or poor elders would do well to look beyond the initial problems (such as poor health or poverty) to examine other issues, such as the availability of family support or adequacy of housing, in developing their strategies to provide assistance. Physicians, for example, sending an older person home after a health crisis may presume the availability of either family caregivers or money to hire surrogates to provide that care. Absence of such support could mean a dangerous situation for the individual and a costly return to the hospital, if not a worse outcome.

Employers shift their retirement policies in response to both government mandates and the economic pressures of the world economy. Currently, the government encourages people to work longer before retiring and is looking ahead to further raising the age of entitlement to full Social Security benefits, while the private sector may offer incentives for early retirement. Families may constrain their childbearing in response to the need for two incomes to meet their needs. Societies cannot develop new (and perhaps badly needed) programs to assist the elderly or any other group unless both economics and political opinion are on their side.

Firming Our Theoretical Foundations

Among the ongoing problems encountered by the study of aging is that most research is not clearly directed by theory (Bengtson, Burgess, & Parrott, 1997). Theoretical development in aging has, according to many experts, lagged behind theoretical development in mainstream disciplines (Passuth & Bengtson, 1988). In fact, Linda George (1995) goes so far as to call the research in aging "theoretically sterile or unsatisfying" (p. S1). Her argument suggests that the field has generated a lot of testable hypotheses and specific conceptual models (what she calls theory with a small t), rather than examining "broad views of fundamental processes underlying social structure and social life," or theory with a capital T (p. S1). The theoretical development in the study of aging has sometimes been parochial, generating specialized, small-scale theories relating to specific points of data of limited concern. In a study of published research in eight leading social-gerontological journals from 1990 to 1994, Bengtson et al. (1997) concluded that 80% of the articles lacked a theoretical framework for their research findings.

Researchers studying the social aspects of aging would do well to look to their disciplinary traditions in history, psychology, or social work for theoretical frames of reference applicable to the needs of the field. Such theoretical frameworks assist in compiling the pieces of the research puzzle, now being generated, into a larger whole. Passuth and Bengtson (1988), among others, advocate examining the dynamic contexts of everyday life in which social aging occurs. Such a contextual view would examine historical, political, and economic aspects of aging as well as the ongoing construction of everyday life among aging individuals and groups (Passuth & Bengtson, 1988; Settersten, 1999).

Perhaps some of the reluctance to theorize on the grand scale derives from the early experience with disengagement theory. Highly controversial when it was introduced, disengagement theory was immediately attacked, including some rather hostile reactions (Achenbaum & Bengtson, 1994). Attacks were based both on scientific criteria and on implicit value positions of researchers oriented toward activity as the successful mode of adaptation to later-life changes. This first major attempt to examine the relationship of the individual to the social world and how that relationship changed with aging may have dissuaded theoretically minded individuals from putting forward a brash or potentially flawed theoretical orientation that might experience a similar fate (Achenbaum & Bengtson, 1994).

Yet another barrier to the development of theory has been the applied origins of the field. Both the "social problems" background of the study of aging and the funding available for research, which tends to focus on policy- or practice-relevant questions, have sometimes turned attention away from theoretical considerations. Theorizing is considered by some to be a waste of valuable time that could be spent problem-solving. Thus, the field, by virtue of its roots and research funding, has turned away from theoretical concerns.

What is lost when we lack theoretical models to organize our knowledge of the changes with aging? In the absence of theory, research provides a set of unrelated bits of knowledge that fail to build a larger picture, support effective interventions, or predict how future cohorts will age differently. Results of research not driven by theory become an array of "factoids"—what Seltzer (1993) calls "itty-bitty" gerontology—which fail to contribute to our understanding of the underlying process of aging. Theories assist us in creating a meaningful, albeit tentative, frameworks for understanding the complexities of the social world. Both research and practice need theories to connect their research findings and make them applicable. As Bengtson and his colleagues (1997) note,

A policymaker would have difficulty supporting a program that does not have clearly stated goals and a plan for how they will be achieved. And it is intellectually irresponsible for a program of research to proceed without a similar set of statements—in short, a theory. (p. S73)

They conclude that there is nothing as practical as a good theory.

Addressing Diversity in Policy and Practice

The older population is becoming more diverse; in sociological terms, the older population is more differentiated by structural factors, such as age, race, ethnicity, social class, and cohort (Calasanti, 1996b). Even though it has always been problematic to discuss "the elderly," it will become increasingly critical to focus on which components of the older population are under consideration. Formulating policy for older adults as a single category may be a thing of the past (Torres-Gil, 1992). The life experiences, and hence the later-life trajectories, of various social groups differ in ways that are obvious but also in more subtle ways.

Can we expect, for example, that a Black woman, aged 85, with a large network of family but little income will have much in common with a newly retired, White professional man who has remained single and childless? Not only do their objective circumstances of aging differ, but also perhaps more important, they may interpret their situations and even the meaning of later life very differently. For example, retirement for the man just described may mean free time, with opportunities to pursue new hobbies, travel, and participate in community service; for the woman, retirement may mean moving from two jobs (one in the home and one for pay) to one, paired with a dramatic reduction in income (Calasanti, 1996a)—clearly not the same meaning at all.

We have already emphasized the changing racial/ethnic profile of the older population. Those planning future social policy or preparing interventions overlook the growth in diversity among older adults, especially among Hispanic and Asian/Pacific Islander groups, at their own peril. Even a local nutrition program will need to recognize the diverse palates of the people it is serving and be responsive to the dietary and cultural needs of these groups (Kayser-Jones, 2002).

Not only must we think about diversity in terms of race, class, ethnicity, gender, education, and similar social structural variables but also in terms of age cohorts (Gibson, 1996). At any given point in time, 60- and 90-year-old cohorts have experienced different slices of history and been differentially shaped by historical events. Baby boomers and their parents and children are good examples. Many parents of baby boomers were part of the "good times generation," coming of age in the strong economy following World War II and experiencing job security and growing pension coverage. Many of their offspring, however, entered a stagnant economy, where job security and pensions were evaporating at the same time as the Watergate scandal reduced their confidence in the political system. Their children, in turn, are moving toward maturity in the age of computers, as a global economy alters employment toward contingent work and outsourcing jobs to far-flung countries, and the Social Security trust fund appears to be endangered. As these three groups age, their outlooks, expectations, and well-being can be expected to differ substantially.

In the face of this growing diversity, we need to reconsider the standard traditionally used as the reference group for older adults: married, middle-class, White men. Because men face shorter life expectancies, divorce is increasing, and ethnic diversity is growing, it will be increasingly unrealistic to use men of the majority culture as the benchmark for how various groups are doing as they age (Gibson, 1996). This tendency to use male experience as the norm casts other groups into the role of "the other," being compared with a standard. Instead, perhaps women's experience should be promoted as the norm, because they represent a growing majority with increasing age (Gibson, 1996), or no group should be considered the standard against which other groups are compared.

Transforming Knowledge To Inform Policy and Practice

Research on aging grew from a tradition of identifying and ameliorating the problems of aging individuals within societies. Now we recognize that not only individuals but entire societies face challenges as their populations grow older. As both societies and individuals work to face these challenges, high-quality information is essential. More than ever before, those formulating policy need to have access to accurate information, not only on current cohorts in later life but also on the differences to be expected in future cohorts.

The policy process often focuses on immediate problems, without much consideration of the long-term view as new and different cohorts move through the age structure of society. As the 1990s came to a close, for example, members of Congress were struggling with ways to modify both Social Security and Medicare to secure their trust funds into the future. Making decisions regarding the best way to reform these and other policies should, in the best of all possible worlds, consider the likely needs of individuals just born, not just individuals already receiving benefits or the cohorts of the baby boom on the horizon of eligibility. Right now, it appears that the policy process is responding mostly to the immediate threat of the large cohorts entering retirement in the next 25 years. But after the baby boomers will come a group of much smaller cohorts prior to the aging of the baby boom echo cohorts. Will the policies enacted now be suitable for them as well? Unfortunately, the policymaking process seldom encourages consideration of these longer-range views.

Researchers, too, have a critical role to play in making research results accessible to the public and to those making policy. As the research process has become more sophisticated and technical, it often becomes more difficult to translate the results of research into language easily comprehensible by nonscientists. Many researchers studying aging are hesitant, given the complexities of the connections among aging, period effects, and cohort differences, to make definitive statements about trends and recommendations to intervene in the most effective fashion. It is incumbent on both scientists and policymakers to work toward a better understanding of the complexities of the others' work and make their own work more accessible.

SUMMARY

The process of aging is not just an individual journey, but also a societal force, developing within a political/historical/economic context that both shapes individuals and their cohorts and, in turn, is shaped and altered by the passage of those age cohorts through the society (Riley, 1987, 1994). The study of aging is the attempt to capture an ever-changing process that affects us all as we move through our individual lives, through the domains of family, work, and the political world.

Your aging will not be like that of your parents or your grandparents. The dynamic interplay between social change and the aging of cohorts, including your cohort, guarantees that aging in the future will be different socially, economically, and (to some degree) physically. Predicting the form that those differences will take, however, is a much more difficult task.

Even if age is a socially constructed phenomenon, and thought by some people therefore to be "unreal," we must recall W. I. Thomas's (1972) wisdom that such phenomena, if perceived as real, are real in their consequences. We have constructed as part of our social world a complex understanding of aging and what it means that extends far beyond the physical parameters and changes experienced by individuals. We organize much of our social lives based on age, with access to opportunities and relationships among individuals constrained by the formal and informal rules of age stratification systems. This reality, which we share as part of our culture, comes to be a system by which society organizes itself and through which individuals develop their lives. Just because it is socially constructed does not mean it isn't a powerful force. When someone encourages an individual to "act their age"—regardless of whether that age is 6 or 66—you are witnessing the power of age as a social construct in operation.

It is not simply for individuals, however, that age is significant. Social life would be chaotic if we lacked some rules and orderliness of events and relationships imposed by the social construct of age. We rely on the rules of the system and build it into our social planning in complex ways. It is unlikely that a completely "age irrelevant" society is on the horizon. Nonetheless, many of the distinctions we make today, between someone who is 16 and 18 or between 63 and 66, for example, are subject to serious question.

We must recognize the power of aging as a concept. Individual and large-scale planning, as we face an aging society, must include flexibility. Social scientists do not have a very good track record of predicting trends far into the future, and the aging of society is one of the most potent trends we face today. One goal of any planning is certain: If you plan, you must plan for change. The future of aging is uncertain; only the fact that we are all aging is firmly guaranteed.

WEB WISE

Association for Gerontology in Higher Education Student Page
http://www.aghe.org/

The Association for Gerontology in Higher Education, the national association for educational institutions in gerontology and geriatrics, has a page of resources for students, accessible from its home page. It includes information on a database (with tailored searches available for a modest fee for students) to identify specific types of educational programs in gerontology and geriatrics nationwide, information on scholarships and fellowships for advanced study in aging and gerontology, and information on careers in aging.

Elderhostel
http://www.elderhostel.org/

Elderhostel has been a source of social activity, travel, and education for older adults for many years. A visit to the Web site demonstrates the richness and diversity of education/travel programs offered and provides a notion of what some adults do in their retirement years. Although courses do carry costs and primarily cater to a middle-class clientele, some scholarships are available. Check out activities located at a wide range of locations throughout the United States and Canada and view some of the courses available in your state or elsewhere through the online catalogs.

Senior Net
http://www.seniornet.org/php/default.php

Senior Net is a non-profit organization of computer-using adults ages 50 or above. The goal is to enhance the lives of those in later life and to share useful knowledge. This lively site holds a lot of information and many links to other useful sites related to active, engaged maturity.

Senior Women Web
http://www.seniorwomen.com

Senior Women Web focuses on issues of specific concern to women. It includes news stories, sections on art, leisure, politics, fitness, and media, including links to other woman-oriented Web sites.

QUESTIONS FOR THOUGHT AND DISCUSSION

1. If you were working for a service provider planning for the future needs of the elderly, what steps would you recommend right away based on what we know about changes in the older population? What specific changes are going to be most important to those planning for service needs?

2. Do we have too many life cycle stages, too few, or just the right number? Since these are socially constructed, it is possible to change them. As the average life expectancy grows, does that mean we should have more stages or should we move toward making age irrelevant to more aspects of society?

3. Now that you are more educated about the complexities of aging, what steps can you take right now to maximize a good old age for yourself, including the avoidance of "usual aging?" Answering this question requires you to consider what makes for successful aging according to your value system.

4. Speculate on the likely changes to later life that may be brought by the large cohorts of the baby boom. What have their cohort experiences suggested about this large age group that may transform later life?Dependency Ratios: 1900–2000 and Projections to 2050

References

Aboderin, I. (2004). Decline in material family support for older people in urban Ghana, Africa: Understanding processes and causes of change. *Journals of Gerontology: Social Sciences, 59,* S128–S137.

Abramson, A., & Silverstein, M. (2004). *Images of aging in America 2004: A summary of selected findings.* Washington, DC: AARP and University of Southern California.

Achenbaum, W. A. (1992). With justice for all? Social Security, symbolic politics, and generational equity. *In Depth, 2*(3), 13–36.

Achenbaum, W. A., & Bengtson, V. L. (1994). Re-engaging the disengagement theory of aging: On the history and assessment of theory development in gerontology. *The Gerontologist, 34*(6), 756–763.

Aday, R. H. (1994). Golden years behind bars: Special programs and facilities for elderly inmates. *Federal Probation, 58*(2), 47–54.

Adelman, R. C. (1995). The Alzheimerization of aging. *The Gerontologist, 35*(4), 526–532.

Administration on Aging. (2001). *Profile of older Americans, 2001.* Washington, DC: Department of Health and Human Services. Retrieved May 2, 2005 from http://aoa.gov/prof/Statistics/profile/2001/2001profile.pdf.

Administration on Aging. (2004). *A profile of older Americans, 2004.* Washington, DC: Department of Health and Human Services. Retrieved May 17, 2005 from http://www.aoa.gov/prof/Statistics/profile.

Agree, E. M., Biddlecom, A. E., Chang, M., & Perez, A. E. (2002). Transfers from older parents to their adult children in Taiwan and the Philippines. *Journal of Cross-Cultural Gerontology, 17,* 269–294.

Akiyama, H., Antonucci, C., & Campbell, R. (1990). Rules of support exchange among two generations of Japanese and American women. In J. Sokolovsky (Ed.), *The cultural context of aging.* New York: Bergin & Garvey.

Alessio, H. (2001). Physiology of human aging. In L. A. Morgan & S. Kunkel (Eds.), *Aging: The social context* (2nd ed., pp. 107–137). Thousand Oaks, CA: Pine Forge Press.

Allen, S., Goldscheider, F., & Ciambone, D. (1999). Gender roles, marital intimacy, and nomination of spouse as primary caregiver. *The Gerontologist, 39*(2), 150–158.

Alwin, D. F., & Krosnick, J. A. (1991). Aging, cohorts, and the stability of sociopolitical orientations over the life span. *American Journal of Sociology, 97*(1), 169–195.

Amato, P., Rezac, S., & Booth, A. (1995). Helping between parents and young adult offspring: The role of parental marital quality, divorce, and remarriage. *Journal of Marriage and the Family, 57*(2), 363–374.

Amer, M. L. (2004). *Membership of the 108th Congress: A profile.* (Publication #RS 21379). Washington, DC: Congressional Research Service, Library of Congress. Retrieved May 22, 2005 from http://www.senate.gov/reference/resources/pdf/RS21379.pdf.

American Association of Retired Persons (AARP). (1995). *Valuing older workers: A study of costs and productivity.* Washington, DC: AARP.

American Association of Retired Persons (AARP). (2005a). *Reimagining America.* Retrieved July 25, 2005, from http://www.2030.org.fr990719.html.

American Association of Retired Persons (AARP). (2005b). *Rock the vote 2005.* Washington, DC: AARP.

American Geriatrics Society/Association of Directors of Geriatrics Academic Programs (AGS/ ADGAP). (2005). *Geriatric medicine: A clinical imperative for an aging population.* Retrieved September 15, 2005, from http://www.americangeriatrics.org/WrittenReport.pdf.

American Geriatrics Society Core Writing Group of the Task Force on the Future of Geriatric Medicine. (2005). Caring for older Americans: The future of geriatric medicine. *Journal of the American Geriatrics Society, 53,* S245–S256.

American Obesity Association. (2002). *AOA fact sheets: Obesity research.* Retrieved April 10, 2006, from http://www.obesity.org/subs/fastfacts/Obesity_Research.shtml.

American Society for Aesthetic Plastic Surgery (ASAPS). (2005). *2005 ASAPS statistics.* Retrieved March 25, 2006, from http://www.surgery.org/press/statistics-2005.php.

Amoss, P. T., & Harrell, S. (Eds.). (1981). *Other ways of growing old: Anthropological perspectives.* Stanford, CA: Stanford University Press.

Andersen, R. M. (1995). Revisiting the behavioral model and access to medical care: Does it matter? *Journal of Health and Social Behavior, 36*(1), 1–10.

Anderson, R. N., & Smith, B. L. (2005). Deaths: Leading causes for 2002. *National Vital Statistics Reports, 53*(17).

Ansello, E. F. (2004). Public policy writ small: Coalitions at the intersection of aging and lifelong disabilities. *Public Policy and Aging Report, 14*(4), 1, 3–6.

Antonucci, T. (1990). Social supports and social relationships. In R. H. Binstock & L. K. George (Eds.). *Handbook of aging and the social sciences* (3rd ed., pp. 205–226). San Diego, CA: Academic Press.

Antonucci, T., & Akiyama, H. (1987). Social networks in adult life and a preliminary examination of the convoy model. *Journal of Gerontology, 42,* 519–527.

Antonucci, T., & Akiyama, H. (1995). Convoys of social relations: Family and friendships within a life-span context. In R. Bleiszner & V.H. Bedford, (Eds.) *Handbook of aging and the family* (pp. 355–371). New York: Greenwood Press.

Applebaum, R. A., & Kunkel, S. (1995). Long-term care for the boomers: A public policy challenge for the 21st century. *Southwest Journal on Aging, 11*(1), 25–34.

Arias, E. (2004). United States life tables 2002. *National Vital Statistics Reports, 53*(6).

Aries, P. (1962). *Centuries of childhood: A social history of family life.* New York: Vintage.

Association of Reproductive Health Professionals. (2002). *Mature sexuality clinical proceedings: Who's doing what?* Retrieved April 20, 2006, from http://www.arhp.org/healthcareproviders/cme/onlinecme/maturecmecp/whosdoingwhat.cfm?ID = 45.

Atchley, R. C. (1976). *The sociology of retirement.* New York: Schenkman.

Atchley, R. C. (1989). A continuity theory of normal aging. *The Gerontologist, 29*(2), 183–190.

Atchley, R. C. (1994). *Social forces and aging* (7th ed.). Belmont, CA: Wadsworth.

Atchley, R. C. (1997) *Social forces and aging* (8th ed.). Belmont, CA: Wadsworth/Thompson Learning.

Atchley, R. C. (2004). *Social forces and aging* (10th ed.). Belmont, CA: Wadsworth/Thompson Learning.

Auster, C. (1996). *The sociology of work: Concepts and cases.* Thousand Oaks, CA: Pine Forge Press.

Bachu, A. (1997). Fertility of American women: June 1995 (Update). *Current Population Reports* (pp. 20–499). Retrieved March 8, 1999 from http://www.census.gov.

Barker, J. C. (2002). Neighbors, friends, and other non-kin caregivers of community-living dependent elders. *Journal of Gerontology: Social Sciences, 57B*(3), S158–S167.

Barnes, P. M., Adams, P. F., & Schiller, J. S. (2003). Summary health statistics for the U.S. population: National Health Interview Survey, 2001. National Center for Health Statistics. *Vital Health Stat 10*(217).

Baron, J. N., & Bielby, W. T. (1985). Organizational barriers to gender equality. In A. Rossi (Ed.), *Gender and the life course* (pp. 233–251). New York: Aldine.

Bass, S. A. (Ed.). (1995). *Older and active: How Americans over 55 are contributing to society.* New Haven, CT: Yale University Press.

Becker, G. (1993). Continuity after a stroke: Implications of life-course disruption in old age. *The Gerontologist, 33*(2), 148–158.

Bedford, V. H. (1989). Understanding the value of siblings in old age: A proposed model. *American Behavioral Scientist, 33,* 33–44.

Bedford, V. H. (1995). Sibling relationships in middle and old age. In R. Bleiszner & V. H. Bedford (Eds.), *Handbook of aging and the family* (pp. 201–222). Westport, CT: Greenwood Press.

Beedon, L., & Wu, K. (2005). Women age 65 and older: Their sources of income. *AARP Research Report publication ID: DD126*. Retrieved August 27, 2005 from http://www.aarp.org/research/socialsecurity/benefits/dd126_women.html.

Benbow, A. E. (2004). Increasing access to reliable information on the World Wide Web: Educational tools for web designers, older adults, and caregivers. In D. C. Burdick & S. Kwon (Eds.), *Gerotechnology: Research and practice in technology and aging* (pp. 86–96). New York: Springer.

Bender, K. A., & Jivan, N. A. (2005). *What makes retirees happy?* (Issue Brief #28). Boston: Center for Retirement Research at Boston College.

Bender, W., & Smith, M. (1997). Population, food, and nutrition. *Population Bulletin, 51*(4). Population Reference Bureau.

Bengtson, V. L., Burgess, E. O., & Parrott, T. M. (1997). Theory, explanation, and a third generation of theoretical development in social gerontology. *Journal of Gerontology: Social Sciences, 52B*, S72–S88.

Bengtson, V. L., Cutler, N. E., Mangen, D. J., & Marshall, V. W. (1985). Generations, cohorts, and relations between age groups. In R. H. Binstock & E. Shanas, (Eds.), *Handbook of aging and the social sciences* (2nd ed., pp. 304–338). San Diego, CA: Academic Press.

Bengtson, V. L., Rosenthal, C., & Burton, L. (1990). Families and aging: Diversity and heterogeneity. In R. H. Binstock & L. K. George, (Eds.), *Handbook of aging and the social sciences* (3rd ed., pp. 263–287). San Diego, CA: Academic Press.

Bernard, J. (1972). *The future of marriage*. New York: World.

Bianchi, S. M., & Spain, D. (1996). Women, work, and family in America. *Population Bulletin, 51*(3), 2–48.

Biggs, S., Lowenstein, A., and Hendricks, J. (2003). *The need for theory: Critical approaches to social gerontology*. Amityville, NY: Baywood.

Binstock. R. H. (1991a). Aging, politics, and public policy. In B. B. Hess & E. W. Markson (Eds.), *Growing old in America* (4th ed., pp. 325–340). New Brunswick, NJ: Transaction.

Binstock, R. H. (1991b). From the Great Society to the aging society—25 years of the Older Americans Act. *Generations, 15*(3), 11–18.

Binstock, R. H. (1992). Aging, disability, and long-term care: The politics of common ground. *Generations, 16*(1), 83–88.

Binstock, R. H. (1994). Changing criteria in old-age programs: The introduction of economic status and need for services. *The Gerontologist, 34*(6), 726–730.

Binstock, R. H. (1995). A new era in the politics of aging: How will the old-age interest groups respond? *Generations, 19*(3), 68–74.

Binstock, R. H. (1997). The 1996 election: Older voters and implications for policies on aging. *The Gerontologist, 37*(1), 15–19.

Birren, J. E., & Schaie, K. W. (Eds.). (2006). *Handbook of the psychology of aging* (6th ed.). San Diego, CA: Academic Press.

Blackmar, F. W. (1908). *The elements of sociology*. New York: Macmillan.

Blazer, D. G. (2006). Successful aging. *American Journal of Geriatric Psychiatry, 14*(1), 2–5.

Blendon, R. J., Brodie, M., Benson, J. M., Neuman, T., Altman, D. E., & Hamel, E. C. (2005). American's agenda in aging for the new Congress. *Public Policy & Aging Report, 15*(1), 1, 20–23.

Blumstein, A. (2001). *Why is crime falling*—Or is it? Retrieved August 22, 2005, from http://www.schmalleger.com/pubs/LS2001–2_1.pdf.

Bongaarts, J., & Zimmer, Z. (2002). Living arrangements of older adults in the developing world: An analysis of demographic and health survey household surveys. *Journal of Gerontology: Social Sciences, 57B*(3), S145–S157.

Borden, K. (1995). Dismantling the pyramid: The why and how of privatizing Social Security. *Social Security privatization*. Washington, DC: Cato Institute.

Borglin, G., Edberg, A. K., & Hallberg, I. R. (2005). The experience of quality of life among older people. *Journal of Aging Studies, 19*, 201–220.

Borzi, P. C. (1993). A congressional response to pensions reform. In R. V. Burkhauser & D. L. Salisbury (Eds.), *Pensions in a changing economy* (pp. 111–112). Washington, DC: Employee Benefit Research Institute.

Botwinick, J. (1978). *Aging and behavior*. New York: Springer.

Bound, J., Scheonbaum, M., & Waidmann, T. (1996). Race differences in labor force attachment and disability status. *The Gerontologist, 36*(3), 311–321.

Brody, E. M. (1981). Women in the middle. *The Gerontologist, 21,* 471–480.

Brody, E. M. (1985). Parent care as normative family stress. *The Gerontologist, 25,* 19–29.

Brody, E. M. (2004). *Women in the middle: Their parent care years.* New York: Springer.

Brubaker, T. H. (1990a). *Family relationships in later life.* Newbury Park, CA: Sage.

Brubaker, T. H. (1990b). Families in later life: A burgeoning research area. *Journal of Marriage and the Family, 52*(4), 959–981.

Bryson, K., & Casper, L. M. (1999). Coresident grandparents and grandchildren. *Current Population Reports* (pp. 23–198). Washington, DC: U.S. Government Printing Office. Retrieved August 13, 2005 from http://www.census.gov.

Burkhauser, R. V., & Quinn, J. F. (1994). Changing policy signals. In M. W. Riley, R. L. Kahn, & A. Foner (Eds.), *Aging and structural lag* (pp. 237–262). New York: Wiley-Interscience.

Burkhauser, R. V., & Smeeding, T. M. (1994). Social Security reform: A budget neutral approach to reducing older women's disproportionate risk of poverty. *Policy Brief No 2/1994.* Syracuse, NY: Syracuse University Center for Policy Research.

Burns, B. J., & Taube, C. (1990). Mental health services in general medical care and in nursing homes. In B. S. Fogel, A. Furino, & G. Gottlieb (Eds.), *Mental health policy for older Americans: Protecting minds at risk* (chap. 4). Washington, DC: American Psychiatric Press.

Burton, L. M. (1996). Age norms, the timing of family role transitions and intergenerational caregiving among aging African American women. *The Gerontologist, 36*(2), 199–208.

Burton, L., & DeVries, C. (1995). Challenges and rewards: African-American grandparents as surrogate parents. In L. Burton (Ed.), *Families and aging* (pp. 101–108). Amityville, NY: Baywood.

Butler, R. N. (1989). Dispelling ageism: The cross-cutting intervention. *Annals of the American Academy of Political and Social Sciences, 503,* 138–147.

Button, J. W. (1992). A sign of generational conflict: The impact of Florida's aging voters on local school and tax referenda. *Social Science Quarterly, 73*(4), 786–797.

Button, J. W., & Rosenbaum, W. (1990). Gray power, gray peril, or gray myth?: The political impact of the aging in local sunbelt politics. *Social Science Quarterly, 71*(1), 25–38.

Byrd, M., & Breuss, T. (1992). Perceptions of sociological and psychological age norms by young, middle-aged, and elderly New Zealanders. *International Journal of Aging and Human Development, 34*(2), 145–163.

Cain, L. D. (1987). Alternative perspectives on the phenomena of human aging: Age stratification and age status. *Journal of Applied Behavioral Science, 23*(2), 277–294.

Calasanti, T. M. (1996a). Gender and life satisfaction in retirement: An assessment of the male model. *Journal of Gerontology: Social Sciences, 51B*(1), S18–S29.

Calasanti, T. M. (1996b). Incorporating diversity: Meaning, levels of research, and implications for theory. *The Gerontologist, 36*(2), 147–156.

Callahan, D. (1987). *Setting limits: Medical goals in an aging society.* New York: Simon & Schuster.

Callis, R. R. (2003). Moving to America—moving to homeownership: 1994–2002. *Current Housing Reports H21/03–1.* Washington, DC: U.S. Census Bureau.

Campbell, A. L. (2005). The non-distinctiveness of senior voters in the 2004 election. *Public Policy & Aging Report, 15*(1), 1, 3–6.

Campbell, R. T. (1988). Integrating conceptualization, design, and analysis in panel studies of the life course. In K. W. Schaie, R. T. Campbell, W. Meredith, & S. C. Rawlings (Eds.), *Methodological issues in aging research* (pp. 43–69). New York: Springer.

Campbell, R. T., & O'Rand, A. M. (1985). Settings and sequences: The heuristics of aging research. In J. E. Birren & V. L. Bengtson (Eds.), *Handbook of aging and the social sciences* (pp. 58–79). New York: Springer.

Cantor, M. H. (1983). Strain among caregivers: A study of experience in the United States. *The Gerontologist, 23,* 597–604.

Cantor, M. H. (1995). Families and caregiving in an aging society. In L. Burton (Ed.), *Families and aging* (pp. 135–144). Amityville, NY: Baywood.

Caplan, C., & Brangan, N. (2004). Out-of-pocket spending on health care by Medicare beneficiaries age 65 and older in 2003. *Data Digest.* Washington, DC: AARP Public Policy Institute.

Caro, F. G., Bass, S. A., & Chen, Y. P. (1993). Introduction: Achieving a productive aging society. In S. A. Bass, F. G. Caro, & Y. P. Chen (Eds.), *Achieving a productive aging society* (pp. 3–25). Westport, CT: Auburn House.

Cash & Counseling. (2006). Retrieved March 10, 2006, from http://www.cashandcounseling.org.

Cauthen, N. K. (2005). *Whose security? What Social Security means to children and families.* New York: National Center for Children in Poverty, Columbia University. Retrieved July 18, 2005, from http://www.nccp.org/pub_wsw05a.html.

Center for Health Communication, Harvard School of Public Health. (2004). *Reinventing aging: Baby boomers and civic engagement.* Boston: Harvard School of Public Health.

Center for Retirement Research. (2004). *Most people don't know the Social Security retirement age is rising.* Boston: Center for Retirement Research at Boston College. Retrieved May 24, 2005, from http://www.bc.edu/crr.

Center on an Aging Society. (2004). *Caregivers of older persons data profile: A decade of informal caregiving.* Washington, DC: Georgetown University. Retreived August 20, 2005, from http://ihcrp.georgetown.edu/agingsociety/pubhtml/caregiver.

Center on Budget Policy and Priorities. (2005). *The number of uninsured Americans continues to rise in 2004.* Retrieved May 8, 2006 from http://www.cbpp.org/8-30-05health.htm.

Centers for Medicare and Medicaid Services. (2006). *Medicare and you* 2006. Retrieved May 10, 2006 from http://www.medicare.gov/publications/pubs/pdf/10050.pdf.

Chappell, N. L. (1990). Aging and social care. In R. H. Binstock & L. K. George, (Eds.), *Handbook of aging and the social sciences* (3rd ed., pp. 483–454). San Diego, CA Academic Press.

Chen, Y.-P. (1994). Equivalent retirement ages' and their implications for Social Security and Medicare financing. *The Gerontologist, 34*(6), 731–735.

Chen, Y.-P., & Leavitt, T. D. (1997). The widening gap between White and minority pension coverage. *Public Policy and Aging Report, 8*(1), 10–11.

Cherlin, A. J. (2004). *Public and private families.* Boston: McGraw-Hill.

Cherlin, A. J., & Furstenberg, F. (1986). *The new American grandparent.* New York: Basic Books.

Cicirelli, V. G. (1991). Sibling relationships in adulthood. *Marriage and Family Review, 16*(3/4), 291–310.

Citro, C., & Michaels, R. (1995). *Measuring poverty: A new approach.* Washington, DC: National Academy Press.

Clarke, E. J., Preston, M., Raksin, J., & Bengtson, V. L. (1999). Types of conflicts and tensions between older parents and adult children. *The Gerontologist, 39*(3), 261–270.

Coale, A. (1964). How a population ages or grows younger. In R. Friedman (Ed.), *Population: The vital revolution* (pp. 47–58). Garden City, NY: Anchor Books.

Cockerham, W. C. (1998). *Medical sociology* (7th ed.). Upper Saddle River, NJ: Prentice-Hall.

Cohen, R. A., & Van Nostrand, J. (1995). Trends in the health of older Americans: United States, 1994. National Center for Health Statistics. *Vital and Health Statistics, 3*(30).

Cohler, B. J. (1983). Autonomy and interdependence in the family of adulthood: A psychological perspective. *The Gerontologist, 23,* 33–39.

Cohler, B. J., & Altergott, K. (1995). The family of the second half of life: Connecting theories and findings. In R. Blieszner & V. H. Bedford (Eds.), *Handbook of aging and the family,* (pp. 59–94). Westport, CT: Greenwood Press.

Cole, T. R. (1992). *The journey of life: A cultural history of aging in America.* New York: Cambridge University Press.

Cole, T. R. (1995). What have we "made" of aging? *Journal of Gerontology: Social Sciences, 50B*(6), S341–S343.

Cole, T. R., & Thomson, B. (2001–2002). Introduction: Aging is going out of style. *Generations, 25*(4), 6–8.

Commonwealth Fund. (1993). *The untapped resource: Final report of the Americans Over 55 at Work Program.* New York: Commonwealth Fund.

Condie, S. J. (1989). Older married couples. In S. J. Bahr & E. T. Peterson (Eds.), *Aging and the family* (pp. 143–158). Lexington, MA: Lexington Books.

Congressional Budget Office. (2004). *Financing long-term care for the elderly.* Retrieved May 2006 from http://www.cbo.gov/ftpdocs/54xx/doc5400/04-26-LongTermCare.pdf.

Connidis, I. A., & Davies, L. (1992). Life transitions and the adult sibling tie: A qualitative study. *Journal of Marriage and the Family, 54,* 972–982.

Cooney, T., & Uhlenberg, P. (1990). The role of divorce in men's relations with their adult children after mid-life. *Journal of Marriage and the Family, 52,* 677–688.

Cooperman, L. F., & Keast, F. D. (1983). *Adjusting to an older work force.* New York: Van Nostrand Reinhold.

Cornman, J. M., & Kingson, E. R. (1996). Trends, issues, perspectives, and values for the aging of the baby boom cohorts. *The Gerontologist, 36*(1), 15–26.

Council of State Governments. (1994). *The book of the states (1994–95 ed.) Vol. 30,* Lexington, KY: Council of State Governments.

Cowgill, D. (1972). A theory of aging in cross-cultural perspective. In D. Cowgill & L. Holmes (Eds.), *Aging and modernization.* New York: Appleton-Century-Crofts.

Crown, W. H., Mutschler, P. H., Schulz, J. H., & Loew, R. (1993). *The economic status of divorced older women.* Waltham, MA: Policy Center on Aging, Brandeis University.

Cruise Lines International Association. (1996). *The cruise industry: An overview.* New York: CLIA.

Crystal, S. (1990). Health economics, old-age politics, and the catastrophic Medicare debate. *Journal of Gerontological Social Work, 15*(3–4), 21–31.

Cumming, E., & Henry, W. H. (1961). *Growing old: The process of disengagement.* New York: Basic Books.

Cutler, N. E. (1969–1970). Generation, maturation, and party affiliation: A cohort analysis. *Public Opinion Quarterly, 33,* 583–588.

Cutler, N. E., & Timmerman, S. (Eds.). (2004–2005). Silver industries. *Generations, 28*(4).

Cutler, S. J. (1995).The methodology of social scientific research in gerontology: Progress and issues. *Journals of Gerontology: Social Sciences, 50B*(2), S63–S64.

Dannefer, D. (1988). What's in a name? An account of the neglect of variability in the study of aging. In J. E. Birren & V. L. Bengtson (Eds.), *Emergent theories of aging* (pp. 356–384). New York: Springer.

Davey, A., Savla, J., and Janke, M. (2004). Antecedents of intergenerational support: Families in context and families as context. In M. Silverstein (Ed.), Intergenerational relations across time and place. *Annual review of gerontology and geriatrics, Vol. 24.* New York: Springer.

Day, C. L. (1990). *What older Americans think.* Princeton, NJ: Princeton University Press.

Day, C. L. (1993a). Public opinion toward costs and benefits of Social Security and Medicare. *Research on Aging, 15*(3), 279–298.

Day, C. L. (1993b). Older Americans' attitudes toward the Medicare Catastrophic Coverage Act of 1988. *Journal of Politics, 55,* 167–177.

Day, J. C. (1996) Population projections of the United States by age, sex, race and Hispanic origin 1995–2050. U.S. Bureau of the Census, *Current population reports, P25–1130.* Retrieved June 12, 2005 from http://www.census.gov/prod/2004pubs/04statab/pop.pdf.

Deatrick, D. (1997). Senior-med: Creating a network to help manage medications. *Generations, 21*(3), 59–60.

Depp, C., & Jeste, V. (2006). Definitions and predictors of successful aging: A comprehensive review of larger quantitative studies. *American Journal of Geriatric Psychiatry, 14*(1), 6–20.

DiGiovanna, A. G. (2000). *Human aging: Biological perspectives.* New York: McGraw- Hill.

Dobson, D. (1983). The elderly as a political force. In W. P. Browne & L. K. Olson (Eds.), *Aging and public policy: The politics of growing old in America* (pp. 123–144). Westport, CT: Greenwood Press.

Doeringer, P. B. (1990). Economic security, labor market flexibility and bridges to retirement. In P. B. Doeringer (Ed.), *Bridges to retirement: Older workers in a changing labor market* (pp. 3–19). Ithaca, NY: Cornell University Press.

Doeringer, P. B., & Terkla, D. G. (1990). Business necessity, bridge jobs, and the non-bureaucratic firm. In P. B. Doeringer (Ed.), *Bridges to retirement: Older workers in a changing labor market* (pp. 146–171). Ithaca, NY: Cornell University Press.

Doka, K. J. (1989). *Disenfranchised grief: Recognizing hidden sorrow.* New York: Lexington Books.

Dowd, J. J. (1975). Aging as exchange: A preface to theory. *Journal of Gerontology, 30,* 585–594.

Dowd, J. J. (1980). *Stratification among the aged.* Monterey, CA: Brooks/Cole.

Dowd, J. J. (1981). Age and inequality: A critique of the age stratification model. *Human Development, 24,* 157–171.

Dube, S. C. (1963). Mens' and women's roles in India: A sociological review. In B. Ward (Ed.), *Women in New Asia* (pp. 174–203). Paris: UNESCO.

Dunlop, D. D., Song, J., Lyons, J. S., Mannheim, J. M., & Chang, R. W. (2003). Racial/ethnic differences in rates of depression among preretirement adults. *American Journal of Public Health, 93*(11), 1945–1952.

Duvall, E. M., & Miller, E. C. (1985). *Marriage and family development* (6th ed.). New York: Harper & Row.

Dwyer, J. W. (1995). The effects of illness on the family. In R. Blieszner & V. H. Bedford (Eds.), *Handbook on aging and the family* (pp. 401–421). New York: Greenwood Press.

East, P. L. (1998). Racial and ethnic differences in girls' sexual, marital, and birth expectations. *Journal of Marriage and the Family, 60*(1), 150–162.

Easterlin, R. A. (1987). *Birth and fortune: The impact of numbers on personal welfare* (2nd ed.). Chicago: University of Chicago Press.

Easterlin, R. A. (1996). Economic and social implications of demographic patterns. In R. H. Binstock & L. K. George (Eds.), *Handbook of aging and the social sciences* (4th ed., pp. 73–83). New York: Academic Press.

Edmonson, B. (1997). The facts of death. *American Demographics*, April, 46–53.

Ehrenreich, B., & English, D. (1990). The sexual politics of sickness. In P. Conrad & D. Kerns (Eds.), *The sociology of health and illness: Critical perspectives* (pp. 270–284). New York: St. Martin's Press.

Ehrlich, R. (Ed.). (2000). *Civic responsibility and higher education*. Oryx Press. Retrieved February 1, 2006, from http://www.nytimes.com/ref/college/collegespecial2/.

Ekerdt, D. J. (1986). The busy ethic: Moral continuity between work and retirement. *The Gerontologist, 26*(3), 239–244.

Ekerdt, D. J. (1998). Entitlements, generational equity, and public-opinion manipulation in Kansas City. *The Gerontologist, 38*(5), 525–536.

Ekerdt, D. J., & DeViney, S. (1990). On defining persons as retired. *Journal of Aging Studies, 4*(3), 211–229.

Ekerdt, D. J., DeViney, S., & and Kosloski, K. (1996). Profiling plans for retirement. *Journal of Gerontology: Social Sciences, 41B*(3), S140–S149.

Elman, C., & O'Rand, A. M. (2004). The race is to the swift: Socioeconomic origins, adult education, and wage attainment. *American Journal of Sociology, 110*(1), 123–160.

Employee Benefit Research Institute. (2004). *Databook*. Retrieved June 22, 2005 from http://www.ebri.org/pdf/publications/books/databook.

Epstein, J. S. (1994). *Adolescents and their music: If it's too loud, you're too old*. New York: Garland.

Erikson, E., Erikson, J. M., & Kivnick, H. (1986). *Vital involvement in old age: The experience of old age in our time*. London: Norton.

Espo, D. (2005, June 16). Senators consider boosting Social Security retirement age to 69. *Detroit News*. Retrieved July 29, 2005 from http://www.detnews.com/2005/politics/0506/16/0pols-217281.htm.

Estes, C. L. (1979). *The aging enterprise*. San Francisco: Jossey-Bass.

Estes, C. L. (1991). The new political economy of aging: Introduction and critique. In M. Minkler & C. L. Estes (Eds.), *Critical perspectives on aging: The political and moral economy of growing old* (pp. 19–36). Amityville, NY: Baywood.

Estes, C. L. (1999). Critical gerontology and the new political economy of aging. In M. Minkler & C. Estes (Eds.), *Critical gerontology: Perspectives from political and moral economy*. Amityville, NY: Baywood.

Estes, C., & Binney, E. (1991). The biomedicalization of aging: Dangers and dilemmas. In M. Minkler & C. L. Estes (Eds.), *Critical perspectives on aging: The political and moral economy of growing old* (pp. 117–134). Amityville, NY: Baywood.

Federal Interagency Forum on Aging-Related Statistics. (2004). *Older Americans 2004: Key indicators of well-being*. Washington, DC: U.S. Government Printing Office.

Ferraro, K. F. (Ed.). (1997). *Gerontology: Perspectives and issues* (2nd ed.). New York: Springer.

Ferraro, K. F., & LaGrange, R. L. (1992). Are older people most afraid of crime? Reconsidering age differences in fear of victimization. *Journal of Gerontology: Social Sciences, 47*(5), S233–S244.

Feuerbach, E. J., & Erdwins, C. J. (1994). Women's retirement: The influence of work history. *Journal of Women and Aging, 6*(3), 69–85.

Fields, G. S., & Mitchell, O. S. (1984). *Retirement, pensions, and Social Security*. Cambridge, MA: MIT Press.

Fields, J., & Casper, L. M. (2001). Americans families and living arrangements. *Current Population Reports P20–537*. Washington, DC: U.S. Bureau of the Census.

Finch, J. F., & Graziano, W. G. (2001). Predicting depression from temperament, personality, and patterns of social relations. *Journal of Personality, 69*, 27–55.

Finley, N. J., Roberts, M. D., & Banahan, B. F. (1988). Motivators and inhibitors of attitudes toward aging parents. *The Gerontologist, 28*(1), 73–78.

Firebaugh, G., & Chen, K. (1995).Vote turnout of Nineteenth Amendment women: The enduring effect of disenfranchisement. *American Journal of Sociology, 100*(4), 972–976.

Flowers, L., Gross, L., Kuo, P., & Sinclair, S. (2005). *State profiles 2005: Reforming the health care system.* Washington, DC: AARP Public Policy Institute.

Fogel, B. S., Gottlieb, G., & Furino, A. (1990). Minds at risk. In B. S. Fogel, A. Furino, & G. Gottlieb (Eds.), *Mental health policy for older Americans: Protecting minds at risk* (chap. 1). Washington, DC: American Psychiatric Press.

Foner, A. (1973). The polity. In M. W. Riley, M. Johnson, and A. Foner, (Eds.), *Aging and society: Vol. 3. A sociology of age stratification* (pp. 115–159). New York: Russell Sage Foundation.

Foner, A. (1996). Age norms and the structure of consciousness: Some final comments. *The Gerontologist, 36*(2), 221–223.

Forbes Magazine. (2005). *Forbes 400 richest people in America.* Retrieved August 5, 2005 from http://www.forbes.com/tool/toolbox/rich400/asp/rich.asp.

Foster, L., Brown, R., Phillips, B., Schore, J., & Carlson, B. (2003). Improving the quality of Medicaid personal assistance through consumer direction. *Health affairs data watch: Medicaid,* March 26.

Frank, J. B. (2002). *The paradox of aging in place in assisted living.* Westport, CT: Bergin & Garvey.

Fredonia Group. (2006). *Anti-aging products to 2009.* Retrieved March 11, 2006, from http://www.biz-lib.com/ZFR69320.html.

Freedman, V. A., Martin, L. G., & Schoeni, R. F. (2002). Recent trends in disability and functioning among older adults in the United States: A systematic review. *Journal of the American Medical Association, 288*(24), 3137–3146.

Freund, P. E., & McGuire, M. B. (1995). *Health, illness, and the social body.* Englewood Cliffs, NJ: Prentice-Hall.

Freund, P. E., & McGuire, M. B. (1999). *Health, illness, and the social body* (3rd ed.). Englewood Cliffs, NJ: Prentice-Hall.

Friedland, R. B., & Summer, L. (1999). *Demography is not destiny.* Washington, DC: National Academy on Aging, Gerontological Society of America.

Friedland, R. B., & Summer, L. (2005). *Demography is not destiny, revisited.* Washington, DC: Center on an Aging Society, Georgetown University Commonwealth Pub # 789.

Fuentes, B. (1991). Bank of America—An advocate for older workers. In *Resourceful aging: Vol. 4. Work/second careers* (pp. 73–75). Washington, DC: American Association of Retired Persons.

Furlong, M. (1997). Creating online community for older adults. *Generations, 21*(3), 33–35.

Gale, W. G., Iwry, M., Munnell, A. H., & Thaler, R. H. (2004). *Improving 401(k) investment performance.* Boston: Center for Retirement Research Issue Brief #26, Boston University.

Gallup Organization. (2005). *May economic poll.* Retrieved July 24, 2005 from http://poll.gallup.com/.

Gatz, M., Bengtson, V. L., & Blum, M. J. (1990). Caregiving families. In J. E. Birren & K. W. Schaie (Eds.), *Handbook of the psychology of aging* (3rd ed.). (pp. 404–426). San Diego, CA: Academic Press.

Gelles, R. J., & Cavanaugh, M. M. (2005). Elder abuse is caused by the perception of stress associated with providing care. In D. R. Loeske, R. J. Gelles, and M. M. Cavanaugh (Eds.), *Current controversies in family violence* (2nd ed.). Thousand Oaks, CA: Sage.

Gendell, M. (2005). *Short work lives, long retirements make saving difficult.* Population Reference Bureau. Retrieved May 10, 2005 from http://www.prb.org/Template.cfm?Section = PRB& template = /ContentManagement/ContentDisplay.cfm&ContentID = 5590.

Gendell, M., & Siegel, J. S. (1992). Trends in retirement age by sex, 1950–2005. *Monthly Labor Review, 115*(7), 22–29.

Gendell, M., & Siegel, J. S. (1996). Trends in retirement age in the United States, 1955–1993, by sex and race. *Journal of Gerontology: Social Sciences, 51B*(3), S132–S139.

George, L. K. (1995). The last half-century of aging research and thoughts for the future. *Journal of Gerontology: Social Sciences, 50B*(1), S1–S3.

George, L. K. (1996). Missing links: The case for a social psychology of the life course. *The Gerontologist, 36*(2), 248–255.

George, L. K. (2003). What life course perspectives offer the study of aging and health. In R. Settersten (Ed.), *Invitation to the life course: Toward new understandings of later life* (pp. 161–188). Amityville, NY: Baywood.

Gerontology Research Group. (2006). Retrieved from http://www.grg.org.

Gewerth, K. E. (1988). Elderly offenders: A review of previous research. In B. McCarthy & R. Langworthy (Eds.), *Older offenders: Perspectives in criminology and criminal justice* (pp. 14–31). New York: Praeger.

Giarrusso, R., Feng, D., and Bengtson, V. L. (2004). Charting the intergenerational-stake over historical and biographical time. In M. Silverstein (Ed.), Intergenerational relations across time and place. *Annual review of gerontology and geriatrics, Vol. 24.* New York: Springer.

Gibson, R. (1996). The black American retirement experience. In J. Quadagno & D. Street (Eds.), *Aging for the twenty-first century* (pp. 309–326). New York: St. Martin's Press.

Glaser, B. G., & Strauss, A. L. (1967). *The discovery of grounded theory: Strategies for qualitative research.* Chicago: Aldine.

Glass, T. (1998). Conjugating the "tenses" of function: Discordance among hypothetical experimental, and enacted function in older adults. *The Gerontologist, 38*(1), 101–112.

Glazer, N. Y. (1993). *Women's paid and unpaid labor.* Philadelphia: Temple University Press.

Glick, P. C. (1977). Updating the life-cycle of the family. *Journal of Marriage and the Family, 39*(1), 5–13.

Goffman, E. (1969). *The presentation of self in everyday life.* London: Allen Lane.

Goldstein, S. (1960). *Consumption patterns of the aged.* Philadelphia: University of Pennsylvania Press.

Goldstein, C., & Beall, C. M. (1983). Modernization and aging in the third and fourth world: Views from the rural hinterland in Nepal. *Human Organization, 1,* 48–49.

Goldstein, J. R., & Kenney, C. T. (2001). Marriage delayed or marriage forgone? New cohort forecasts of first marriage for U.S. women. *American Sociological Review, 66*(4), 506–519.

Goss, S. C. (1997). *Comparison of financial effects of advisory council plans to modify the OASDI Program.* Retrieved April 24, 2000, from http://www.ssa.gov./search97cgi.

Goyal, R. S. (1989). Some aspects of aging in India. In R. N. Pati & B. Jena (Eds.), *Aged in India: Sociodemographic dimensions.* New Delhi, India: Ashish.

Gross, C. P., Anderson, G. F., & Powe, N. R. (1999). The relation between funding by the National Institutes of Health and the burden of disease. *New England Journal of Medicine, 340,* 1881–1886.

Grove, L. (1996, April 8). The 100-year-old senator? Some fans, foes say quit. Strom Thurmond says no. *Washington Post.*

Guillemard, A. M. (1996). The trend toward early labor force withdrawal and the reorganization of the life course: A cross-national analysis. In J. Quadagno & D. Street (Eds.), *Aging for the twenty-first century* (pp. 167–176). New York: St. Martin's Press.

Gupta, G. R. (1976). Love, arranged marriage, and the Indian social structure. *Journal of Comparative Family Studies, 7,* 75–85.

Guy, R. F., & Erdner, R. A. (1993). Retirement: An emerging challenge for women. In R. Kastenbaum (Ed.), *Encyclopedia of adult development* (pp. 405–409). Phoenix, AZ: Oryx Press.

Hagburg, B. (1995). The individual's life history as a formative experience to aging. In B. K. Haight & J. D. Webster (Eds.), *The art and science of reminiscing* (pp. 61–76). Washington, DC: Taylor & Francis.

Hagestad, G. O. (2003). Interdependent lives and relationships in changing times: A life course view of families and aging. In R. Settersten (Ed.), *Invitation to the life course: Toward new understandings of later life* (pp. 135–160). Amityville, NY: Baywood.

Hamil-Luker, J., & Uhlenberg, P. (2002). Later life education in the 1990s: Increasing involvement and continuing disparity. *Journal of Gerontology: Social Sciences, 57B*(6), S324–S331.

Hardy, M. A., Hazelrigg, L. E., & Quadagno, J. (1996). *Ending a career in the auto industry: Thirty and out.* New York: Plenum.

Hardy, M. A., & Quadagno, J. (1995). Satisfaction with early retirement: Making choices in the auto industry. *Journal of Gerontology: Social Sciences, 50*(4), S217–S228.

Hareven, T. K. (1993). Family and generational relations in the later years: A historical perspective. In. L. Burton (Ed.) *Families and aging* (pp. 7–22). Amityville, NY: Baywood.

Hareven, T. K. (1994). Family change and historical change: An uneasy relationship. In M. W. Riley, R. L. Kane, & A. Foner (Eds.), *Aging and structural lag* (pp. 130–150). New York: Wiley-Interscience.

Hareven, T. K. (1995). Historical perspectives on the family and aging. In R. Blieszner & V. H. Bedford (Eds.), *Handbook of aging and the family* (pp. 13–31). Westport, CT: Greenwood Press.

Harrington Meyer, M. (1996). Making claims as workers or wives: The distribution of Social Security benefits. *American Sociological Review, 61,* 449–465.

Harris, S. B. (1995). Spouse abuse in the elderly: Is it spouse abuse grown old? (Doctoral dissertation, Cornell University, 1995). *Dissertation Abstracts International, 45,* 13–31.

Hayflick, L. (2001–2002). Anti-aging medicine: Hype, hope, and reality. *Generations, 25*(4), 20–25.

Hayward, M. D., Friedman, S., & Chen, S. (1996). Race inequalities in men's retirement. *Journal of Gerontology: Social Sciences, 51B*(1), S1–S10.

Hazelrigg, L. (1997). On the importance of age. In M. A. Hardy (Ed.), *Studying aging and social change* (pp. 93–128). Thousand Oaks, CA: Sage.

HCFA (Health Care Financing Administration). (1992). *Health care financing review: Medicare and Medicaid statistical supplement.* Baltimore: U.S. Department of Health and Human Services.

He, W., Sengupta, M., Velkoff, V., & DeBarros, K. (2005). 65+ in the United States: 2005. *Current Population Reports, P23–209.* Washington, DC: U.S. Government Printing Office.

Health and Retirement Study. (2006). Retrieved July 21, 2005 from http://hrsonline.isr.umich.edu.

Healthy People 2010. (2006). Retrieved 12/10/2005, from http://www.healthypeople.gov.

Helton, D. R. (1997, April). A look at how Kentuckians in Knox County once treated the dead. *Kentucky Explorer,* 34–39.

Hendricks, J. (1992). Generations and the generation of theory in social gerontology. *International Journal of Aging and Human Development, 35*(1), 31–47.

Hendricks, J., & Cutler, S. (2003). Leisure in life course perspective. In. R. Settersten (Ed.), *Invitation to the life course: Toward new understandings of later life* (pp. 107–134). Amityville, NY: Baywood.

Henretta, J. C. (2003). Social structure and age-based careers. In M. W. Riley, R. L. Kahn, & A. Foner (Eds.). *Age and structural lag* (pp. 57–79). New York: Wiley-Interscience.

Herd, P. (2005). Ensuring a minimum: Social Security reform and women. *The Gerontologist, 45*(1), 12–25.

Herz, D. E. (1995), Work after early retirement: An increasing trend among men. *Monthly Labor Review, 118*(4), 13–20.

Hess, B. B., & Waring, J. H. (1978). Changing patterns of aging and family bonds in later life. *Family Coordinator, 27,* 303–314.

Hill, R. (1965). Decision making and the family life cycle. In E. Shanas & G. F. Streib (Eds.) *Social structure and the family: Generational relations* (pp. 114–126). Englewood Cliffs, NJ: Prentice-Hall.

Hill, R. (1970). *Family development in three generations.* Cambridge, MA: Schenkman.

Hillier, S., & Barrow, G. (1999). *Aging, the individual, and society* (7th ed.). Belmont, CA: Wadsworth Press.

Hobbs, F. B., & Damon, B. L. (1996). 65+ in the United States. *Current Population Reports, P-23,* No. 190. Washington, DC: U.S. Government Printing Office.

Hochschild, A. R. (1975). Disengagement theory: A critique and proposal. *American Sociological Review, 14*(5), 553–569.

Hogan, D. P., & Astone, N. M. (1986). The transition to adulthood. *Annual Review of Sociology, 12,* 109–130.

Hogan, D. P., Eggebeen, D. J., & Clogg, C. C. (1993). The structure of intergenerational exchanges in American families. *American Journal of Sociology, 98*(6), 1428–1458.

Hogarth, J. M. (1991). Involving older persons in the labor force: An agenda for the future. In *Resourceful aging: Vol. 4. Work/second careers* (pp. 101–108). Washington, DC: American Association of Retired Persons.

Holden, K. C., & Kuo, H.-H. D. (1996). Complex marital histories and economic well-being: The continuing legacy of divorce and widowhood as the HRS cohort approaches retirement. *The Gerontologist, 36*(3), 383–390.

Holstein, M. (1995). The normative case: Chronological age and public policy. *Generations, 19*(3), 11–14.

Holstein, M., & Minkler, M. (1991). The short life and painful death of the Medicare Catastrophic Coverage Act. In M. Minkler & C. L. Estes (Eds.), *Critical perspectives on aging: The political and moral economy of growing old* (pp. 189–204). Amityville, NY: Baywood.

Holtz-Eakin, D., & Smeeding, T. M. (1994). Income, wealth, and intergenerational economic relations of the aged. In L. G. Martin & S. H. Preston (Eds.), *Demography of aging* (pp. 102–145). Washington, DC: National Academy Press.

Horowitz, A. (1985a). Family caregiving to the frail elderly. *Annual Review of Gerontology and Geriatrics, 6,* 194–246.

Horowitz, A. (1985b). Sons and daughters as caregivers to older parents: Differences in role performance and consequences. *The Gerontologist, 25*(6), 612–617.

Hoskins, D. D. (1992). Developments and trends in Social Security, 1990–1992: Overview of principal trends. *Social Security Bulletin, 55*(4), 36–42.

Hoyert, D. L., Heron, M. P., Murphy, S. L., & Kung H. C. (2006). Deaths: Final data for 2003. *National Vital Statistics Report, 54*(13).

HSBC/AgeWave. (2005). *The future of retirement in a world of rising life expectancies.* Retrieved from http://www.hsbc.com/public/groupsite/retirement_future/en.

Hu, Y., & Goldman, M. (1990). Mortality differentials by marital status: An international comparison. *Demography, 27*(2), 223–250.

Hudson, R. (1978). The "graying" of the federal budget and its consequences for old-age policy. *The Gerontologist, 18,* 428–440.

Hudson, R. (1996). The changing face of aging politics. *The Gerontologist, 36*(1), 33–35.

Hudson, R. B. (2005). *The new politics of old age policy.* Baltimore: Johns Hopkins University Press.

Hunt, G. G. (1997). Cleveland free-net Alzheimer's forum. *Generations, 21*(3), 37.

Huyck, M. H. (1995). Marriage and close relationships of the marital kind. In R. Blieszner & V. H. Bedford (Eds.), *Handbook of aging and the family* (pp. 181–200). Westport, CT: Greenwood Press.

Ikels, C. (1993). Chinese kinship and the state: Shaping of policy for the elderly. In G. L. Maddox & M. P. Lawton (Eds.), *Annual review of gerontology and geriatrics: Focus on kinship, aging, and social change* (Vol. 13. pp. 123–146). New York: Springer.

Infoplease. (2003). *2003 median annual earnings by race and sex.* Retrieved May 9, 2005 from http://www.infoplease.com/ipa/A0197814.html.

Jackson, J. S., & Gibson, R. C. (1985). Work and retirement among the black elderly. In Z. S. Blau (Ed.), *Work, retirement, and social policy* (pp. 193–222). Greenwich, CT: JAI Press.

Jacobs, B. (1990). Aging and politics. In R. H. Binstock & L. K. George (Eds.), *Handbook of aging and the social sciences* (3rd ed., pp. 349–361). San Diego, CA: Academic Press.

Jacobs, L. R., & Burns, M. (2005). Don't lump seniors. *Public Policy & Aging Report, 15*(1): 7–9.

James, J. B., and P. Wink. (2006). The crown of life: Dynamics of the early post-retirement period. *Annual review of gerontology and geriatrics, Vol. 26.* New York: Springer.

Jarrett, W. H. (1985). Caregiving within kinship systems: Is affection really necessary? *The Gerontologist, 25*(1), 5–20.

Johnson, C. L. (1995a). Divorce and reconstituted families: Effects on the older generation. In L. Burton (Ed.), *Families and aging* (pp. 33–41). Amityville, NY: Baywood.

Johnson, C. L. (1995b). Cultural diversity in the late-life family. In R. Blieszner & V. H. Bedford (Eds.), *Handbook of aging and the family* (pp. 307–331). Westport, CT: Greenwood Press.

Johnson, E. H. (1988). Care for elderly inmates: Conflicting concerns and purposes in prisons. In B. McCarthy & R. Langworthy (Eds.), *Older offenders: Perspectives in criminology and criminal justice* (pp. 157–163). New York: Praeger.

Johnson, E. S., & Williamson, J. B. (1987). Retirement in the United States. In K. S. Markides & C. L. Copper (Eds.), *Retirement in industrialized societies* (pp. 9–41). New York: Wiley.

Johnson, R. W., & Favreault, M. M. (2004). Economic status in later life among women who raised children outside of marriage. *Journal of Gerontology: Social Sciences, 59B*(6), S315–S323.

Johnson, R. W., & Schaner, S. G. (2005). Value of unpaid activities by older Americans tops $160 billion per year. *Perspectives on productive aging.* Washington, DC: Urban Institute.

Johnson, R. W., Uccello, C. E., & Goldwyn, J. H. (2005). Who forgoes survivor protection in employer-sponsored pension annuities? *The Gerontologist, 45*(1), 26–35.

Jones, T. W. (1996). Strengthening the current Social Security system. *Public Policy and Aging Report, 7*(3), 1, 3–6.

Kahn, J. R., & Mason, W. M. (1987). Political alienation, cohort size, and the Easterlin hypothesis. *American Sociological Review, 52*(2), 155–169.

Kahn, R. (1994). Opportunities, aspirations, and goodness of fit. In M. W. Riley, R. L. Kahn, & A. Foner (Eds.), *Aging and structural lag* (pp. 37–53). New York: Wiley-Interscience.

Kaiser Family Foundation. (2005). *Medicare fact sheet: Medicare at a glance.* Publication number 1066–08. Retrieved April 18, 2006, from www.kkf.org.

Kaiser Family Foundation. (2006). *Trends and indicators in the changing care marketplace.* Publication number 7031. Retrieved April 2, 2006, from www.kff.org/insurance/7031.

Kane, J. N. (1993). *Facts about the presidents.* New York: Wilson.

Kane, R. A. (2004). Coalitions between aging and disability interests: Potential effects on choice and control for older people. *Public Policy and Aging Report, 14*(4), 15–18.

Kane, R. A., & Kane, R. L. (1987). *Long-term care: Principles, programs, and policies.* New York: Springer.

Kane, R. A., Kane, R. L., & Ladd, R. C. (1998). *The heart of long-term care.* New York: Oxford University Press.

Kasl, S. V. (1995). Strategies in research on health and aging: Looking beyond secondary data analysis. *Journal of Gerontology: Social Sciences, 50*(4), S191–S193.

Kassner, E. (2006). Medicaid and long-term services and supports for older people. *Research report.* Washington, DC: AARP Public Policy Institute.

Kastenbaum, R. (1993). Disengagement theory. In R. Kastenbaum (Ed.), *Encyclopedia of adult development* (pp. 126–130). Phoenix, AZ: Oryx Press.

Katz, S., Downs, T., Cash, H., & Grotz, R. (1970). Progress in the development of the Index of ADL. *The Gerontologist, 10*(1), 20–30.

Kayser-Jones, J. (2002). The experience of dying: An ethnographic nursing home study. *The Gerontologist, 42*(3), 11–19.

Kelley, C. L., & Charness, N. (1995). Issues in training older adults to use computers. *Behaviour & Information Technology, 14*(2), 107–120.

Kennedy, G. E. (1990). College students' expectations of grandparent and grandchild role behaviors. *The Gerontologist, 30*(1), 43–48.

Kent, M. M., & Haub, C. (2005). Global demographic divide. *Population Bulletin, 60*(4). Washington, DC: Population Reference Bureau.

Kim, J. E., & Moen, P. (2002). Retirement transitions, gender, and psychological well-being: A life-course, ecological model. *Journal of Gerontology: Psychological Sciences, 57B*(3), P212–P222.

Kimmel, D. C. (1993). The families of older gay men and lesbians. In L. Burton (Ed.), *Families and aging* (pp. 75–79). Amityville, NY: Baywood.

Kingson, E. R. (1994). Testing the boundaries of universality: What's mean? What's not? *The Gerontologist, 34*(6), 736–742.

Kingson, E. R., Hirshorn, B. A., & Cornman, J. M. (1986). *Ties that bind: The interdependence of generations.* Washington, DC: Seven Locks Press.

Kinsella, K., & Gist, Y. (1995). *Older workers, retirement, and pensions.* Washington, DC: U.S. Bureau of the Census.

Kinsella, K., & Phillips, D. R. (2005). Global aging: The challenge of success. *Population Bulletin, 60*(1), 3–42.

Kinsella, K., & Taeuber, C. M. (1993). *An aging world II.* Washington, DC: U.S. Bureau of the Census.

Kinsella, K., & Velkoff, V. (2001). *An aging world: 2001.* U.S. Census Bureau Series P95/01–1. Washington, DC: U.S. Government Printing Office.

Klaus, P. (2005). *Crimes against persons age 65 or older, 1993–2002.* Special report: Bureau of Justice Statistics. Retrieved August 21, 2005 from http://www.ojp.usdoj.gov/bjs/abstract/cpa6502.htm.

Kmart pharmacists win $2.17 million in age-discrimination case. (1995, August 5). *Detroit News.*

Kneese, A., & Cooper, C. L. (1993). Demography, resources, and the environment: Further considerations. In *Aging of the U.S. population: Economic and environmental implications.* (pp. 61–68). Washington, DC: American Association of Retired Persons.

Kobayashi, K. M., Martin-Matthews, A., Rosenthal, C. J., & Matthews, S. (2001). *The timing and duration of women's life course events: A study of mothers with at least two children.* Hamilton, Ontario: Research Institute for Quantitative Studies in Economics and Population, McMaster University.

Kochanek, K. D., Murphy, S. L., Anderson, R. N., & Scott C. (2004). Deaths: Final data for 2002. *National Vital Statistics Reports, 53*(5).

Kohli, M. (1994). Work and retirement: A comparative perspective. In M. W. Riley, R. L. Kahn, & A. Foner (Eds.), *Aging and structural lag* (pp. 80–106). New York: Wiley-Interscience.

Korczyk, S. M. (2004). *Is early retirement ending?* Washington, DC: AARP Public Policy Institute. Retrieved June 25, 2006 from http://www.aarp.org/ppi.

Kovar, M. G., & Lawton, M. P. (1994). Functional disability: Activities and instrumental activities of daily living. In *Annual review of gerontology and geriatrics: Focus on assessment techniques* (Vol. 14). New York: Springer.

Krach, C., & Velkoff, V. (1999). Centenarians in the United States. *Current Population Reports* P23–199RV.

Kramer, B. J. (1997). Gain in the caregiving experience: Where are we? What next? *The Gerontologist, 37*, 218–232.

Kranczer, S. (1994). Outlook for U.S. population growth. *Statistical Bulletin, 75*(4), 19–26.

Krause, N. (2001). Social support. In R. Binstock & L. George (Eds.), *Handbook of aging and the social sciences* (5th ed., pp. 273–294). San Diego, CA: Academic Press.

Krause, N., & Rook, K. S. (2003). Negative interaction in late life: Issues in the stability and generalizability of conflict across relationships. *Journal of Gerontology: Psychological Sciences, 58B*, P88–P99.

Ku, L., & Guyer, J. (2001). *Medicaid spending: Rising again, but not to crisis levels.* Center on Budget and Policy Priorities. Retrieved March 2, 2006 from http://www.cbpp.org/4-20-01health.pdf.

Kubler-Ross, E. (1969). *On death and dying.* New York: Macmillan.

Kuhn, T. S. (1996). *The structure of scientific revolutions* (3rd ed.). Chicago: University of Chicago Press.

Kunkel, S., & Atchley, R. C. (1996). Why gender matters: Being female is not the same as not being male. *American Journal of Preventive Medicine, 12*(5), 294–295.

Kunkel, S., & Nelson, I. (2005). Consumer direction: Changing the landscape of long-term care. *Public Policy & Aging Report, 15*(4), 13–16.

Kunkel, S., & Subedi, J. (1996). Aging in south Asia: How "imperative" is the demographic imperative? In Minichiello, V., Chappell, N., Kendig, H., & Walker, A.(Eds.), *Sociology of aging* (pp. 459–466). Melbourne, Australia: International Sociological Association, Toth Publishing.

Kunkel, S., and Wellin, V. (2006). *Consumer voice and choice in long-term care.* New York: Springer.

Lashbrook, J. (1996). Promotional timetables: An exploratory investigation of age norms for promotional expectations and their associations with job well-being. *The Gerontologist, 36*(2), 189–198.

Laslett, P. (1991). *A fresh map of life: The emergence of the third age.* Cambridge, MA: Harvard University Press.

Lassey, M., Lassey, W., & Jinks, M. (1997). *Health care systems around the world.* Upper Saddle River, NJ: Prentice-Hall.

Laub, J. H., Nagin, D. S., & Sampson, R. J. (1998). Trajectories of change in criminal offending: good marriages and the desistance process. *American Sociological Review, 63* (April), 225–238.

Lave, J. (1996). Rethinking Medicare. *Generations, 20*(2), 19–23.

LaViest, T. A. (1995). Data sources for aging research on racial and ethnic groups. *The Gerontologist, 35*(3), 328–339.

Lawrence, B. S. (1996). Organizational age norms: Why is it so hard to know one when you see one? *The Gerontologist, 36*(2), 209–220.

Lawton, M. P. (1986). *Environment and aging.* Classics in Aging Reprinted Series 1, Vol. 1. New York: Center for the Study of Aging.

Lawton, M. P., & Herzog, A. R. (1989). Introduction. In M. P. Lawton & A. R. Herzog (Eds.), *Special research methods for gerontology* (pp. v–viii). Amityville, NY: Baywood.

Lawton, M. P., Moss, M., Kleban, M. H., Glicksman, A., & Rovine, A. (1991). A two-factor model of caregiving appraisal and psychological well-being. *Journal of Gerontology: Psychological Sciences, 46*, P181–P189.

Lee, G. R. (1988). Marital satisfaction in later life: The effects of nonmarital roles. *Journal of Marriage and the Family, 50*(3), 775–783.

Lee, R., & Haaga, J. (2002). Government spending in an older America. *Population Reference Bureau Reports on America, 3*(1).

Leiberman, M. A., & Tobin, S. S. (1976). *Last home for the aged.* San Francisco: Jossey-Bass.

Lemon, B. W., Bengtson, V. L., & Peterson, J. A. (1972). An exploration of the activity theory of aging: Activity types and life expectation among in-movers to a retirement community. *Journal of Gerontology, 27*, 511–523.

Leonesio, M. V., Vaughn, D. R., & Wixon, B. (2000). Early retirees under Social Security: Health status and economic resources. Washington, DC: Social Security Administration. Retrieved June 26, 2005 from http://www.ssa.gov/policy/docs/workingpapers/wp86.pdf.

Levine, R., Sato, S., Hashimoto, T., & Verma, J. (1995). Love and marriage in eleven cultures. *Journal of Cross-Cultural Psychology, 26*, 554–571.

Liang, J., Krause, N., & Bennett, J. (2001). Social exchange and well-being: Is giving better than receiving? *Psychology and Aging, 16*, 511–523.

Liang, J., & Lawrence, R. H. (1989). Secondary analysis of surveys in gerontological research. In M. P. Lawton & A. R. Herzog (Eds.), *Special research methods for gerontology* (pp. 31–61). Amityville, NY: Baywood.

Lichstenstein, J., & Wu, K. B. (2000). *Pension and IRA coverage among boomer, pre-boomer and older workers.* Washington, DC: AARP Public Policy Institute. Retrieved July 12, 2005 from http://www.aarp.org/policy.

Lindquist, L. A., & Golub, R. M. (2004). Cruise ship care: A proposed alternative to assisted living facilities. *Journal of the American Geriatrics Society, 52*(11), 1951.

Linton, R. (1942). Age and sex categories. *American Sociological Review, 7,* 589–603.

Litwak, E. (1960). Geographic mobility and extended family cohesion. *American Sociological Review, 25,* 385–394.

Litwak, E. (1965). Extended kin relations in an industrial society. In E. Shanas & G. Streib (Eds.), *Social structure and the family: Generational relations* (pp. 290–323). Englewood Cliffs, NJ: Prentice-Hall.

Long-Foley, K., Tung, H., & Mutran, E. J. (2002). Self-gain and self-loss among African American and White caregivers. *Journal of Gerontology: Social Sciences, 57B*(1), S14–S22.

Longino, C. F., Jr. (1990). Geographical distribution and migration. In R. H. Binstock & L. K. George (Eds.), *Handbook of aging and the social sciences* (3rd ed., pp. 45–63). San Diego, CA: Academic Press.

Lopata, H. Z. (1979). *Women as widows: Support systems.* New York: Elsevier.

Lueschler, K., & Pillemer, K. (1998). Intergenerational ambivalence: A new approach to the study of parent–child relations in later life. *Journal of Marriage and the Family, 60*(2), 413–425.

Lund, D. A., Caserta, M. S., Dimond, M. F., & Shaffer, S. K. (1989). Competencies, tasks of daily living, and adjustments to spousal bereavement in later life. In D. A. Lund (Ed.), *Older bereaved spouses* (pp. 135–152). New York: Hemisphere.

Lynch, S. M., Brown, J. S., & Harmsen, K. G. (2003). The effect of altering ADL thresholds on active life expectancy estimates for older persons. *Journal of Gerontology: Social Sciences, 58,* S171–S178.

Machemer, R. (1992). *The news in the biology of aging: The good, the bad, and the confusing.* Paper presented at annual meeting of the Association for Gerontology in Higher Education. Baltimore, MD.

Macionis, J. J. (1997). *Sociology.* Upper Saddle River, NJ: Prentice-Hall.

Maddox, G. L. (1968). Retirement as a social event in the United States. In B. L. Neugarten (Ed.), *Middle age and aging* (pp. 357–365). Chicago: University of Chicago Press.

Maddox, G. L., & Lawton, M. P. (1988). Varieties of aging. *Annual review of gerontology and geriatrics, Vol. 8.* New York: Springer.

Maddox, G. L., & Lawton, M. P. (Eds.). (1993). *Annual review of gerontology and geriatrics: Focus on kinship, aging, and social change.* New York: Springer.

Mannheim, K. (1952a). *Ideology and utopia.* New York: Harcourt, Brace & World.

Mannheim, K. (1952b). *Essays on the sociology of knowledge* (P. Kecskemeti, Ed.). New York: Oxford University Press.

Markides, K. S., Liang, J., & Jackson, J. S. (1990). Race, ethnicity, and aging: Conceptual and methodological issues. In R. H. Binstock & L. K. George (Eds.), *Handbook of aging and the social sciences* (3rd ed., pp. 112–129). San Diego, CA: Academic Press.

Marmour, T. R., Mashaw, J. L., & Harvey, P. L. (1990). *America's misunderstood welfare state: Persistent myths, enduring realities.* New York: Basic Books.

Martin, G. M. (2000). Genetic influences on late-life diseases. *Generations, 24*(1), 8–11.

Martin, L., & Kinsella, K. (1994). Research in the demography of aging in developing countries. In L. Martin & S. Preston (Eds.), *Demography of aging.* Washington, DC: National Academic Press.

Martin, P. J. (1995). *Sounds and society: Themes in the sociology of music.* Manchester, England: Manchester University Press.

Matras, J. (1990). *Dependency, obligations, and entitlements: A new sociology of aging, the life course, and the elderly.* Englewood Cliffs, NJ: Prentice-Hall.

Matthews, S. (2002). *Sisters and brothers/daughters and sons: Meeting the needs of old parents.* Bloomington, IN: Unlimited.

Matthews, A. M. & Rosenthal, C. J. (1993). Balancing work and family in an aging society: The Canadian experience. In G. L. Maddox and M. P. Lawton (Eds.) *Annual review of gerontology and geriatrics: Focus on kinship, aging and social change* (pp. 96–119). New York: Springer.

McAuley, J. (1987). *Applied research in gerontology.* New York: Van Nostrand-Reinhold.

McConatha, D., McConatha, J. T., & Dermigny, R. (1994). The use of interactive computer services to enhance the quality of life for long-term care residents. *The Gerontologist, 34*(4), 553–556.

McConnell, S. R. (1983). Age discrimination in employment. In H. S. Parnes (Ed.), *Policy issues in work and retirement* (pp. 159–196). Kalamazoo, MI: W. E. Upjohn Institute.

McConnell, S., & Beitler, D. (1991). The Older Americans Act after 25 years: An overview. *Generations, 15*(3), 5–10.

McCrea, F. B. (1983). The politics of menopause: The "discovery" of a deficiency disease. *Social Problems, 31*(1), 111–123.

McFalls, J. A. (1998). Population: A lively introduction. *Population Bulletin, 53*(3).Washington, DC: Population Reference Bureau.

McGarry, K., & Schoeni, R. F. (2005). Widow(er) poverty and out-of-pocket medical expenditures near the end of life. *Journal of Gerontology: Social Sciences, 60B*(3), S160–S168.

McKinlay, J., & McKinlay, S. (1990). Medical measures and the decline of mortality. In P. Conrad & R. Kerns (Eds.), *The sociology of health and illness: Critical perspectives* (pp. 10–23). New York: St. Martin's Press.

McNaught, W. (1994). Realizing the potential: Some examples. In M. W. Riley, R. L. Kahn, & A. Foner (Eds.), *Aging and structural lag* (pp. 219–236). New York: Wiley-Interscience.

Mehdizadeh, S. A., Nelson, I. M., & Applebaum, R. A. (2006). Nursing home use in Ohio: Who stays, who pays? Scripps Gerontology Center Brief Report. Retrieved April 22, 2006, from http://casnov1.cas.muohio.edu/scripps/publications/NHUse.html.

Mehdizadeh, S., Kunkel, S., and Ritchey, P. (2001). *Projections of Ohio's older disabled population: 2015 to 2050.* Retrieved May 5, 2005 from http://casnov1.cas.muohio.edu/scripps/publications/Sum_ProjectionsPop.html.

Metlife Mature Market Institute. (2001). *Toward a national caregiving agenda: Empowering family caregivers in America.* Metlife Research Center. Retrieved August 22, 2005 from http://www.metlife.com.

Meyer, J. A., & Greenwood, D. (1997). Back to the future: Poverty among the elderly in the twenty-first century. *Public Policy and Aging Report, 8*(1), 1, 17–20.

Miech, R. A., & Shanahan, M. J. (2000). Socioeconomic status and depression over the life course. *Journal of Health and Social Behavior, 41*(2), 137–161.

Miller, B., McFall, S., & Campbell, R. T. (1994). Changes in sources of community long-term care among African-American and White frail older persons. *Journal of Gerontology: Social Sciences, 49*(1), S14–S24.

Miller, D. (1985). The Economic Equity Act of 1985. *Washington Social Legislation Bulletin, 29,* 61–64.

Miller, S. (1991). Days Inns recruits older workers. In *Resourceful aging: Vol. 4. Work/second careers* (pp. 65–67). Washington, DC: American Association of Retired Persons.

Mills, C. W. (1959). *The sociological imagination.* New York: Oxford University Press.

Minkler, M. (1991a). "Generational Equity" and the new victim blaming. In M. Minkler & C. L. Estes (Eds.), *Critical perspectives on aging: The political and moral economy of growing old* (pp. 67–80). Amityville, NY: Baywood.

Minkler, M. (1991b). Gold in gray: Reflections on business discovery of the elderly market. In M. Minkler & C. L. Estes (Eds.), *Critical perspectives on aging: The political and moral economy of growing old* (pp. 81–93). Amityville, NY: Baywood.

Minkler, M., & Fuller-Thompson, E. (2005). African American grandparents raising grandchildren: A national study using the Census 2000 American Community Survey. *Journal of Gerontology: Social Sciences, 60B*(2), S82–S92.

Mitchell, J., & Register, J. C. (1984). An exploration of family interaction with the elderly by race, socioeconomic status, and residence. *The Gerontologist, 24*(1), 48–54.

Moen, P. (1994). Women, work and family: A sociological perspective on changing roles. In M. W. Riley, R. L. Kahn, & A. Foner (Eds.), *Aging and structural lag* (pp. 151–170). New York: Wiley-Interscience.

Moen, P., Dempster-McClain, D., & Williams, R. M. (1989). Social integration and longevity: An event history analysis of women's roles and resilience. *American Sociological Review, 54,* 635–647.

Moller, D. W. (1996). *Confronting death.* New York: Oxford University Press.

Mollica, R., & Johnson-Lamarche, H. (2005) *State Residential and Assisted Living Policy: 2004.* Portland, ME: National Academy for State Health Policy. Retrieved April 22, 2006, from http://aspe.hhs.gov/daltcp/reports/04alcom.htm.

Moody, H. R. (1992). *Ethics in an aging society.* Baltimore: Johns Hopkins University Press.

Moody, H. R. (1993). Overview: What is critical gerontology and why is it important? In T. R. Cole, W. A. Achenbaum, P. L. Jakobi, & R. Kastenbaum (Eds.), *Voices and visions of aging: Toward a critical gerontology* (pp. xv–xli). New York: Springer.

Moody, H. R. (2001–2002). Who's afraid of life extension. *Generations, 25*(4), 33–37.

Moon, M., & Smeeding, T. M. (1989). Can the elderly really afford long term care? In S. Sullivan & M. E. Lewin (Eds.), *The care of tomorrow's elderly: Encouraging initiatives and reshaping public programs* (pp. 137–160). Washington, DC: University Press of America.

Moore, P. (1985). *Disguised.* Waco, TX: Word Books.

Morgan, D. L. (1998). Facts and figures about the baby boom. *Generations* (Spring), 10–15.

Morgan, L. A. (1984). Changes in family interaction following widowhood. *Journal of Marriage and the Family, 46*(2), 323–332.

Morgan, L. A. (1991). Economic security of older women: Issues and trends for the future. In B. B. Hess & E. W. Markson (Eds.), *Growing old in America* (4th ed., pp. 275–292). New Brunswick, NJ: Transaction.

Morgan, L. A., Gruber-Baldini, A. L., & Magaziner, J. (2001). Resident characteristics. In S. I. Zimmerman, P. D. Sloane, & J. K. Eckert (Eds.), *Assisted living: Residential care in transition* (pp. 144–172). Baltimore: Johns Hopkins University Press.

Morrell, R. W., Mayhorn, C. B., & Echt, K. V. (2004). Why older adults use or do not use the internet. In D. C. Burdick & S. Kwon (Eds.) *Gerotechnology: Research and practice in technology and aging* (pp. 71–85). New York: Springer.

Munnell, A. H. (2004). *A bird's eye view of the Social Security debate.* Boston: Center for Retirement Research Issue Brief #25, Boston College.

Munnell, A. H. (2005). *Social Security's financial outlook: The 2005 update and a look back.* Boston: Center for Retirement Research, Boston University.

Mutchler, J. E., Burr, J. A., Pienta, A. M., & Massagli, M. P. (1997). Pathways to labor force exit: Work transitions and work instability. *Journal of Gerontology: Social Sciences, 52B*(1), S4–S12.

Mutran, E. (1985). Intergenerational family support among Blacks and Whites: Responses to culture or to socioeconomic differences. *Journal of Gerontology, 40*(3), 382–389.

Myers, G. C. (1990). Demography of aging. In R. H. Binstock & L. K. George (Eds.), *Handbook of aging and the social sciences* (3rd ed., pp. 19–44). San Diego, CA: Academic Press.

Myers, S. L., & Chung, C. (1996). Racial differences in home ownership and home equity among preretirement-aged households. *The Gerontologist, 36*(3), 350–360.

Myles, J. F. (1983). Conflict, crisis, and the future of old age security. *Millbank Memorial Fund Quarterly/Health and Society, 61,* 462–472.

Myles, J. F. (1984). *Old age in the welfare state: The political economy of public pensions.* Boston: Little, Brown.

Myles, J. F. (1989). *Old age and the welfare state: The political economy of public pension* (2nd ed.). Lawrence: University Press of Kansas.

Myles, J. F. (1996). Social Security and support of the elderly: The western experience. In J. Quadagno & D. Street (Eds.), *Aging for the twenty-first century* (pp. 381–397). New York: St. Martin's Press.

Myles, J. F., & Quadagno, J. (1995). Generational equity and Social Security reform. *Aging Research & Policy Report, 3*(5), 12–16.

Nathanson, C. A. (1990). The gender-mortality differential in developed countries: Demographic and sociocultural dimensions. In M. Ory & H. Warner (Eds.), *Gender, health and longevity: Multidisciplinary perspectives* (pp. 3–24). New York: Springer.

National Alliance for Caregiving. (1997). *Family caregiving in the U.S.: Findings from a national survey.* Bethesda, MD: NAC and AARP.

National Center for Health Statistics. (1989). Advance report on final mortality statistics, 1987. *Monthly Vital Statistics, 38*(5), 1–48.

National Coalition on Health Care. (2006). *Health care costs.* Retrieved April 2006 from http://www.nchc.org/facts/cost.shtml.

National Election Studies. (2004). *The NES guide to public opinion and electoral behavior.* Ann Arbor: University of Michigan, Center for Political Studies. Retrieved from http://www.umich.edu/~nes/nesguide/nesguide.htm.

Nelson, I. M. (2002). Continuing care retirement communities. In D. Ekerdt (Ed.), *Encyclopedia of aging.* New York: Macmillan.

Nesselroade, J. R. (1988). Sampling and generalizability: Adult development and aging research issues examined within the general methodological framework of selection. In K. W. Schaie, R. T. Campbell,

W. Meredith, & S. C. Rawlings (Eds.), *Methodological issues in aging research* (pp. 13–42). New York: Springer.

Neugarten, B. L., & Datan, N. (1973). Sociological perspectives on the life cycle. In P. B. Baltes & K. W. Schaie (Eds.), *Life-span developmental psychology* (pp. 53–71). New York: Academic Press.

Neugarten, B. L., Moore, J., & Lowe, J. (1965). Age norms, age constraints, and adult socialization. *American Journal of Sociology, 70*, 710–717.

Neugarten, B. L., Moore, J., & Lowe, J. (1968). Age norms, age constraints, and adult socialization. In B. L. Neugarten (Ed.), *Middle age and aging* (pp. 22–28). Chicago: University of Chicago Press.

Newcomer, R., & Preston, S. (1994). Relationship between acute care and nursing unit use in two continuing care retirement communities. *Research on Aging, 16*(3), 280–300.

Nieswiadomy, M., & Rubin, R. M. (1995). Change in expenditure patterns of retirees: 1972–1973 and 1986–1987. *Journal of Gerontology: Social Sciences, 50*(5), S275–S290.

Office of the Federal Register. (1995). *The United States government manual 1995/1996*. Washington, DC: U.S. Government Printing Office.

O'Brien, R., Stockard, J., and Isaacson, L. (1999). The enduring effects of cohort characteristics on age-specific homicide rates, 1960–1995. *American Journal of Sociology 104*(4), 1061–1095.

O'Rand, A. M. (1990). Stratification and the life course. In R. H. Binstock & L. K. George (Eds.), *Handbook of aging and the social sciences* (3rd ed., pp. 130–148), San Diego, CA: Academic Press.

O'Rand, A. M. (1996). The precious and the precocious: Understanding cumulative disadvantage and cumulative advantage over the life course. *The Gerontologist, 36*(2), 230–238.

Organisation for Economic Co-Operation and Development. (2000). *Employment outlook 2000*. Paris: OECD.

Palmore, E. (2005). Three decades of research on ageism. *Generations, 29*(3), 87–90.

Pandya, S. (2005). *Caregiving in the United States*. Washington, DC: AARP Policy Institute. Retrieved August 13, 2005 from http://www.aarp.org/research.

Parsons, T. (1959). The social structure of the family. In R. Anshen (Ed.), *The family: Its function and destiny* (2nd ed., pp. 241–274). New York: Harper & Row.

Parsons, T., & Bales, R. F. (1955). *Family socialization and process*. New York: Free Press.

Passuth, P. M., & Bengtson, V. L. (1988). Sociological theories of aging: Current perspectives and future directions. In J. E. Birren & V. L. Bengtson (Eds.), *Emergent theories of aging* (pp. 333–355). New York: Springer.

Paulin, G. D. (2000). Expenditure patterns of older American, 1984–97. *Monthly Labor Review, 123* (May), 3–28.

Pavalko, E. K., & Elder Jr., G. H. (1990). World War II and divorce: A life-course perspective. *American Journal of Sociology, 95*(5), 1213–1234.

Pearlin, L. I., Aneshensel, C. S., Mullan, J. T., & Whitlach, C. J. (1996). Caregiving and its social support. In R. H. Binstock & L. K. George (Eds.), *Handbook of aging and the social sciences* (pp. 283–325). New York: Academic Press.

Pension Rights Center. (2005) *The pension underfunding "crisis": Should you be worried?* Retrieved July 27, 2005 from http://www.pensionrights.org.

Peterson, S. A., & Somit, A. (1994). *The political behavior of older Americans*. New York: Garland.

Pew Research Center. (2003). *Evenly divided and increasingly polarized: 2004 political landscape*. Washington, DC: Pew Research Center for the People and the Press. Retrieved May 21, 2005 from http://people-press.org/reports/display.php3?PageID = 750.

Pillemer, K., and Suitor, J. J. (2004). Ambivalence in intergenerational relations over the life-course. In M. Silverstein (Ed.), Intergenerational relations across time and place. *Annual review of gerontology and geriatrics, Vol. 24*. New York: Springer.

Pineo, P. C. (1961). Disenchantment in the later years of marriage. *Marriage and Family Living, 23*, 3–11.

Plakans, A. (1994). The democratization of unstructured time in western societies: A historical overview. In M. W. Riley, R. L. Kahn, & A. Foner (Eds.), *Aging and structural lag* (pp. 107–129). New York: Wiley-Interscience.

Post, J. A. (1996). Internet resources on aging: Seniors on the net. *The Gerontologist, 36*(5), 565–569.

Preston, S., Elo, I., & Rosenwaike, I. (1996). African-American mortality at older ages: Results of a matching study. *Demography, 33*, 193–209.

Quadagno, J. (1982). *Aging in early industrial society*. New York: Academic Press.

Quadagno, J. (1988). *The transformation of old age security: Class and politics in the American welfare state*. Chicago: University of Chicago Press.

Quadagno, J. (1989). Generational equity and the politics of the welfare state. *Politics and Society, 17,* 353–376.

Quadagno, J. (1991). Generational equity and the politics of the welfare state. In B. B. Hess & E. W. Markson (Eds.), *Growing old in America* (4th ed., pp. 341–351). New Brunswick, NJ: Transaction.

Quadagno, J. (1996). Social Security and the myth of the entitlement "crisis." *The Gerontologist, 36*(3), 391–399.

Queen, S., Pappas, G., Harden, W., & Fisher G. (1994). The widening gap between socioeconomic status and mortality. *Statistical Bulletin, 75*(2), 31–35.

Quinn, J. F. (1987). The economic status of the elderly: Beware the mean. *Review of Income and Wealth, 33,* 63–82.

Quinn, J. F. (1993). *Poverty and income security among older persons: Overview of proceedings.* Syracuse, NY: National Academy on Aging.

Quinn, J. F., & Burkahauser, R. V. (1990). Work and retirement. In R. H. Binstock & L. K. George (Eds.), *Handbook of aging and the social sciences* (3rd ed., pp. 307–327). San Diego, CA: Academic Press.

Quinn, J. F., & Kozy, M. (1996). The role of bridge jobs in the retirement transition: Gender, race, and ethnicity. *The Gerontologist, 15*(3), 363–372.

Quinn, J. F., & Smeeding, T. M. (1993). The present and future economic well-being of the aged. In R. V. Burkhauser & D. L. Salisbury (Eds.), *Pensions in a changing economy* (pp. 5–18). Washington, DC: Employee Benefit Research Institute.

Quirk, D. (1991). An agenda for the nineties and beyond. *Generations, 15*(3), 23–26.

Radner, D. B. (1993). Economic well-being of the old: Family unit income and household wealth. *Social Security Bulletin, 56*(1), 3–19.

Rank, M. R., & Hirschi, T. A. (1999). Estimating the proportion of Americans ever experiencing poverty during their elderly years. *Journal of Gerontology: Social Sciences, 54B*(4), S184–S193.

Redford, L. J., & Whitten, P. (1997). Ensuring access to care in rural areas: The role of communication technology. *Generations, 21*(3), 19–23.

Reinhardt, U. E., Hussey, P.S., & Anderson, G. F. (2004). U.S. health care spending in an international context. *Health Affairs, 23*(3), 10–25.

Reitzes, D. C., Mutran, E. J., & Fernandez, M. E. (1996). Does retirement hurt well-being? Factors influencing self-esteem and depression among retirees and workers. *The Gerontologist, 36*(5), 649–656.

Reno, V. P. (1993). The role of pensions in retirement income. In R. V. Burkhauser & D. L. Salisbury (Eds.), *Pensions in a changing economy* (pp. 19–32). Washington, DC: Employee Benefit Research Institute.

Reno, V. P. (2005). How Social Security works. *Generations, 29*(1), 23–26.

Reskin, B., & Padavic, I. (1994). *Women and men at work.* Thousand Oaks, CA: Pine Forge Press.

Reynolds, S. L., Crimmins, E. M., & Saito, Y. (1998). Cohort differences in disability and disease presence. *The Gerontologist, 38*(5), 578–590.

Reynolds, S. L., Saito, Y., & Crimmins, E. M. (2005). The impact of obesity on active life expectancy in older American men and women. *The Gerontologist, 45,* 438–444.

Riley, M. W. (1983). The family in an aging society: A matrix of latent relationships. *Journal of Family Issues, 4,* 439–454.

Riley, M. W. (1987). On the significance of age in sociology. *American Sociological Review, 52,* 1–14.

Riley, M. W. (1994). Aging and society: Past, present, and future. *The Gerontologist, 34*(4), 436–446.

Riley, M. W. (1996). Discussion: What does it all mean? *The Gerontologist, 36*(2), 256–258.

Riley M. W., Johnson, M., & Foner, A. (1973). *Aging and society: Vol. 3. A sociology of age stratification.* New York: Russell Sage Foundation.

Riley, M. W., Kahn, R. L., & Foner, A. (Eds.). (1994). *Aging and structural lag.* New York: Wiley-Interscience.

Riley, M. W., & Riley, J. (1994). Age integration and the lives of older people. *The Gerontologist, 34,* 110–115.

Rix, S. E. (1991). Making resourceful aging a reality. In *Resourceful aging: Vol. 4. Work/second careers* (pp. 85–91). Washington, DC: American Association of Retired Persons.

Rix, S. E., & Williamson, J. B. (1998). *Social Security reform: How might women fare?* Washington, DC: AARP Public Policy Institute.

Roberto, K. A. (1990). Grandparent and grandchild relationships. In T. H. Brubaker (Ed.), *Family relationships in later life* (2nd ed., pp. 100–112). Newbury Park, CA: Sage.

Robertson, A. (1991). The politics of Alzheimer's disease: A case study in apocalyptic demography. In M. Minkler & C. Estes (Eds.), *Critical perspectives on aging: The political and moral economy of growing old* (pp. 135–152). Amityville, NY: Baywood.

Robert Wood Johnson Foundation. (2005). *Working but uninsured.* Retrieved February 6, 2006, from http://rwjf.org/newsroom/newsreleasesdetail.

Rogers, R. (1995). Marriage, sex and mortality. *Journal of Marriage and the Family, 57*(2), 515–526.

Rogers, W. A., Mayhorn, C. B., & Fisk, A. D. (2004). Technology in everyday life for older adults. In D. C. Burdick & S. Kwon (Eds.), *Gerotechnology: Research and practice in technology and aging* (pp. 3–17). New York: Springer.

Rogot, E., Sorlie, P. D., & Johnson, N. J. (1992). Life expectancy by employment status, income, and education in the National Longitudinal Mortality Study. *Public Health Report, 107,* 457–461.

Rosen, B., & Jerdee, T. H. (1985). *Older employees: New roles for valued resources.* Homewood, IL: Dow Jones-Irwin.

Rosenbaum, W. A., & Button, J. W. (1992). Perceptions of intergenerational conflict: The politics of young vs. old in Florida. *Journal of Aging Studies, 6*(4), 385–396.

Rosenmayr, L., & Kockeis, E. (1963). Propositions for a sociological theory of action and the family. *International Social Science Journal, 15,* 410–426.

Rosenthal, C. J., Matthews, S. H., & Marshall, V. W. (1991). Is parent care normative? The experiences of a sample of middle-aged women. In B. B. Hess & E. Markson (Eds.), *Growing old in America* (pp. 427–440). New Brunswick, NJ: Transaction.

Rosow, I. (1985). Status and role change through the life cycle. In R. H. Binstock & E. Shanas (Eds.), *Handbook of aging and the social sciences* (2nd ed.). New York: Van Nostrand-Reinhold.

Rossi, P. H., Lipsey, M. L., & Freeman, H. E. (2004). *Evaluation: A systematic approach* (7th ed.). Thousand Oaks, CA: Sage.

Rostein, G. (1999, July 6). The promise of longer life grows, but eternal youth remains out of reach. *Pittsburgh Post-Gazette.*

Rowe, J. W., & Kahn, R. L. (1997). Successful aging. *The Gerontologist, 37*(4), 433–440.

Rowe, J. W., & Kahn, R. L. (1998). *Successful aging.* New York: Pantheon Books.

Ruhm, C. J. (1990). Career jobs, bridge employment, and retirement. In P. B. Doeringer (Ed.), *Bridges to retirement: Older workers in a changing labor market* (pp. 92–107). Ithaca, NY: Cornell University Press.

Ruhm, C. J. (1996). Gender differences in employment behavior during late middle age. *Journal of Gerontology: Social Sciences, 51B*(1), S11–S17.

Rupert, P. (1991). Contingent work options: Promise or peril for older workers. In *Resourceful aging: Vol. 4. Work/second careers* (pp. 51–53). Washington, DC: American Association of Retired Persons.

Russell, A., & McWhirter, N. (1987). *1988 Guinness book of world records.* New York: Bantam Books.

Ryan, E. B., Szectman, B., & Bodkin, J. (1992). Attitudes toward younger and older adults learning to use computers. *Journal of Gerontology: Psychological Science, 47*(2), P96–P101.

Ryder, N. B. (1965). The cohort as a concept in the study of social change. *American Sociological Review, 30,* 843–861.

Sacramento Bee. (2006). *Health facts.* Retrieved March 18, 2006, from http://www.sacbee.com/marketguide/cosmetic_health/facts.

Salisbury, D. L. (1993). Policy implications of changes in employer pension protection. In R. V. Burkhauser & D. L. Salisbury (Eds.), *Pensions in a changing economy* (pp. 41–58). Washington, DC: Employee Benefit Research Institute.

Salthouse, T. (2006). Theoretical issues in the psychology of aging. In J. Birren & K. W. Schaie (Eds.), *Handbook of the psychology of aging* (6th ed., pp. 3–13). San Diego, CA: Academic Press.

Saluter, A. F. (1996). Marital status and living arrangements: March 1994, U.S. Bureau of the Census, *Current Population Reports, Series P-20,* No. 484. Washington, DC: U.S. Government Printing Office.

Sandell, S. H., & Iams, H. M. (1997). Reducing women's poverty by shifting Social Security benefits from retired couples to widows. *Journal of Policy Analysis and Management, 16*(2), 279–297.

Sankar, A., & Gubrium, J. (1994). Introduction. In J. Gubrium & A. Sankar (Eds.), *Qualitative methods in aging research* (pp. vii–xvii). Thousand Oaks, CA: Sage.

Schachter-Shalomi, Z., & Miller, R. S. (1995). *From age-ing to sage-ing: A profound new vision of grow-ing older.* New York: Warner Books.

Schaie, K. W., & Hertzog, C. (1982). Longitudinal methods. In B. B. Woman (Ed.), *Handbook of de-velopmental psychology* (pp. 91–115). Englewood Cliffs, NJ: Prentice-Hall.

Schmittroth, L. (1991). *Statistical record of women worldwide.* Detroit, MI: Gale Research.

Schoenborn, C., Vickerie, J., & Powell-Griner, E. (2006). Health characteristics of adults 55 years of age and over: United States 2000–2003. *Advance Data from Vital and Health Statistics,* No. 370.

Schultz, K. S., Morton, K. R., & Weckerle, J. R. (1998). The influence of push and pull factors on voluntary and involuntary early retirees' retirement decision and adjustment. *Journal of Vocational Behavior, 53,* 45–57.

Schulz, J. H. (1986). Voodoo economics and the aging society. In Brandeis University, *Of Current Interest from the Policy Center on Aging, 6*(2).

Schulz, J. H. (1992). *The economics of aging* (5th ed.). New York: Auburn House.

Schulz, J. H., & Myles, J. (1990). Old age pensions: A comparative perspective. In R. H. Binstock & L. K. George (Eds.). *Handbook of aging and the social sciences* (3rd ed., pp. 398–414). San Diego, CA: Academic Press.

Schulz, R., Visintainer, P., & Williamson, G. M. (1990). Psychiatric and physical morbidity effects of caregiving. *Journals of Gerontology, 45,* 181–191.

Schumacher, J. G., Eckert, J. K., Zimmerman, S., Carder, P., & Wright, A. (2005). Physician care in assisted living: A qualitative study. *Journal of the American Medical Directors Association, 6,* 1, 34–45.

Schuman, H., & Scott, J. (1989). Generations and collective memories. *American Sociological Review, 54*(3), 359–381.

Schutt, R. K. (2004). *Investigating the social world* (4th ed.). Thousand Oaks, CA: Pine Forge Press.

Schwartz, G. E. (1982). Testing the biopsychosocial model: The ultimate challenge facing behavioral medicine? *Journal of Consulting and Clinical Psychology, 50*(6), 1040–1053.

Scialfa, C. T., Ho, G., & Laberge, J. (2004). Perceptual aspects of gerontechnology. In D. C. Burdick & S. Kwon (Eds.), *Gerotechnology: Research and practice in technology and aging* (pp. 18–41). New York: Springer.

Scott, J. P. (1990). Sibling interaction in later life. In T. H. Brubaker (Ed.), *Family relationships in later life* (2nd ed., pp. 86–99). Newbury Park, CA: Sage.

Scrutton, S. (1996). Ageism: The foundation of age discrimination. In J. Quadagno & D. Street (Eds.), *Aging for the twenty-first century* (pp. 141–154). New York: St. Martin's Press.

Sears, D. O. (1983). The persistence of early political predispositions: The roles of attitude ob-ject and life stage. In L. Wheeler (Ed.), *Review of personality and social psychology, Vol. 4* (pp. 79–116). Thousand Oaks, CA: Sage.

Seltzer, M. M., & Greenberg. J. S. (1999). The caregiving context: The intersection of social and individual influences in the experience of family caregiving. In C. D. Ryff & V. W. Marshall (Eds.), *The self and society in aging processes* (pp. 362–397). New York: Springer.

Senior Journal. (2003). Almost half of U.S. domestic spending in 2002 for Social Security, Medicare and Medicaid. Retrieved May 15, 2005 from http://www.seniorjournal.com/NEWS/Features/3–06–4almost.htm.

Settersten, R. A., & Hagestad, G. O. (1996a). What's the latest? Cultural age deadlines for family transitions. *The Gerontologist, 36*(2), 178–188.

Settersten, R. A., & Hagestad, G. O. (1996b). What's the latest? II: Cultural age deadlines for educational and work transitions. *The Gerontologist, 36*(5), 602–613.

Settersten, R. A. (1999). *Lives in time and place: Problems and promises of developmental science.* Ami-tyville, NY: Baywood.

Settersten, R. A. (2003). Propositions and controversies in life-course scholarship. In. R. Settersten (Ed.), *Invitation to the life course: Toward new understandings of later life* (pp. 15–45). Amityville, NY: Baywood.

Settersten, R. A. (2005a). Toward a stronger partnership between life-course sociology and life-span psychology. *Research in Human Development, 2*(1&2), 25–41.

Settersten, R. A. (2005b). Linking the two ends of life: What gerontology can learn from childhood studies. *Journal of Gerontology: Social Sciences, 60B*(4), S173–S180.

Setton, D. (2000). Cyber granny. *Forbes, 165*(12), 40–41.

Shanas, E. (1967). Family help patterns and social class in three countries. *Journal of Marriage and the Family, 29*(2), 257–266.

Shanas, E. (1979a). Social myth as hypothesis: The case of family relations of old people. *The Gerontologist, 19,* 3–9.

Shanas, E. (1979b). The family as a social support system in old age. *The Gerontologist, 19,* 169–174.

Shatzkin, K. (1995, October 22). Twilight behind bars. *Baltimore Sun,* 1B.

Shea, D. G., Miles, T., & Hayward, M. (1996). The health-wealth connection: Racial differences. *The Gerontologist, 36*(3), 342–349.

Shuey, K., & Hardy, M. (2003). Assistance to aging parents and parents-in-law: Does lineage affect family allocation decisions? *Journal of Marriage and the Family, 65,* 418–431.

Silverstein, M. (2004). Intergenerational relations across time and place. *Annual review of gerontology and geriatrics, Vol. 24.* New York: Springer.

Silverstein, M. (2006). Intergenerational family transfers in social context. In R. H. Binstock & L. K. George (Eds.), *Handbook of aging and the social sciences* (6th ed., pp.166–181). Burlington, MA: Academic Press.

Silverstein, M., Angelelli, J. J., & Parrott, T. M. (2001). Changing attitudes toward aging policy in the United States during the 1980s and 1990s: A cohort analysis. *Journal of Gerontology: Social Sciences, 56B*(1), S36–S43.

Silverstein, M., Conroy, S. J., Wang, H., Giarrusso, R., & Bengtson, V. L. (2002). Reciprocity in parent-child relations over the adult life course. *Journal of Gerontology: Social Sciences, 57B*(1), S3–S13.

Silverstein, M., Parrott, T. M., & Bengtson, V. L. (1995). Factors that predispose middle-aged sons and daughters to provide social support to older parents. *Journal of Marriage and the Family, 57*(2), 465–475.

Simmons, C. H., Vom Kolke, A., & Hideko, S. (1986). Attitudes toward romantic love among American, German, and Japanese students. *Journal of Social Psychology, 126*(3), 327–336.

Slevin, K. F., & Wingrove, C. R. (1995). Women in retirement: A review and critique of empirical research since 1976. *Sociological Inquiry, 65*(1), 1–21.

Sloane, P. D., Zimmerman, S., Williams, C. S., Reed, P. S., Gill, K. S., & Preisser, J. S. (2005). Evaluating the quality of life of long-term care residents with dementia. *The Gerontologist, 45*(1), 37–49.

Smeeding, T. M. (1990). Economic status of the elderly. In R. H. Binstock & L. K. George (Eds.), *Handbook of aging and the social sciences* (3rd ed., pp. 362–381). New York: Academic Press.

Smeeding, T. M., Estes, C. L., & Glasse, L. (1999). Social Security in the 21st century: More than deficits: Strengthening security for women. *Gerontology News* (August, special insert), 1–8.

Social Security Administration. (1994). *Income of the aged chartbook, 1992.* SSA Publication #13-11727. Washington, DC: U.S. Department of Health and Human Services.

Social Security Administration. (1995). *Fast facts and figures about Social Security.* SSA Publication #13–11785. Washington, DC: U.S. Department of Health and Human Services.

Social Security Administration. (2004a). *Income of the aged chartbook 2002.* Retrieved June 28, 2005 from http://www.ssa.gov/policy/docs/chartbooks/income_aged/2002/iac02.pdf.

Social Security Administration. (2004b). *Exempt amounts under the earnings test.* Retrieved July 12, 2005 from http://www.ssa.gov/OACT/COLA/rtea.html.

Social Security Administration. (2004c). *Annual statistical supplement.* Available internet: Retrieved June 26, 2005 from http://www.ssa.gov/policy/docs/statcomps/supplement/2004/6b.pdf.

Social Security Administration. (2004d). *SSI federal payment amounts.* Retrieved July 12, 2005 from http://www.ssa.gov/OACT/COLA/SSI.html.

Social Security Administration. (2005). *Social Security and Medicare benefits.* Actuarial Publications (2/11/2005). Retrieved June 26, 2005 from http://www.ssa.gov/OACT/STATS/table4a4.html.

Stansfield, S. A. (1999). Social support and social cohesion. In J. Marmot & R. Wilkinson (Eds.), *Determinants of health* (pp. 155–178). Oxford, England: Oxford University Press.

Starr, P. (1988). Social Security and the American public household. In T. R. Marmour & J. L. Mashaw (Eds.), *Social Security: beyond the rhetoric of crisis* (pp. 119–148). Princeton, NJ: Princeton University Press.

Steffensmeier, D. J., Allan, E. A., Harer, M. D., & Streifel, C. (1989). Age and the distribution of crime. *American Journal of Sociology, 94*(4), 803–831.

Steinmetz, S. K. (1988). *Duty bound: Elder abuse and family care.* Newbury Park, CA: Sage.

Steinmetz, S. K. (2005). Elder abuse is caused by the deviance and dependence of abusive caregivers. In D. R. Loeske, R. J. Gelles, & M. M. Cavanaugh (Eds.). *Current controversies in family violence* (2nd ed.). Thousand Oaks, CA: Sage.

Stone, R., Caffertata, G. L., & Sangl, J. (1987). Caregivers of the frail elderly: A national profile. *The Gerontologist, 27*(5), 616–626.

Strate, J. M., Parish, C. J., Elder, C. D., & Ford III, C. (1989). Life span civic development and voting participation. *American Political Science Review, 83*(2), 443–464.

Street, D. (1993). Maintaining the status quo: The impact of old-age interest groups on the Medicare Catastrophic Care Act of 1988. *Social Problems, 40,* 431–444.

Suitor, J. J., &. Pillemer, K. (1993). Support and interpersonal stress in the social networks of married daughters caring for parents with dementia. *Journal of Gerontology: Social Sciences, 48,* S1–S8.

Suitor, J. J., Pillemer, K., Keeton, S., & Robison, J. (1994). Aged parents and aging children: Determinants of relationship quality. In R. Blieszner & V. H. Bedford (Eds.), *Handbook of aging and the family* (pp. 223–242). Westport, CT: Greenwood Press.

Sussmann, M. B. (1985). The family life of old people. In R. H. Binstock & E. Shanas (Eds.), *Handbook of aging and the social sciences* (2nd ed., pp. 415–449). New York: Van Nostrand Reinhold.

Sussmann, M. B., & Burchinal, L. (1968). Kin family network: Unheralded structure in current conceptualizations of family functioning. In B. L. Neugarten (Ed.), *Middle age and aging* (pp. 247–25). Chicago: University of Chicago Press.

Sweeney, M. M. (2002). Two decades of family change: The shifting economic foundations of marriage. *American Sociological Review, 67*(1), 132–147.

Szanton, P. (1993). Implications of an aging population: Predictions, doubts, and questions. In *Aging of the U.S. population: Economic and environmental implications* (pp. 69–76). Washington, DC: American Association of Retired Persons.

Szinovacz, M. E., & Davey, A. (2004). Retirement transitions and spouse disability: Effects on depressive symptoms. *Journal of Gerontology: Social Sciences, 59B*(6), S333–S342.

Szinovacz, M. E., & Davey, A. (2005). Predictors of perceptions of involuntary retirement. *The Gerontologist, 45*(1), 36–47.

Szinovacz, M. E., & Ekerdt, D. J. (1996). Families and retirement. In R. Blieszner & V. H. Bedford (Eds.), *Aging and the family: Theory and research* (pp. 373–400). Westport, CT: Praeger.

Szinovacz, M. E., & Washo, C. (1992). Gender differences in exposure to life events and adaptation to retirement. *Journal of Gerontology: Social Sciences, 47*(4), S191–S196.

Thomas, W. H. (2004). *What are old people for?* Acton, MA: Vander Wyk & Burnham.

Thomas, W. I. (1972 [1931]). Definition of the situation. In J. G. Mannis & B. L. Meltzer (Eds.) *Symbolic interaction (rev. ed.)* (pp.331–336). Boston: Allyn & Bacon.

Thompson, L., & Walker, A. (1987). Mothers as mediators of intimacy between grandmothers and their young adult granddaughters. *Family Relation, 36,* 72–77.

Thompson, W. S., & Whelpton, P. K. (1933). *Population trends in the United States.* New York: McGraw-Hill.

Tornstam, L. (1997). Gerotranscendence: The contemplative dimension of aging. *Journal of Aging Studies, 11*(2), 143–154.

Tornstam, L. (2005). *Gerotranscendence: A developmental theory of positive aging.* New York: Springer.

Torres-Gil, F. M. (1992). *The new aging: Politics and change in America.* Westport, CT: Auburn House.

Torres-Gil, F. M. (1998). Policy, politics, aging: Crossroads in the 1990s. In J. S. Steckenrider & T. M. Parrott (Eds.), *New directions in old-age policies* (pp. 75–88). Albany: State University of New York Press.

Tout, K. (1989). *Aging in developing countries.* New York: Oxford University Press.

Townsend, P. (1968). The emergence of the four-generation family in industrial society. In B. L. Neugarten (Ed.), *Middle age and aging* (pp. 255–257). Chicago: University of Chicago Press.

Treas, J. (1995). Older Americans in the 1990s and beyond. *Population Bulletin, 50*(2), 2–46.

Uhlenberg, P. (1993). Demographic change and kin relationships in later life. In G. L. Maddox & M. P. Lawton (Eds.), *Annual review of gerontology and geriatrics: Focus on kinship, aging, and social change, Vol. 13* (pp. 219–238). New York: Springer.

Uhlenberg, P. (1996). Mutual attraction: Demography and life-course analysis. *The Gerontologist, 36*(2), 226–229.

Uhlenberg, P., Cooney, T., & Boyd, R. (1990). Divorce for women after midlife. *Journal of Gerontology: Social Sciences, 45*(1), S3–S11.

United Nations. (2002). *World population ageing: 1950–2050.* Department of Economic and Social Affairs, Population Division. New York: United Nations.

United Nations. (2003). *International plan of action on ageing.* Retrieved October 25, 2005, from http://www.un.org/esa/socdev/ageing/ageipaal.htm.

U.S. Bureau of the Census. (1975). *Statistical abstract of the United States.* Washington, DC: U.S. Government Printing Office.

U.S. Bureau of the Census. (1976). *Historical statistics of the United States, colonial times to 1970.* Washington, DC: U.S. Government Printing Office.

U.S. Bureau of the Census. (1977). *Statistical abstract of the United States.* Washington, DC: U.S. Government Printing Office.

U.S. Bureau of the Census (1985). *Statistical abstract of the United States.* Washington, DC: U.S. Government Printing Office.

U.S. Bureau of the Census. (1987). *Statistical abstract of the United States.* Washington, DC: U.S. Government Printing Office.

U.S. Bureau of the Census. (1991a). Marital status and living arrangements: March 1990. *Current Population Reports, P-20,* No. 450. Washington, DC: U.S. Government Printing Office.

U.S. Bureau of the Census. (1991b). *Global aging: Comparative indicators and future trends.* Washington, DC: U.S. Department of Commerce.

U.S. Bureau of the Census. (1992b). Voting and registration in the election of November 1992. *Current population reports, P20–466.* Retrieved April 24, 2000 from www.census.gov/population/socdemo/voting/history/vot04.txt-3k-Supplemental Result.

U.S. Bureau of the Census. (1993). *Statistical abstract of the United States: 1993.* Washington, DC: U.S. Government Printing Office.

U.S. Bureau of the Census. (1995). *Statistical abstract of the United States.* Washington, DC: U.S. Government Printing Office.

U.S. Bureau of the Census. (1996a). Population projections of the United States by age, sex, race and Hispanic origin: 1995–2050. *Current population reports, P-25,* No. 1130. Washington, DC: U.S. Government Printing Office.

U.S. Bureau of the Census. (1996b). *Statistical abstract of the United States.* Washington, DC: U.S. Government Printing Office.

U.S. Bureau of the Census. (1997). *Statistical abstract of the United States.* Washington, DC: U.S. Government Printing Office.

U.S. Bureau of the Census. (1998). Money income in the United States: 1998. *Current population reports, 60–206.* Washington, DC: U.S. Government Printing Office.

U.S. Bureau of the Census. (2001). *Employment size of employer firms 2001.* Retrieved May 2, 2005 from http://www.census.gov/epcd/www/smallbus.html.

U.S. Bureau of the Census. (2003a). *Annual demographic survey, March supplement.* Retrieved August 24, 2004 from http://pubdb3.census.gov/macro/032004/pov/new01_100_01.htm.

U.S. Bureau of the Census. (2003b). Net worth and asset ownership of households: 1998 and 2000. *Current population reports, P70–88.* Washington, DC: U.S. Government Printing Office.

U.S. Bureau of the Census. (2004a). *US interim projections by age, sex, race, and Hispanic origin.* Retrieved October 8, 2005, from http//www.census.gov/ipc/www/usinterimproj.

U.S. Bureau of the Census. (2004b). *Historical income tables.* Retrieved July 8, 2005 from http://www.census.gov/hhes/www/income/histinc/h10ar.html.

U.S. Bureau of the Census (2005a). *Statistical abstract of the United States 2004–2005.* Retrieved July 11, 2005 from http://www.census.gov/prod/2004pubs/04statab/socinsur.pdf.

U.S. Bureau of the Census. (2005b). *International data base population pyramids.* Retrieved November 1, 2005, from http://www.census.gov/ipc/www/idbnew.html.

U.S. Bureau of the Census. (2005c). *Poverty thresholds 2005.* Retrieved September 3, 2005 from http://www.census.gov/hhes/www/poverty/threshld/thres05.html.

U.S. Department of Health and Human Services, Centers for Disease Control and Prevention, National Center for Health Statistics. (2005). *Health, United States 2005, special excerpt: Trend tables on 65 and older population.* Washington, D.C.: U.S Government Printing Office.

U.S. Department of Justice, Federal Bureau of Investigation. (2006). *Crimes in the U.S., 2004.* Retrieved 03/03/2006 from http://www.fbi.gov/ucr/cius_04/persons_arrested/table_38-43.html.

U.S. Department of Justice, Federal Bureau of Prisons. (1989). Looking ahead—The future BOP population and their costly health care needs. *Research Bulletin,* January, 1–5.

U.S. Department of Labor, Bureau of Labor Statistics. (2001). *Contingent and alternative employment arrangements, February 2001.* Retrieved June 8, 2005 from http://www.bls.gov/news.release/conemp.nr0.htm.

U.S. Department of Labor, Bureau of Labor Statistics. (2004a). *Economic and employment projections: 2002–2012.* Retrieved June 9, 2005 from http://www.bls.gov/news.release/ecopro.nr0.htm.

U.S. Department of Labor, Bureau of Labor Statistics. (2004b). *Projections: Civilian labor force 2002–2012.* Retrieved June 9, 2005 from ftp://ftp.bls.gov/pub/special.requests/ep/labor.force/clfa0212.txt.

U.S. Department of Labor, Bureau of Labor Statistics. (2005). *Employment and earnings, January 2004.* Retrieved July 8, 2005 from http://www.bls.gov/cps/cpsa2004.pdf.

U.S. Senate Special Committee on Aging. (1991). *Aging America: Trends and projections.* Washington, DC: U.S. Department of Health and Human Services.

Vaillant, C. O. & Vaillant, G. A. (1993). Is the u-curve of marital satisfaction an illusion? A 40 year study of marriage. *Journal of Marriage & Family, 55*(1), 230–239.

Van der Maas, P. J. (1988). Aging and public health. In J. Schroots, J. Birren, & A. Svanborg (Eds.), *Health and aging: Perspectives and prospects* (pp. 95–115). The Netherlands: Swets and Zeitlinger.

Vastag, B. (2001). Easing the elderly online in search of health information. *Journal of the American Medical Association, 285*(12), 1563–1564.

Velkoff, V. (2000). Centenarians in the United States, 1990 and beyond. *Statistical Bulletin, 81*(1), 2–9.

Verbrugge, L. M. (1990). The twain meet: Empirical explanations of sex differences in health and mortality. In M. Ory & H. Warner (Eds.), *Gender, health and longevity: Multidisciplinary perspectives* (pp. 159–200). New York: Springer.

Vinton, L. (1991). Abused older women: Battered women or abused elders? *Journal of Women and Aging, 3*(3), 5–19.

Vitez, M. (1995, November 29). Ripeness is all, in centenarians as in cheeses. *The Sun,* 5E.

Waldfogel, J. (1997). The effects of children on women's wages. *American Sociological Review, 62,* 209–217.

Waldron, I. (1993). Recent trends in sex mortality ratios for adults in developed countries. *Social Science and Medicine, 36*(4), 451–462.

Walker, A. J., Martin, S., & Jones, L. L. (1992). The benefits and costs of caregiving and care receiving for daughters and mothers. *Journal of Gerontology: Social Sciences, 47,* S130–S139.

Wallace, H. (1996). *Family violence: Legal, medical and social perspectives.* Needham Heights, MA: Allyn and Bacon.

Wallace, S. P., Williamson, J. B., Lung, R. G., & Powell, L. A. (1991). A lamb in wolf's clothing? The reality of senior power and social policy. In M. Minkler & C. L. Estes (Eds.), *Critical perspectives on aging: The political and moral economy of growing old* (pp. 95–114). Amityville, NY: Baywood.

Ward, R., Logan, J., & Spitze, G. (1992). The influence of parent and child needs on coresidence in middle and later life. *Journal of Marriage and the Family, 54*(1), 209–221.

Ware, J., Bayliss, M., Rogers, W., & Kosinski, M. (1996). Differences in four-year health outcomes for elderly and poor, chronically ill patients treated in HMO and fee-for-service systems. *Journal of the American Medical Association, 276*(13), 1039–1047.

Weaver D. A. (1994). The work and retirement decisions of older women: A literature review. *Social Security Bulletin, 57*(1), 3–24.

Weaver, D. A. (1997). The economic well-being of Social Security beneficiaries, with an emphasis on divorced beneficiaries. *Social Security Bulletin, 60*(4), 3–17.

Weeks, J. R. (1994). *Population: An introduction to concepts and issues.* Belmont, CA: Wadsworth.

Weishaus, S., & Field, D. (1988). A half century of marriage: Continuity or change? *Journal of Marriage and the Family, 50*(3), 763–774.

Welford, A. T. (1993). Work capacity across the adult years. In R. Kastenbaum (Ed.), *Encyclopedia of adult development* (pp. 541–552). Phoenix, AZ: Oryx Press.

Wellman, B., & Wortley, S. (1989). Brothers' keepers: Situating kinship relations in broader networks of social support. *Sociological Perspectives, 32,* 273–306.

Wells, T. (1998). *Changes in occupational sex segregation during the 1980s and 1990s.* Madison: Center for Demography and Ecology, University of Wisconsin.

White, H., McConnell, E., Clipp, E., Bynum, L., Teague, C., Navas, L., Craven, S., & Halbrecht, H. (1999). Surfing the net in later life: A review of the literature and pilot study of computer use and quality of life. *Journal of Applied Gerontology, 18*(3), 358–378.

White, L., & Edwards, N. (1990). Emptying the nest and parental well-being: An analysis of national panel data. *American Sociological Review, 55*(2), 235–242.

White, L., & Peterson, D. (1995). The retreat from marriage: Its effect on unmarried children's exchange with parents. *Journal of Marriage and the Family, 57*(2), 428–434.

White, L. K., & Reidman, A. (1992). When the Brady Bunch grows up: Step/half- and full sibling relationships in adulthood. *Journal of Marriage and the Family, 54*, 197–208.

Wiley, D., & Bortz, W. (1996). Sexuality and aging—Usual and successful. *Journals of Gerontology, 51A*, M142–M146.

Winship, C., & Harding, D. (2004). *A general strategy for the identification of age, period, cohort models: A mechanism based approach.* Retrieved 07/20/2005, from http://www.qmp.isr.umich.edu/ASAMConference/Papers/WinshipHardingAPC.pdf.

Wolff, J. L., & Agree, E. M. (2004). Depression among recipients of informal care: The effects of reciprocity, respect, and adequacy of support. *Journal of Gerontology: Social Sciences, 59B*, S173–S180.

Women's Initiative. (1993). *Women, pensions and divorce: Small reforms that could make a big difference.* Washington, DC: American Association of Retired Persons.

World Health Organization. (2006). *World Health Organization mortality database.* Retrieved June 18, 2005, from http://www3.who.int/whosis/mort/table1_process.cfm.

Wu, K. B. (2005). *How Social Security keeps older persons out of poverty across developed countries.* Washington, DC: AARP Public Policy Institute. Retrieved August 28, 2005 from http://www.aarp.org/ppi.

Wynne. E. A. (1991). Will the young support the old? In B. B. Hess & E. W. Markson (Eds.), *Growing old in America* (4th ed., pp. 507–623). New Brunswick, NJ: Transaction Books.

Yaukey, D. (1985). *Demography: The study of human population.* Prospect Heights, IL: Waveland Press.

Zepelin, H., Sills, R. A., & Heath, H. W. (1986–1987). Is age becoming irrelevant? An exploratory study of perceived age norms. *International Journal of Aging and Human Development, 24*(4), 241–256.

Zimmerman, S., Sloane, P. D., Eckert, J. K., Gruber-Baldini, A., Morgan, A. L., Hebel, J. R., Magaziner, J., Stearns, S. C., & Chen, C. K. (2005). How good is assisted living? Findings and implications from an outcomes study. *Journal of Gerontology: Social Sciences, 60B*(4), S195–S204.

Index